LONG TERM HEALTH CARE

Long Term Health Care

Providing a Spectrum of Services to the Aged

PHILIP W. BRICKNER, M.D.

ANTHONY J. LECHICH, M.D.

ROBERTA LIPSMAN, M.S.S.W.

LINDA K. SCHARER, M.U.P.

Basic Books, Inc., Publishers   *New York*

Material from Philip W. Brickner, *Home Health Care for the Aged* (New York: Appleton-Century-Crofts, 1978) reprinted with permission.

Library of Congress Cataloging-in-Publication Data

Long term health care.

   Bibliographical notes: p. 310.
   Includes index.
   1. Aged—Long term care—United States.
2. Aged—Home care—United States.   3. Aged—
Health and hygiene—United States.   I. Brickner,
Philip W., 1928-   .   [DNLM: 1. Health
Services for the Aged—United States.   2. Long
Term Care—in old aged.   WT 30 L8489]
RA564.8.L67   1987   362.1'6'0880565   87–47743
ISBN   0–465–04220–1

This book is dedicated to

Sister Teresita Duque, R.N.

Sister of Charity of
Saint Vincent De Paul

Cofounder of the
Chelsea-Village Program

Contents

BIOGRAPHICAL NOTES   X

ACKNOWLEDGMENTS   xii

PREFACE   xiv

PART ONE: INTRODUCTION

1   The Long Term Care Spectrum   3
    The Magnitude of the Problem 4 / Consequences of Increased Life
    Expectancy 5 / Establishing a Spectrum of Long Term Care
    Services 8 / Needed: An Orderly Approach 10 / How Did We Get
    into This Situation? 12 / Areas Requiring Immediate Attention
    19 / The Nursing Home: Is There a Way Out? 22

2   Financing Long Term Care for the Aged   25
    Government Sources of Long Term Care Funds 26 / Medicaid
    26 / Medicare 35 / Other Sources of Government Funds
    40 / Private Sources of Long Term Care Funds 45 / Solutions:
    Approaches to Financing Long Term Care 53

PART TWO: CLINICAL CONCERNS

3 Health, Disease, and Functional Ability   59
   Intrinsic Factors: Physical and Psychological Characteristics
   60 / Extrinsic Factors: The Environment, People Who Help, and
   Community Resources 64 / Integrating Health, Disease, and
   Functional Ability: Case Examples 71

4 Dementia   81
   Defining Dementia 83 / The Historical Background of Dementias
   84 / Alzheimer's Disease 85 / Multi-Infarct Dementia
   99 / Subcortical Dementias 101 / Treatable Dementias
   103 / Therapeutic Approaches to Dementias 112

5 Alcoholism and Older People   117
   Diagnosis of Alcoholism 120 / Characteristics of Older Drinkers
   122 / Definition of Terms 129 / Consequences of Alcoholism in
   Older People 131 / Physical Dependence, Tolerance, and
   Withdrawal Symptoms 139 / Approaches to Treatment
   140 / Conclusion 145

PART THREE: HOME CARE

6 Long Term Home Health Care   149
   Definition of Terms 151 / Values and Significance of Long Term
   Home Health Care 153 / Exemplary Long Term Home Health Care
   Programs 154 / The Nursing Home Without Walls: New York
   State's Long Term Home Health Care Program 155 / Long Term
   Home Care Demonstrations: Medicare and Medicaid Waivers
   158 / Conclusion 171

7 Paraprofessional Workers   173
   Historical Background 174 / A Changing, Growing Field
   174 / Definition of Terms 176 / Specific Paraprofessional Functions
   178 / Standards for Paraprofessionals 181 / Training 182 / Ethical
   Matters 184 / Building Morale 188 / Sources of Funding 190

8 Informal Supports   198
   Informal Supporters 199 / Families and Friends Give Help
   203 / Impact on Caregivers 204 / Giving Help to Natural
   Supporters 206 / Friends 210 / An Overview of Informal Supports
   211 / Volunteers 212 / Conclusion 219

Contents

PART FOUR: AUGMENTING THE LONG TERM CARE SYSTEM

 9 Day Care, Foster Care, Hospice, and Respite   223
    Adult Day Care 224 / Foster Care 230 / Hospice Care
    235 / Respite 237 / Conclusion 241

10 Housing   242
    The Significance of Housing in a Long Term Care Spectrum
    243 / Solutions: What Elderly People Want 247 / The Housing
    Spectrum 248 / A Quick History of Housing for the Elderly
    249 / Rural Housing Policy 251 / Finding a Solution
    251 / Conclusion 263

11 The Nursing Home   265
    History 268 / Transfer Trauma 274 / Quality of Life in the
    Nursing Home 275 / Administration and Organization 276 / The
    Medical Director 279 / The Teaching Nursing Home
    280 / Questions of Ethics 281

12 Trends and Forecasts   286
    The Demographic Imperative 287 / Attitudes About Aging
    288 / Training in Gerontology 290 / Policy 291 / Access to Services
    291 / Allocation of Resources 293 / Program Development
    294 / Legislation 299 / Financing the Long Term Care Spectrum
    307 / Conclusion 309

NOTES   310

INDEX   361

Biographical Notes

Philip W. Brickner, M.D., received his medical degree from Columbia University College of Physicians and Surgeons. After completing his postgraduate training in internal medicine, he joined the staff of St. Vincent's Hospital and Medical Center of New York, where he managed the hospital's affiliation with the Village Nursing Home. When the hospital established a Department of Community Medicine in 1974, Dr. Brickner became its first director, a position he has held to date. The department is responsible for the development and conduct of the hospital's community-based health care programs. Among these are the Chelsea-Village Program and the PRIDE Long Term Home Health Care Institute, both of which focus on care of the frail elderly at home. The department has also conducted one of New York's Nursing Home Without Walls programs since 1979, one of the initial nine pilot efforts in the state. Dr. Brickner has written widely on care of the elderly. Among his other books are *Care of the Nursing Home Patient* (1971) and *Home Health Care for the Aged* (1978). He was a New York State Delegate to the 1981 White House Conference on Aging.

Anthony J. Lechich, M.D., attended the State University of New York, Downstate, where he received his medical degree. Following completion of residency training in internal medicine, he joined the Departments of Community Medicine and Medicine at St. Vincent's Hospital and Medical Center of New York. He has participated in all aspects of long term care of the aged, including home health care (through his service as a physician on the Chelsea-Village Program), clinical responsibility (at the Village Nursing Home, where he has also been a board member since 1979), ambulatory care, teaching of house officers, and planning for a geriatric training program at the hospital. Dr. Lechich was an alternate delegate to the 1981

White House Conference on Aging. Since 1985 he has been medical director of the Kateri Residence, a 520-bed skilled nursing facility in New York City.

Roberta Lipsman, M.S.S.W., received her bachelor's degree from Smith College and her master's degree in social work planning and administration from Columbia University. She became the first coordinator of New York State's Enriched Housing for the Elderly Program. Later, as its first director, she shared in the development of the PRIDE Long Term Home Health Care Institute at St. Vincent's Hospital and Medical Center of New York, and initiated its *Journal of Long Term Care.* Subsequently, as a staff member to Senator John Glenn on the United States Senate Special Committee on Aging, Ms. Lipsman continued work on policy development in the fields of housing and long term care. In 1984 she became deputy director of Community Counseling Center, Portland, Maine, and was a delegate to the 1986 Maine State Conference on Aging.

Linda K. Scharer, M.U.P., graduated with a bachelor's degree from Connecticut College and holds a master's degree in urban planning from New York University. Since 1977 she has been on the staff of the Department of Community Medicine at St. Vincent's Hospital and Medical Center of New York, and is now the assistant director of the department. Her responsibilities include liaison with community and governmental agencies, program development and administration in the area of long term home health care, consulting in this field, and supervision of placement of master's degree students within the department. Ms. Scharer serves on the Committee for the New York Community Trust Center on Aging, is a member of the editorial board of the *PRIDE Institute Journal of Long Term Home Health Care,* and has written on the subject of informal supports for the aged.

Acknowledgments

Our work in the field of care for the elderly and our opportunities to learn have flourished largely through the encouragement and support of the administration and personnel of St. Vincent's Hospital and Medical Center of New York. We are especially grateful to the late Sister Anthony Marie FitzMaurice, Sister Evelyn M. Schneider, and Sister Margaret Sweeney, presidents of the hospital in recent years, for their nurturing of our efforts. We owe particular thanks as well to other individuals, past and present, within the administration and staff: Sister Marian Catherine Muldoon, Mary Hart, Albert Samis, Gary Horan, Tom McGourty, John Fales, Jack Koretsky, Rita Conyers, John Ferguson, Joe Corcoran, Roger Weaving, Martin Spector, Claudia Zocki, Jeff Davis, Mary Ann Maisonett, Bill Devitt, Sylvia Gray, Angel Vergez, Candi Ramos, Ray Scardapane, Anthony Formato, Joe English, Mick McGarvey, the late William J. Grace, Jim Mazzara, Joe Hoffman, Ted Druhot, Lambert King, Sister Karen Helfenstein, Agnes Frank, John Dolan, Peter Ghiorse, Mark Ackermann, Dan Sorrenti, the late Hazel Halloran, Suzanne Kohut, Dorothy Murray, Annita Treacy, Barbara Conanan, Marianne Savarese, Al Elvy, Carl Nolte, Bart Price, Sister Mary T. Boyle, Ralph O'Connell, Sam Sverdlick, Anne Boland, Father Jefferson Hammer, Tommy Ball, Thomas Johns, Julio Martinez, Sister Patrice Murphy, Charlotte Natale, Andrew Portelli, Carol Zipse, Walter Harkin, Dorothy Conley, Bill Wilson, Paul Savage, Frances Rodriguez, Virginia Sweeny, Mary Jean O'Brien, Stephan Koblick, Thomas Detrano, Margaret Tangeman, Lauren Finn, Jill Koproski, Sister Gilmary Simmons, the late Sister Regina McAvoy, and Carol Coven.

Our colleagues of the Chelsea-Village Program, the Long Term Home Health Care Program, and the PRIDE Long Term Home Health Care Institute, all within the hospital's Department of Community Medicine, have shared their skills, energy, and empathy with us over the past fifteen years: Margaret Amato, Richard Beck, Jessica Blumert, Linda Brandt, Joel Brauser, Alex Bruton, Ray Bucko, Dorothy Calvani, Robert Campion, Claire Carlo, Brenda Carter, Edith Chanin, Ellen Cohen, Loretta Conley, Michael Conroy, Eleanor Davis, Joseph DeFillippi, Barbara DiCicco-Bloom, Bridget Downes, Daniel DuCoffe, William P. Duggan, Richard Epstein, Carol Ewig, Thomas Flannery, Jan Fogelquist, Kate Gaffney, Michael Garvey, Jeffrey Gimbel, Roslynn Glicksman, Robert Goldberg, Tom Gradler, Jody Greco, Gina Gregory, Ellen Harnett, Elizabeth Healy, Claire Henry, Deborah Hillman, Sister Margaret Rose Ibe, Yoel Isenberg, Jeffery Jahre, James Janeski, Bernee Kapili, Faith Karkowski, Ellen Katsorhis, Arthur Kaufman, David Kaufman, F. Russell Kellogg, Sharon Kiely, Priscilla Kistler, Richard Lander, Louis Larca, Richard LaRocco, Helene Lee, Mary Ann Lee, Pearl Lefkowitz, Betsy Litsas, Lila McConnell, Hugh McDonald, James McEnrue, Carol McGarvey, Samuel Madeira, Michael Makowski, Katherine Marino, Rowena Martinez-Pita, Margaret Mason, Susan Maturlo, Nancy Mellow, Chris Mills, Mary Ann Mosher, Jane Mossberg, Anthony Mure, Margaret Murphy, Jeffrey Naiditch, Zorquina Naranjo, Mark Nathanson, Edward Navarro, Jeffrey Nichols, John Novello, Ellen Olsen, Barbara Olvany, John Oppenheimer, Susan Palermo, Ellen Quirke, Jane Reilly, Kevin Reilly, Gloria Rich, Marilyn Rogers, Terry Rogers, Nancy Roistacher, Gladys Rosado, Wilfredo Royo, Barbara Ruether, Michael Sarg, Brian Scanlan, Anne Schroeder, Lorette Shea, Marc Sherman, Richard Sherwin, Howard Siegel, Irma Stahl, Jeffrey Stall, Laura Starita, J. Reed Sterrett, Sister Mary Sugrue, Jane Taylor, Gabriel Torres, Lorraine Tosiello, Patricia Trossman, Janet Varon, Christine Vitarella, Fredda Vladeck, Ira Wagner, Edward Walker, Priscilla Wallack, Floyd Warren, Duane Webb, Carol Weber, Jacqueline Weir, Steven Werlin, Richard Westfall, Kathy Lynne Woodson, Lois Young, and Kathryn Zunich.

We acknowledge with gratitude the advice and assistance over many years of persons outside the hospital, in our community and across the country: Mark J. Appleman, Ann Berson, Janice Caldwell, Marjorie Cantor, James Capalino, Ronald Docksai, Louis Gary, Orrin Hatch, Chris Jennings, Al Kaplan, Edward I. Koch, Diane Lifsey, Tommy Lipscomb, Tommy Loeb, Anthony Mangiaracina, Evelyn Mathis, Mary Mayer, Barbara Michaels, Joe Michaels, Arthur Milton, Guy Molinari, Budd Norris, Manfred Ohrenstein, Lawrence Orton, Carol O'Shaughnessy, Bill Passannante, Richard Price, Nancy Rankin, Meg Reed, Janet Sainer, Al Schwarz, David Sundwall, Phil Toia, Ronald Wickham, and Burk Zanft.

We owe thanks to George Greenberg, Ph.D., Peter Davies, M.D., and Jeffrey Wilkins, M.D., who gave expert readings to chapters 2, 4, and 5, respectively. Their advice and guidance is deeply appreciated. Any errors of fact, omission, or commission remain, however, the responsibility of the authors.

We are grateful to Daniel Beaudoin and Darcy Guhl for assistance in preparation of the manuscript, Patricia Ambrosino for word processing, Michele Salcedo and Marian Malakoff for editing, Robert Markel for agenting, and, with particular emphasis, Judy Greissman of Basic Books.

On a personal level, thanks to Alice Brickner, Maria Lechich, Eric Wright, and Lawrence Scharer, without whom . . .

Preface

The number of older people in our population is growing explosively, and will continue to do so over the next fifty years. Unfortunately, our country lacks a coherent policy to meet the long term care needs of the elderly, even though considerable practical experience and scholarly analysis are available. Substantial data are scattered through diverse disciplines, including medicine, nursing, gerontology, social services, and the behavioral and biological sciences. However, these resources are not integrated and therefore are poorly understood and assimilated. This book attempts a systematic compilation and evaluation of information about older persons' long term care needs and how they may best be met. We hope to define the necessary components of a national policy, one that will lead to development of a spectrum of long term care services for the aged.

Our society is poised at a moment of critical decision. It is possible to plan for care of the aged in a humane and caring spirit, with prudent use of resources and encouragement of maximum possible independence. Alternatively, we can abdicate the hard work of policy formulation and then find that growing numbers of the elderly, without adequate health services and deprived of social support, are packed into institutions or suffering in their homes without help.

Our own work with the aged spans more than two decades and provides the background for this book. We have created and conducted long term home health care programs and engaged in care of older persons in skilled nursing facilities; helped formulate relevant legislation in Washington, D.C., and Albany, New York; consulted with hospitals and community agencies regarding practical aspects of project development; carried out clinical studies of the frail elderly; and, since 1982, published a professional journal in the field of long term care.

St. Vincent's Hospital established the Chelsea-Village Program in New York City in 1973, one of the first hospital-based long term home health care programs in the United States. Our deep involvement in this program has been especially educational. To date, we have shared in the lives of more than fifteen hundred homebound persons. Their average age is eighty-three. Two-thirds live alone. All are chronically disabled. We have learned about the nature of disease among the very old, the extent of health and extended care benefits available to them, and the variable limits of family assistance. We have learned to recognize the individuality of each of our patients and the invalidity of measuring their worth by chronology. We have been particularly struck by their urgent desire to remain in their own homes and out of institutions.

Much of the information we offer derives from the experience of others. We have learned from many individuals, including professionals, family members of older persons, and especially from the aged themselves throughout the country. Among our most striking lessons is the degree of complexity hidden within the subject of long term care. The vast and shifting range of physical ability, intellectual capacity, and social settings of those whom we consider old requires sophistication in program design. Another lesson learned, one of grave human and ethical value, is that all of us, at any age, should remain free to make our own major life decisions, a stand that must ever be supported and strengthened or we are all at risk.

Through these experiences we have recognized the need for new directions in national policy that will permit fulfillment of these goals. It is our central purpose to share these insights with others.

In this book we discuss the program components, history, and financing of a long term care spectrum and the health status and functional ability of the elderly. We also review trends and forecasts leading to policy recommendations. Among the clinical concerns faced by the aged, we have chosen to consider in depth dementia and alcohol abuse. The dementias, including particularly Alzheimer's disease, have become common, well-recognized, and pressing issues. However, there now exists the need to define with clarity the various syndromes, and in particular to recognize those forms of dementia that are treatable. Alcohol abuse in the elderly, on the other hand, often remains hidden and unacknowledged. The ability to perceive that a problem exists in an individual case requires raising the general level of sensitivity to the possibility of the diagnosis. Abuse of alcohol is a genuine difficulty for significant numbers of the aged and is relatively easily treated.

We have striven to be scientifically accurate, current, and objective; yet we assert a distinct viewpoint in regard to the health and social service needs of the frail aged in our country and to the principles of policy development that should follow. We are not, in a fundamental sense, neutral. Rather, we are firmly committed to achieving all that is feasible so that the elderly may be independent and in control. We are also committed realists. Our country's current fiscal state restricts the various conceivable approaches, and government, in any case, cannot be the sole source of funds. All the more reason, therefore, that we should press to maximize the intelligent use of those resources that are available.

We have written this book for a diverse audience, in addition to those currently involved in care of old people. We hope that students and other practitioners in the health professions will be stimulated by it to work with the aged. We wish to encourage older persons themselves, and their family members, to become aware of and to seek available options for care, and to share with others the effort to develop needed community services. We intend to inspire those in the legislative and executive branches of government to grapple with the imperative need for creation of far-seeing, logical, prudent, and caring policy.

Composer and pianist Eubie Blake said, at the celebration of his ninety-sixth birthday, "If I'd known I was going to live so long I would have taken better care of myself." This degree of serenity and wry humor is given to few. However, most older persons, with a bit of assistance, can have better care and at the least maintain a free and independent life. Others, if given more defined and consistent help, can avoid institutional placement. Only a few of the elderly—the most disabled, isolated, and helpless—need a nursing home.

Philip W. Brickner
Anthony J. Lechich
Roberta Lipsman
Linda K. Scharer

PART ONE

INTRODUCTION

Chapter 1

The Long Term Care Spectrum

Caring for the needs of older people in this nation is now a subject of major human and financial significance. About five thousand persons in the United States turn sixty-five every day, and about thirty-five hundred that age or older die.[1] The proportion and gross number of the elderly in our population are steadily increasing,[2] and that growth is expected to continue unabated well into the next half century.[3,4] We face a tidal wave of the aging.

Our policies regarding long term health and social services for older people are poorly organized, often fail to meet the needs of those who require assistance, and are wasteful, costly, and cruel. To the extent that a focus is discernible, it is one based on a predisposition toward institutional placement. As a result, and because noninstitutional forms of long term care are stultified, frail elderly persons are often forced to leave their homes against their wishes, at substantial dollar and personal costs to themselves, their families, and the larger community.

In the United States today, there is a paucity of options for care of the elderly. Financial and demographic considerations will increasingly demand the creation of a comprehensive spectrum of programs for the aged. Our current set of choices is too narrow, too rigid in eligibility, and is not sufficiently flexible to accommodate growth and change. Therefore it is in the broad interests of our country that a long term care spectrum for the aged be created.

This book defines a basis for such a long term care spectrum. It explains why diverse service options for the elderly are an effective and financially rational response to today's needs and tomorrow's demands; and it illustrates methods of developing and implementing programs consistent with this strategy. We discuss demographic and cost analyses, an evolving role for government, the absolute need to defend the individual rights of elderly persons, problems with current programs, and clinical disorders of the aged that may impact particularly on long term care, such as dementia and alcohol abuse. All policy designers must recognize that services should be tailored to individual need and that older people are entitled to make their own choices, their own major life decisions.

Old age is honored only on condition that it defends itself, maintains its rights, is subservient to no one, and to the last breath rules over its own domain.

—CICERO, QUOTING CATO, in *Old Age XI*

Gerontologist George Maddox was the first to use the apposite term demographic imperative[5] to indicate the potential pressures the numerical growth of the elderly might place on our health and social service systems. The challenge is substantial, particularly in regard to care for those older persons who are very old, frail, and disabled. We must:

Understand the magnitude of the problem. Beyond mere demographic studies, the degree to which older people need help to remain independent must be analyzed. Funding and cost issues, age cohort distinctions and expectations,[6] and technical and personnel resources all must be considered. We should be able to define the needs of our aged population in terms of their degree of dependence on others.[7]

Establish a spectrum of service programs. Today we still focus far too much on institutionalization[8] despite recent growth in homemaker and home aide businesses.[9] Once a spectrum is in place, it will become increasingly important to *distinguish clearly the clinical disorders of very old people.* Only then can we move toward proper diagnosis and treatment. The medical causes of frailty and homeboundedness are the concern here, and there is a particular need to recognize the chronicity of many illnesses in the aged.

THE MAGNITUDE OF THE PROBLEM

Money for long term care of the frail aged flows toward institutions. Other options are starved because our norms now dictate that form follows finance.[10] This institutional emphasis continues despite recent amendments to Medicare law[11] and new attempts to restrict nursing home placement to the most helpless.[12]

Based on 1980 census figures, about 5 percent of persons aged sixty-five and older live in chronic care institutions such as nursing homes; about 10 percent of those over seventy-five are so placed.[13] By the year 2000, the number of those aged sixty-five and over will have doubled and those of greatly advanced age, defined as aged eighty-five and more, quadrupled.[14] (See table 1.1.)

If we continue to use our current placement policies, to meet the nursing home requirements of our population we would need to increase the number of chronic care beds from the 1980 figure of 1.22 million to 1.69 million in 1990, 2.19 million in 2000, and 2.99 million by 2020.[15] The cost of this bricks-and-mortar approach would reach $76 billion a year by 1990 and would continue to rise. In contrast, in 1982 we spent only $27 billion on nursing home costs.[16]

Thus, unless we move toward doubling the stock of chronic care beds, there will be no room at the nursing home; yet the dollar cost of such an approach is prohibitive.

The social costs of incarcerating increased numbers of the aged must also be calculated. Some older persons welcome institutional placement, but most do not. Most prefer a life of independence.

The following quotation from the case record of a seventy-six-year-old disabled woman makes the point:

Why should I go to a nursing home? You see my shrine over there? When I wake up at night, I sit in my rocker and say my rosary. When I feel like it, I can go to the kitchen and make myself a cup of tea. [She looked around her sparsely furnished apartment.] Do you see this furniture and this rug? They're mine, and I worked hard for them. Why should I give them up? No. I will have no part of a nursing home.[17]

It is on the most frail and disabled older people, growing in number, great in need, that attention must be focused, and it is here that the major opportunity for financial and social gains exists.

CONSEQUENCES OF INCREASED LIFE EXPECTANCY

As more people reach what is now the potential human life-span, the proportion of the very old among the general population will grow.[18] (See table 1.2.) Critical questions then arise: If people live longer, will their

TABLE 1.1

The Growth of the Older Population, Actual and Projected: 1900–2050
(Numbers in Thousands)

Year	Total Population, All Ages No.	%	55 Years and Over No.	%	55 to 64 Years No.	%	65 to 74 Years No.	%	75 to 84 Years No.	%	85 Years and Over No.	%	65 Years and Over No.	%
1900	76,303	100	7,093	9.3	4,009	5.3	2,189	2.9	772	1.0	123	0.2	3,084	4.0
1910	91,972	100	9,004	9.8	5,054	5.5	2,793	3.0	989	1.1	167	.2	3,950	4.3
1920	105,711	100	11,465	10.8	6,532	6.2	3,464	3.3	1,259	1.2	210	.2	4,933	4.7
1930	122,775	100	15,031	12.2	8,397	6.8	4,721	3.8	1,641	1.3	272	.2	6,634	5.4
1940	131,669	100	19,591	14.9	10,572	8.0	6,375	4.8	2,278	1.7	365	.3	9,019	6.8
1950	150,697	100	25,565	17.0	13,295	8.8	8,415	5.6	3,278	2.2	577	.4	12,270	8.1
1960	179,323	100	32,132	17.9	15,572	8.7	10,997	6.1	4,633	2.6	929	.5	16,560	9.2
1970	203,302	100	38,588	19.0	18,608	9.2	12,447	6.1	6,124	3.0	1,409	.7	19,980	9.8
1980	226,505	100	47,244	20.9	21,700	9.6	15,578	6.9	7,727	3.4	2,240	1.0	25,544	11.3
1990	249,731	100	52,889	21.2	21,090	8.4	18,054	7.2	10,284	4.1	3,461	1.4	31,799	12.7
2000	267,990	100	58,815	21.9	23,779	8.9	17,693	6.6	12,207	4.6	5,136	1.9	35,036	13.1
2010	283,141	100	74,097	26.2	34,828	12.3	20,279	7.2	12,172	4.3	6,818	2.4	39,269	13.9
2020	296,339	100	91,629	30.9	40,243	13.6	29,769	10.0	14,280	4.8	7,337	2.5	51,386	17.3
2030	304,330	100	98,310	32.3	33,965	11.2	34,416	11.3	21,128	6.9	8,801	2.9	64,345	21.1
2040	307,952	100	101,307	32.9	34,664	11.3	29,168	9.5	24,529	8.0	12,946	4.2	66,643	21.6
2050	308,856	100	104,337	33.8	37,276	12.1	30,022	9.7	20,976	6.8	16,063	5.2	67,061	21.7

SOURCE: U.S. Bureau of the Census. 1982 October. Decennial Censuses of Population, 1900–1980, and Projections of the Population of the United States: 1982–2050 (Advance Report). *Current Population Reports*, ser. P-25, no. 922. Projections are middle series.

increased years be generally productive and healthy, or will the positive qualities of life be thwarted by chronic illness? Will these people be functional or disabled?

A study issued by the Federal Council on Aging[19] indicates that 1 percent of all people under forty-five are unable to carry on significant major activity important to daily life, due to chronic disabling conditions. For those forty-five to sixty-four, the figure is 6 percent. Table 1.3 illustrates further the correlation between aging and decrease in functional ability to perform.

The correlation can also be measured in terms of activities of daily living (ADL). ADL include, for instance, bathing, dressing, eating, and moving from supine to erect position or from bed to chair. Efforts have been made to analyze the functional well-being of older people through ADL testing. In an exemplary Massachusetts study,[20] results show that people sixty-five to seventy years of age could expect to average 10 more years of ADL independence. For those eighty-five or older, the expectation was 2.9 years. The period of independent activity tended to be shorter for poor people and longer for women.

TABLE 1.2

Life Expectancies at Birth and
Age 65 by Sex and Calendar Year

Calendar Year	Male At Birth	Male At Age 65	Female At Birth	Female At Age 65
1900	46.56	11.35	49.07	12.01
1910	50.20	11.38	53.67	12.10
1920	54.59	11.81	56.33	12.34
1930	58.01	11.38	61.36	12.91
1940	60.89	11.92	65.34	13.42
1950	65.33	12.81	70.90	15.07
1960	66.58	12.91	73.19	15.89
1970	67.05	13.14	74.80	17.12
1980	69.85	14.02	77.53	18.35
1990	72.29	15.11	79.85	19.92
2000	73.42	15.71	81.05	20.81
2010	73.93	16.08	81.62	21.27
2020	74.42	16.45	82.18	21.73
2030	74.90	16.81	82.74	22.18
2040	75.37	17.18	83.29	22.64
2050	75.84	17.55	83.84	23.11

SOURCE: Social Security Administration, Office of the Actuary, 1982 September, cited in U.S. Senate Special Committee on Aging in conjunction with the American Association of Retired Persons (1984). *Aging America: Trends and Projections.* PL 3377(584), Washington, DC.

TABLE 1.3

*Age Relationship to
Loss of Ability to Perform
Major Activity*

Age Group	Percent Unable to Perform Major Activity
65 to 74 years	14
75 to 84	20
85 and over	31

SOURCE: Federal Council on Aging. (1981). *The need for long term care: Information and issues.* Washington, DC: U.S. Dept. of Health and Human Services, Office of Human Development Services.

Using these measures, specific populations at high risk for loss of independent activity can be sought and available resources targeted. Further, this type of analysis permits us to focus attention on indicators of the quality of life rather than on expected time of death. Our natural desire for long life can be placed in a more sophisticated perspective: each person's life spent in maximum possible independence.

ESTABLISHING A SPECTRUM
OF LONG TERM CARE SERVICES

No genuine system of long term care for the aged exists, as such, in this country. Instead we live with a set of anachronistic and uncoordinated programs, policies, and funding methods. We envision the creation of a spectrum of services that would address the current individual requirements of older people, allow the easy transition from one program to another as needs change, and use available funds prudently. The components of such a system include institutions such as nursing homes, home care, paraprofessional services such as care by aides, respite and day care programs, hospice services, foster care, and designed housing.

The basic elements already exist in the United States. Some, such as nursing homes and other institutions, are well known in all their ramifications. Others, such as paraprofessional services, are not available in some geographic areas and are funded irregularly. Still others, including respite care, various housing options, and long term home health care, remain largely experimental. Of all the components in a spectrum of care services, some require strengthening; others, more control. Coordination among the various components is largely absent.

When a systematic approach to the problem is taken, a range of options will become available. Where feasible, relatively inexpensive services can be used to meet minimum essential requirements of the aged; costly nursing homes should be reserved for those who truly need twenty-four-hour-a-day care and are willing to be institutionalized. Older people should be free to move between programs of varying comprehensiveness and cost as their health and social requirements require. A day care program for older persons, for instance, might allow them to live with working adult offspring. If day care were not available, a nursing home might be the only alternative placement available.

We should seek the least restrictive form of care that is appropriate. This principle allows for maximum individual responsibility and decreases dependency and infantilization of older people. The story of Maria L. is a case in point:

Maria, a childless widow, lived alone in a walk-up tenement building in the lower Manhattan neighborhood where she had spent her whole life. When she was seventy-five, she was referred to a long term health care program by a social worker from a local senior citizens' center. At the first visit to her apartment, the health care team discovered that Maria was legally blind because of irreversible retinal disease. She suffered also from marked osteoarthritis, with persistent low back and shoulder pain, and reactive depression. She managed to cook and clean by sheer rote memory. Her main complaint: "If I could only see—I would give up everything to get my eyes back. If I only had my eyes, I'd fly; I'd be richer than Rockefeller!"

Maria's only relatives lived in Arizona. Concerned about her well-being and distressed by her isolated and homebound condition, they proposed to place her in a nursing home. But Maria tenaciously adhered to her resolve: "No. No. No. I want my home—however small and humble it is, it's mine!" Regular telephone calls from the team's social worker allayed the family's fears.

During the six years Maria was seen by the team, she developed further significant medical problems, including gallstones with intermittent abdominal pain. She refused surgery for this condition, but her other ailments were handled successfully. About a year after Maria was first visited, the social worker, familiar with gross symptoms of diseases common among the elderly, noted that Maria was short of breath. She alerted the nurse and physician who promptly placed Maria under treatment for heart failure. Shortly afterward, the social worker arranged for minor renovations in Maria's apartment to help her manage at home with less physical exertion. Two years later symptoms of diabetes mellitus were noted, and Maria was hospitalized for institution of insulin treatment. Team visits continued during her hospital stay, and when Maria returned home, the nurse organized her insulin therapy. Prefilled syringes were stocked in the refrigerator, and Maria learned to inject herself. Maria died in 1984, when she was eighty-one, of carcinoma of the gall bladder. Her single source of contentment and pride was her ability to remain independent and at home. Until the final days of her malignancy, through her own determination and the combined skills of the health care team, she managed to maintain her life-sustaining goals. In this case, effective teamwork—regular assessments, shared responsibility, frequent interaction, and seasoned trust among team members—yielded a special advantage.[21]

The person at risk must be the focus of every program. Often there is distortion to serve interests of staff members rather than those of clients. Government functionaries make decisions (or fail to do so) to serve agency or personal ends. The term professional narcissism is apt.[22]

NEEDED: AN ORDERLY APPROACH

No coherent program for long term care planning exists. We must abandon the patchwork quality that has dominated our thinking in favor of an orderly and systematic approach that includes an understanding and clarification of:

1. *Definitions of long term care.* Here confusion abounds. For instance, para-professional workers may be called homemakers, home health aides, housekeepers, and even homemaker/home health aides.[23] Functions overlap, rates of pay vary indiscriminately, and job descriptions include arbitrary lists of permitted tasks and rigid hours of work. Or look at terms like nursing home, retirement home, foster home, skilled nursing facility, health-related facility, and boarding house.[24] Some institutions and programs receive full government support; some, partial; some, none at all.
2. *An evolutionary role for government.* The American form of government, based so strongly on the will of the people as implemented by elected representatives, has tended to respond to crisis. Too often long-range planning to meet anticipated social needs has evaded us. Now, however, through demographic data and projections, we have an unusual opportunity to perceive the future. It will be wise to evolve, prudently yet promptly, the creation of long term care options. Otherwise we will lack effective means of providing adequate services to our people. Crises are costly.
3. *The validity of asserting individual rights.* Insofar as it is possible in our complex world, full of demanding people, we work toward allowing

choices.[25] This country, with its diverse populations, speaks with many loud voices. Clichéd thinking and stereotyping abound, and too often the weakest are not heard. While in recent decades older people generally have been well served—through Medicare and the Social Security laws, for instance—the frailest among them have not. Major life decisions for aged people are made by others—their children, employees of institutions, health professionals. It is our task to protect the rights of the weak. Otherwise we are all potentially at risk.

4. *The room for choices.* Our tendency to perceive institutional placement as the logical consequence of old age and weakness persists, and too often the value of encouraging older people to make choices for themselves is ignored. Thus the frail elderly face the classic Hobson's choice: no choice at all.[26]

5. *Recognition of the gaps and overlaps in existing programs.* The irregular, often unfocused manner in which programs for the aged have evolved has resulted in serious inadequacies in service. On the other hand, resources to help the frail aged may be available locally but may lack coordination. Meals-on-Wheels, Friendly Visitors, a senior citizens' center, and transportation services may all exist, but they are useless to an older, isolated, or confused person without a case manager to integrate the service effort. This issue is a consequence of, and is compounded by, uncoordinated legislation. The sheer number of federal efforts—for instance, Title XVIII of the Social Security Act (Medicare), Title XIX (Medicaid), Title XX (the Older Americans Act), each with its own eligibility requirements—suggests the degree of confusion that prevails. This situation has been compounded by recent federal legislation amending Medicare law, including the Tax Equity and Fiscal Responsibility Act of 1982 (TEFRA), the Social Security Amendments of 1983, the Deficit Reduction Act of 1984, the Balanced Budget and Deficit Control Act of 1985 (also known as the Gramm-Rudman-Hollings Act), and the Consolidated Omnibus Reconciliation Act of 1985, or COBRA.[27] The great variety of state and local programs only adds to the difficulty. Gaps and overlaps are the inevitable consequences of uncoordinated legislative effort.

HOW DID WE GET INTO THIS SITUATION?

The past has made the present.

—REBECCA WEST, *Black Lamb and Grey Falcon*

How did we come to accept institutions as the best way to care for the frail aged and, at the same time, find that we can neither build nor pay for enough nursing homes to satisfy future needs? Why have we pressed for long term institutional placement when the very people targeted for such care resist and resent the idea?

In the eighteenth and early nineteenth centuries, perceptions of old age were ambiguous, but the tendency of our society to shun the elderly was present even then. During the nineteenth century the practice of dumping poor older people and younger paupers together into almshouses grew. It then became easy to think of the aged, in general, as helpless and dependent on the charity of others. The attitudes of nineteenth-century physicians about life force and vital energy encouraged this view. Each human being was believed to be born with a limited quantity of vital energy; as it was consumed, the body became an empty husk, devoid, finally, of life force. It was logical, then, for advanced age to signify inevitable physical and mental decline, and older people themselves were perceived as disabled and useless.

These views challenged more ancient concepts of aged people as the repository of society's wisdom. Instead, enforced retirement became the only sane and kind social policy for most older people in order to sustain "the feeble germ of life that still remains."[28] It followed that it was pointless to treat the diseases of the aged. The notion of dependent superannuation developed, a view that has led directly to our current model of old-age dependency, advocacy of institutional care for aged paupers, and state financing of the arrangements.

But at the same time that these general concepts were being translated into policy, individual and local efforts in opposition to institutional placement were growing. In fact, since colonial days Americans have tried to develop creative ways of providing health care at home. Unfortunately, past efforts were just as marred by the absence of a long term approach as are today's.

In 1796 the Boston Dispensary created a service that gave the impoverished sick the option of care at home rather than in the hospital. As Allen Spiegel of Downstate Medical Center and Gerard Domanowski of Massachusetts General Hospital point out,[29] hospitals of that era were akin to pesthouses, where the old and homeless went to die. The rich were treated at home by their own physicians. Thus home care for poor people was an enlightened concept. The overseers of the Boston program wished to see that "those who have seen better days may be comforted without being humiliated."[30]

Shame in the face of need was a concern that Lillian Wald and Mary Brewster faced in the 1890s. Their efforts to help care for immigrant mothers and their infants on the Lower East Side of New York were at first hampered by the reluctance of the poor themselves to consider help. "And these women did not try to uplift them or sentimentalize over them or offer them charity. . . . Practically the only concrete help they could give was nursing care for the sick."[31] The Visiting Nurse Service of New York was born of this small beginning. During the early 1900s, the number of visiting nurse agencies in the northeastern United States grew significantly.[32] These home health programs expanded to include nutrition and social services; occupational, physical, and speech therapy; as well as homemaker and home health aide care.

As a matter of good business, the insurance industry soon began to recognize home care as a factor. In 1909 the Metropolitan Life Insurance Company offered home health services to its policy holders; the John Hancock Insurance Company provided similar coverage.[33] This benefit became so popular that by 1928 Metropolitan employed more than five hundred home care nurses and had contractual relationships with almost one thousand visiting nurse agencies around the country. These programs were phased out at the beginning of World War II, when hospitals became more widely used and inpatient insurance coverage grew broadly available.

In 1942 Michael Reese Hospital in Chicago and in 1947 Montefiore Hospital in New York founded the country's first major hospital-based home care programs, efforts that have served as prototypes.[34] The rationale behind this concept, as developed by Dr. E. M. Bluestone and Dr. Martin Cherkasky at Montefiore, was expressed succinctly: "it must be clearly understood that the hospital bed is not the 'natural habitat' of a sick human being and that the alternatives to hospitalization not only may be economical of beds and money but may be beneficial as well as comforting to the patient."[35]

As perceived by Bluestone and Cherkasky, patients could be divided into two groups. Some required the specialized facilities of the acute care hospital. Others, however, while also needing medical and nursing services, could have this care provided at home. They remained hospitalized only because their poverty prevented them from obtaining the services of a private physician.[36]

In the years since 1947, the common sense and intellectual validity behind the Montefiore concept have led to the creation of a network of home care programs emanating from hospitals across the country.[37] However, as these programs gradually became subject to government control, they were permitted to function only after certification by state authorities, a process that continues to date.[38] Certification has the virtue of controlling costs through strict admission rules for patients, limiting services through the so-called skilled nursing and intermittent care requirements, and insisting on a maximum stay of approximately three to six weeks. But these very requirements render hospital home care programs powerless to meet a significant need: *long term* care at home for the frail aged, with assistance from both paraprofessionals and professional health workers.

Evidence documenting this unmet need is found in the list of referral sources for one of the few longstanding hospital-based programs in the country that concentrates on the chronically disabled and frail homebound aged, the Chelsea-Village Program at St. Vincent's Hospital and Medical Center of New York. According to its fourteen-year report, of more than fifteen hundred patients under care during these years, almost 5 percent were referred from the hospital's own excellent certified home care programs.[39] More than 7 percent came from the rolls of the Visiting Nurse Service of New York, a certified agency that is forced to function under the same set of arbitrary restrictions as the hospital home care program. These two certified agencies were required to give up care of their patients, because Medicare reimbursement ran out.

LEGISLATIVE HISTORY

Formal attempts on the part of government to develop a basis for long term care services can be traced to the Social Security Act of 1935. As policy analyst Peter Fox has pointed out, this legislation

> established the cash welfare payments for the old age, dependent children, and blind categories. It also prohibited payments to "inmates of public institutions," which provided an impetus for placing people in private profit-oriented board and care homes rather than county service systems. These homes formed part of the provider-base when nursing home benefits subsequently were explicitly adopted.[40]

In 1950 states were permitted for the first time to pay health service costs for individuals receiving welfare benefits. Prior to this date, care for this group was a local responsibility and dealt with haphazardly. The Hill-Burton Act, as amended in 1954, authorized funding through grants for nursing home construction in the not-for-profit sector. This critical development set a precedent for public support of nursing homes and is recognized as the initial impetus for the major and explosive growth of these institutions, both public and proprietary, during the third quarter of the twentieth century.[41]

In 1960 the Kerr-Mills amendments to the Social Security Act provided federal funds, with matched state money, for health services to the aged poor. Thus the concept of medical indigency was recognized in federal legislation. In large part the funds made available through this bill were used to house old people in nursing homes.

In 1964 Medicare was a new concept in health care funding for this country. For the first time a significant portion of the population, largely persons aged sixty-five years and more, received entitlement to health insurance protection on a basis other than indigency. Medicare is paid for by each individual through deductions from Social Security benefits.[42] At present no means test is required for eligibility, although fiscal pressures on the program may ultimately alter this basic principle.

Ironically, long term health care needs of the elderly receive minimal support under Medicare. This insurance program provides benefits instead largely for *acute* hospital inpatient care and for physician's fees, a concept established in the original legislation and regulations that remains unaltered today. Yet the demographic changes we have noted strongly support the view that *chronic* health care needs of the elderly are substantial, increasing, and unmet.

Medicaid, developed in 1965 as amendments to the Social Security Act, is more a compilation and summary of prior health care financing legislation than a new concept. These amendments incorporated funding to pay health care costs of the poor through a relationship to the welfare system. Medicaid is therefore strictly limited to those who pass a means test, and is supported by tax levy funds of federal, state, and some local governments. The Medicaid legislation resulted in a broadened definition of medical indigency, implementation of payment for health care costs of all persons receiving welfare support, and stressed nursing home placement for eligible individuals, thus enhancing our country's proinstitutional bias for care of the frail elderly.

THE PATCHWORK OF TODAY

The impact of this legislative history, through the distortions it has imposed on health care planning and funding, is substantial. The economy of the country and the welfare of the frail aged have been placed at unnecessary risk. Although there are a number of government-sponsored efforts—local, state, and federal—related to long term care, no single agency has control, and the inevitable consequence is overlap and discontinuity.

Characteristic of today's situation are reimbursement regulations that emphasize institutional care and legislation that sanctions the separation of social and nursing services from physician services in the home. The mandated Part A of Medicare covers hospital costs and services only, including nurses and social workers. The optional Part B pays for private physician care, both in hospital and at home. Medicaid generally maintains this distinction in a most peculiar way: while theoretically all professional services at home may be covered, in at least one major state (New York) the fee for a visiting nurse's visit is more than $70, while a physician's visit is $7 or less, a fee insufficient to pay for the cost of service. This effectively freezes out medical care at home for Medicaid patients. Visits from social workers are not paid for at all. Similar legislative and regulatory distinctions apply in other government-supported programs, including the various titles of the Older Americans Act and nutrition programs.

There is marked geographic variability in reimbursement. The government divides authority between central and local forces. Medicaid law and regulations, for instance, vary in policy and funding among the fifty states. Further, because of differences in Medicaid regulations, building codes, lobbying forces, and population density of the aged, the number of nursing home beds differs markedly from state to state and seems often to be unrelated to need. For instance, in 1983, Arizona had about twenty-two such beds per one thousand elderly people, compared to eighty-nine in Wisconsin. (See table 1.4.)

Paraprofessional service providers may be lacking in rural areas. In crowded cities, however, where many patients can be reached fairly quickly, home health aide companies are competing for business.

Medicaid eligibility varies by state regulation and is based on income and family size. Since local initiative is so important in establishing the nature of Medicaid programs, enormous variety exists across the country. The role of the fiscal intermediaries, like Blue Cross, and the ability of functionaries at various levels of government to inhibit or expand services by interpretation have a major impact on service delivery as well.

As Bruce Vladeck, president of the United Hospital Fund of New York, points out,[43] revisions in nursing home surveillance suggested in 1984 in the final report of President Reagan's Deregulation Task Force[44] calls for a reduction in federal support for state enforcement and inspection activities. A decreased total dollar flow to the states for these purposes would result, and it is reasonable to suppose that states would be reluctant to substitute their own monies. A prompt diminution in quality of nursing home services is likely to follow.

These points illustrate our country's inherent crisis-oriented approach to critical issues involving health care, with a consequent lag in ability to meet the population's changing needs. Other causes also contribute. These include desire to simplify regulations, fear of open-ended funding, and liberal nursing home entry standards.

The Desire for Simplified Regulation and Administration

Legislators and regulators who attempt to exercise their mandated authority over budgets often try to simplify a system. One set of rules that

TABLE 1.4
Nursing Home Beds Per 1,000
Age 65 and Older in 1983

By State		By Number	
Alabama	46	Arizona	22
Alaska	58	Florida	24
Arizona	22	West Virginia	28
Arkansas	62	Hawaii	29
California	43	Nevada	30
Colorado	67	North Carolina	33
Connecticut	66	New Jersey	34
Delaware	66	District of Columbia	35
District of Columbia	35	New Mexico	35
Florida	24	South Carolina	40
Georgia	65	Virginia	41
Hawaii	29	California	43
Idaho	44	New York	43
Illinois	66	Idaho	44
Indiana	80	Kentucky	44
Iowa	84	Utah	45
Kansas	83	Alabama	46
Kentucky	44	Mississippi	46
Louisiana	63	Oregon	46
Maine	62	Pennsylvania	48
Maryland	53	Tennessee	48
Massachusetts	60	Michigan	49
Michigan	49	Vermont	50
Minnesota	88	Wyoming	52
Mississippi	46	Maryland	53
Missouri	67	Alaska	58
Montana	68	Washington	58
Nebraska	87	Ohio	59
Nevada	30	Massachusetts	60
New Hampshire	63	Arkansas	62
New Jersey	34	Maine	62
New Mexico	35	Louisiana	63
New York	43	New Hampshire	63
North Carolina	33	Georgia	65
North Dakota	79	Connecticut	66
Ohio	59	Delaware	66
Oklahoma	76	Illinois	66
Oregon	46	Colorado	67
Pennsylvania	48	Missouri	67
Rhode Island	68	Rhode Island	68
South Carolina	40	Texas	69
South Dakota	81	Oklahoma	76
Tennessee	48	North Dakota	79
Texas	69	Indiana	80
Utah	45	South Dakota	81
Vermont	50	Kansas	83
Virginia	41	Iowa	84
Washington	58	Nebraska	87
West Virginia	28	Minnesota	88
Wisconsin	89	Montana	88
Wyoming	52	Wisconsin	89

SOURCE: *Improving the quality of care in nursing homes.* (1986). Washington, DC: Institute of Medicine.

lumps all aged recipients of government-sponsored care into a single, institutionally based program is attractive to them. This reasoning allows regulators to force the system into previously existing and familiar formulas.

For example, regulations promulgated for the long term home health care program in New York State (the Nursing Home Without Walls) were found to be a virtual copy of those used for preexisting certified home care programs. Because the new program differed significantly in terms of patient needs and staffing from the old home care programs, the certification regulations actually inhibited the goals of the Nursing Home Without Walls. This fact mattered less to the regulators than the comfort level achieved by using ill-fitting, old but familiar regulations.

Such an approach permits regulators to appear to have control over spending and is easy to administer. It avoids the taking of risks and sustains contact with providers already known, rather than attempting development of relations with innovators.

Fear of Open-ended Funding

People in government have, quite properly, grown to fear new spending programs, such as the chronic renal dialysis program,[45] that lack built-in cost limits. Attempts to add a home health care entitlement provision to Medicare have failed, to date, because estimates of growth in Medicare costs are already frightening.

A careful study by the General Accounting Office in 1982 evaluated the add-on costs of a Medicare home care entitlement. Although this report did not cite dollar figures, it recognized that new demands would arise and would require payment:

> Two to three times as many chronically ill elderly live in the community as live in nursing homes. Making home health care services more widely available might mean that some people living in the community who are eligible for the additional services might use them because they are as disabled as some nursing home residents. The additional services would probably be beneficial to them but would also increase the overall health care costs because of the larger client population.[46]

Liberal Nursing Home Entry Standards

Entry into a nursing home is comparatively easy if long term care is needed, especially for those with cash. This remains true despite current efforts to restrict entry for persons who are not seriously disabled. It is harder to put together the varied elements necessary for care of a frail and disabled person at home.

The nursing home industry, a coherent entity since the 1940s, is a big and growing business. From the industry's viewpoint, the value of lobbying government to develop favorable legislation or to obstruct potentially harmful new developments is obvious; and this effort has been reasonably successful.[47]

Although the proprietary home care industry has started to lobby, few other components within the long term care spectrum apply pressure to government. Agencies that sell the services of homemakers and other paraprofessional workers and permanent equipment are now able to bill Medicare and Medicaid for reimbursement under certain limited conditions; and they are vigorously championing the concept of carrying out advanced technological functions at home for disabled people. The new battle is related to methods of reimbursement for such functions as chronic oxygen treatment, intravenous cancer chemotherapy, and total parenteral nutrition.

In contrast, other entities within the potential long term care spectrum have no clout. Hospice alone has achieved a legislative breakthrough[48] but remains hampered by inadequate funding. There are no serious lobbying efforts by long term home health care programs, day care centers, or respite services. There is no major industry or substantial profit to be protected.

AREAS REQUIRING IMMEDIATE ATTENTION

No solution to the problem of adequate care for the nation's frail elderly on a sustained basis will be found without proper and immediate attention to the important and pernicious problems inherent in our health care system: rising costs, inadequate hospital discharge planning, and hospital overstay.

COST CONTROL

Control of public cost for long term care is a proper concern. Particularly in a field where needs are large, growing, and unmet, the fear of unanticipated add-ons is legitimate. Nonetheless, long term care programs must be broadly affordable. Methods of payment must vary according to individual need and ability to pay.

It is our nation's task to develop the resources to finance long term care that are adequate, yet not excessive, and to create realistic control mechanisms that are workable, logical, and humane. An essential element in the fiscal plans for the long term care spectrum is careful, prudent use of available funds. Various approaches to control public cost have been developed. These include capitation plans, entitlement programs, and block grants.

In *capitation plans,* a program is paid a given sum for total care of a population of specific size. No cost overrun can occur in this situation, and government budget allocations can be controlled. As with all health maintenance organizations (HMOs), the potential problem of insufficient or poor service must be recognized. The Social/Health Maintenance Organization, now in the demonstration stage, is an interesting example of a capitation program.[49]

Governments at all levels allocate funds that filter down to patients as a right, by regulation. Medicare and Medicaid have functioned in principle as *entitlement programs,* and serious concerns over costs have developed. However, the possibility of permitting individuals some discretionary choice in the use of their entitlement funds is as yet untried. This concept might allow people to opt for various service programs on the long term care spectrum and thus in some instances avoid institutional placement.

A potential problem in entitlement programs is the tendency of the executive branch to thwart legislative intent. An example is the present status of the long term home health care program (Nursing Home Without Walls) in New York State. Although it was designed by State Senator Tarky Lombardi as a Medicaid entitlement program, it has been implemented by the executive branch, through its regulatory powers, as a set of geographically limited efforts, inconsistently covering various parts of the state. Many people who should be eligible are left out.

Through *block grants,* the government makes money available for various programs, usually as demonstrations or examples, rather than for universal use. These grants encourage experimentation and new initiatives, but services are available only in a few areas of the country and for short periods of time.

The costs of new long term care approaches are not well understood. Perhaps the one clear point is that current funding methods are inadequate to meet service needs. It is generally accepted that public expenditures will be limited, that the gap will have to be filled through other means.[50] These might be:[51]

1. *Increased income for the elderly.* This approach appears unlikely to work. The sole, broadly structured means of implementing it—the Social Security system—is inadequate for the purpose.

2. *Changes in employee fringe benefits.* Instead of a life insurance policy, employees might be able to choose an annuity applied to a long term care benefit.[52] A revised form of individual retirement account (IRA) could also be developed to be called upon solely for payment of long term care needs.

3. *Growth of the reverse mortgage concept.* In this process, also termed home

equity conversion, older people can arrange to use the equity they own in their homes to buy an annuity.[53]

4. *Long term care insurance.* A comprehensive, broadly attractive set of insurance benefits for the elderly could encompass a wide range of services—the long term care spectrum.

DISCHARGE PLANNING

The importance of proper discharge planning from hospitals and community sites has become increasingly evident since October 1983, when the Diagnosis-Related Group (DRG) legislation, an attempt by the federal government to control Medicare costs, went into effect.[54] This bill, Public Law 87-21, the Social Security Amendments of 1983, provides for fixed reimbursement to hospitals for care of Medicare patients based on the patients' diagnosis.

The critical issues that must be considered are financial (who pays for care in hospitals beyond DRG-approved days?), placement (where can people go when they leave acute care beds but are too ill to care for themselves?), and ethical (who decides among the needs of human beings, institutions, and government?).

DRG regulations directly affect the long term care system by removing the buffer of a hospital stay as a temporary option in the care of the chronically disabled. Thoughtful planning for safe care may be affected severely.[55] Prospective payment systems such as DRGs are designed to offer economic incentive for restraint in use of resources and to increase efficiency, without at the same time diminishing access to care or harming the quality of services.[56] Yet we are at risk of failing to achieve the necessary balance.

HOSPITAL OVERSTAY

Hospital overstay is the paradigm of resource abuse, manipulation of helpless people, and misuse of money. Costs in an acute care hospital, while variable, are in the range of several hundred dollars per day. Nursing home costs are one-fourth that amount or less.

Attempts have been made to understand the national magnitude of hospital overstay,[57] but their accuracy is doubtful because of the range of factors that must be included: the number of hospital beds occupied by patients certified for discharge on a given day; the number of empty nursing home beds on that day; the degree of the patients' disability; the nature of insurance coverage each person holds—largely Medicare or

Medicaid—and whether private funds are available, plus difficulties in determining insurance eligibility; and whether the patients have, in fact, expressed willingness to accept nursing home placement.

The American Association of Professional Standards Review Organizations conducted a one-day survey in 1980, covering the entire country.[58] The survey showed that the percentage of acute hospital beds holding patients who no longer needed hospital care ranged from 7.26 percent in New York to 0.4 percent in Arizona. At that time, Arizona was the only state that did not participate in the Medicaid program.[59]

Reports from across the country, some dating back to the mid-1970s,[60] suggest why prospective payment systems such as DRGs have been imposed. These studies estimated that Medicare and Medicaid paid each year for between 1.0 million and 9.2 million days of acute inpatient hospital care in cases where chronic institutional placement was indicated. Today Medicare outlays for such patients are controlled by DRGs; similar regulations to limit Medicaid, Blue Cross, and commercial insurance expenses surely will follow.

It seems absolutely rational to keep patients out of hospital beds when such placement is not required, but other resources must be available to maintain humane and affordable care. This is not the case today. A comparison with the fate of the chronically mentally ill is pertinent. In the early 1960s the community psychiatry movement, in association with civil rights activists and with the ready compliance of state governments, worked to remove patients from state mental hospitals. It was believed that, through the use of new medications, a set of community-based resources such as clinics and halfway houses could replace the harsh institutional life for many patients. Today state hospitals house about 130,000 individuals across the fifty states, compared to more than 550,000 in 1955.[61] Where are these people now? Many live in the shelters of our large cities, on the streets and riverbanks, in bus and train stations, under bridges and viaducts. Why? Removing them from the hospital was simple and cheap. Replacing hospital care with community-based resources was complex, costly, and difficult to accomplish. Are we bound to repeat this experience, with the frail aged as the victims?

THE NURSING HOME:
IS THERE A WAY OUT?

Is it possible to leave a nursing home once one is admitted? Can residents graduate into the real world of independent living? Or are long term institutions more likely to be storage facilities for the aged, where they are safely packed away or forgotten? Believable information on this subject is sparse.

Attempts have been made to assess the potential, rather than the likelihood, of discharge from such institutions.[62] A broad review of more than twenty-five thousand nursing home patients in Detroit noted in 1974 that only 2 percent were receiving skilled nursing services from staff members.[63] An earlier study in Massachusetts reviewed the status of one hundred nursing home residents and found that twenty-three could function safely at home with occasional visits by a nurse and that fourteen needed no help at all.[64] An analysis by the United States Bureau of the Census in 1978 made a similar point.[65] More than 1 million persons over age sixty-five living in chronic care institutions were surveyed; 16.3 percent were found to need no assistance.

Pilot efforts now underway in three states, designed to limit nursing home placement only to the sickest applicants,[66] may alter this phenomenon. Paul Willging, Executive vice-president of the American Health Care Association, points out, however, that it may not be simple to depopulate nursing homes: "Data suggesting that a large proportion of nursing home residents do not belong in nursing homes is 10–15 years old. Since that time, the nature of the nursing home patient has changed dramatically. . . . Today, the average patient is 83 years old, and has at least four limitations in the basic activities of daily living."[67]

It is true that some aged people now in nursing homes could live successfully at home;[68] the secret to achieving this goal lies more in avoiding institutions to begin with than in trying vainly to remove people after placement. Institutionalization itself frequently causes confusion and consequent physical failure.[69] The fate of patients becomes increasingly fixed. The longer they remain in the nursing home, the less likely they are to ever leave alive.

A major resource for helping older people avoid placement in the first place is strong support from family, friends, and volunteers in the community.[70] These people must be actively involved in making posthospitalization arrangements for their aged friends and relatives.

Planning for long term care is a combined task of the patient, professional staff members of a hospital, community agencies, and natural supporters. Planning should start before a crisis and utilize all available resources. Unfortunately, when the case becomes challenging, health care planners too often resort to the nursing home. This pattern is rooted partly in habit, partly in the reality that nursing homes are often the only option available after hospital discharge.

Proper case management is the controlling factor in achieving effective discharge planning. As hospital administrator Harriet Dronska points out: "A good case manager must be a generalist who understands national law, state reimbursement rules, neighborhood culture, local policy, individual and family dynamics, and the specifics of the needed service delivery system."[71]

Various models of case management exist. In all circumstances, however, helping patients to achieve proper care when they are old and disabled is taxing. It is often a plodding, even tedious process, requiring the persistent gathering of information and negotiation. But the potential payoff, in terms of good care, fiscal common sense, and human dignity for the aged, is significant.

Chapter 2

Financing Long Term Care for the Aged

Broad economic circumstances have a complex effect on long term care services. Policies created during the years of expansion in spending on health care, the late 1960s and the early 1970s, do not thrive in today's economy. A firm understanding has grown that public expenditures in the field of long term care must be limited and that any gap must be filled by private monies. Whatever the mix of funding sources, it seems clear that government will remain the support of some services; that society's prime concern should be with the destitute elderly; that new ideas must be developed and tried; and that the middle-income elderly should not be driven from their homes or forced into total financial dependency because of their long term care needs.

Acute health care expenses for the elderly are covered reasonably well by Medicaid and Medicare, and coverage for certain catastrophic expenses may be added.[1] Supplementary insurance policies and various sources of personal income—including pensions, Social Security payments, investments, and means-tested welfare programs—usually pay any remainder.

Support of long term care is another matter. For most people, the only programs available are for nursing home placements paid for by Medicaid and spotty coverage of some home care services. Medicare is explicitly barred from paying for long term care. How can our country support the essentials?

GOVERNMENT SOURCES
OF LONG TERM CARE FUNDS

As analyst Carol O'Shaughnessy and her associates at the Congressional Research Service, Library of Congress, point out, "at least 80 federal programs assist persons with long-term care problems, either directly or indirectly through cash assistance, in-kind transfers, or the provision of goods and services."[2] The variety of government-supported services for the aged—state and local as well as federal—has produced confusion, overlaps, and gaps. Since 1965 government financing of health services has focused on institutional care, through Medicare and Medicaid. Modestly supported social services have appeared as well, including adult day care, nutrition programs, homemaker and chore services, senior centers, and transportation. The natural function of these services is to help elderly people remain independent in the community.

Regrettably, the systems for health insurance and social services are not coordinated.

The major problem that has evolved is the control of expenditures for acute care services and the allocation of resources between institutional and social services. The allocation problem is a result of the complex set of eligibility criteria, benefit structures, regulatory requirements, and organized vested interests. Controlling both systems has become a Herculean task. New legislative initiatives manipulate very small pieces of the total health insurance and social service network. The outcome has been a patchwork of health insurance and social service programs serving select constituencies without a common policy objective.[3]

The major sources of government support for long term care are summarized in table 2.1.

MEDICAID

Medicaid was created in 1965 under Title XIX of the Social Security Act. It is a means-tested program through which the federal government shares costs with the states to give health care services to the poor. To receive chronic care benefits, people are required virtually to exhaust their financial assets, often being left with barely enough to pay for a funeral. The spend-down provisions vary by state. In 1983, for example, a single person in Rhode Island could earn $4,600 yearly and be eligible, while in Tennessee, an income above $1,404 created ineligibility.[4] About 16 percent of

TABLE 2.1

Government Expenditures—Long Term Care Services for the Elderly

Program	Total Budget	Fiscal Year	For All Components of the Long Term Care Spectrum	For Long Term Care Institutions	For Home Care and Related Services
Medicaid	$33.895 billion	1984	$15.665 billion	$14.8 billion—skilled nursing facilities, intermediate care facilities, intermediate care facilities for mental retardation	$865 million—of this, $765 million for home care services, $100 million for waivered services
Medicare	$61.3 billion	1984	$2.445 billion	$545 million—skilled nursing facilities	$1.9 billion—home and home-related services [3.1% of entire Medicare budget for 1984]
			Note that all Medicare services listed here, both for institutional and home care, are of brief duration, limited by regulation to about six weeks (see text)		
Supplemental Security Income (SSI)	$2.24 billion, combined federal and state contributions. Federal: approx. $1.12 billion; states: approx. $1.12 billion in recent years.	Variable from year to year (see text)	Federal: $370 million for skilled nursing facilities; states: Unknown amount for home health services	Federal: $370 million for skilled nursing facilities	States: Unknown amount (see text)

TABLE 2.1 *(Continued)*

Program	Total Budget	Fiscal Year	For All Components of the Long Term Care Spectrum	For Long Term Care Institutions	For Home Care and Related Services
Older Americans Act (Title III)	$766 million. Of this, $666 million from federal funds, $100 million [15%] from states.	1985	$766 million	–	$67.9 million—Meals-on-Wheels; $336 million—congregate meals; $265 million—supportive services, of which $66.25 million for in-home care $555 million
Social Services Block Grant (Title XX)	Federal: $2.7 billion; states: $1.3 billion; total: $4.0 billion	1985	$555 million	–	$555 million
Veterans Administration	$26.387 billion	1985	$830 million	Total: $708 million. $265 million—community homes, $395 million—VA-owned nursing homes, $48 million—state-run facilities	Total: $122 million. $96 million—domiciliary care; $12 million—state-run facilities; $14 million—hospital-based home care

SOURCE: Davis, K., Rowland, D. (1986). Medicare Policy. Baltimore, MD: Johns Hopkins Univ. Press; Gornick, M., Greenberg, J.N., and Eggers, P.W. (1985, Dec.) Twenty years of Medicare and Medicaid. HCFA Annual Supplement. Office of the Actuary, HCFA. Data from the Medicaid Statistics Branch. In *Health Care Financing Review*, (1985 Suppl.); Office of Financial and Actuarial Analysis, HCFA. (1984). State Medicaid Tables for Fiscal Year 1984. Baltimore, MD: U.S. Dept. of Health and Human Services; Personal communication, George Greenberg, Ph.D., (1986, Oct. 10). Compiled from unpublished program data, U.S. Dept. of Health and Human Services.

Medicaid enrollees are aged sixty-five and older (about 4 million persons). They account for approximately 36 percent of expenditures.[5]

Medicaid's beneficiaries are poor, have not paid for their benefits through their own cash contributions through years of work, and may be perceived pejoratively and stereotypically as hapless, ineffectual, and undeserving. Unlike Medicare, Medicaid has no effective people's lobby: "[The public sees] the Medicare program as a 'medically successful' albeit costly effort. However, the public has felt a gnawing dissatisfaction with the Medicaid program, because expenditures that were grudgingly budgeted to begin with have not yielded similarly enhanced health outcomes."[6] It is noteworthy that Medicaid is protected from budget reductions under the 1985 Gramm-Rudman-Hollings Act as part of the safety net designed to protect the weakest and poorest, while Medicare is not.[7]

The portion of state Medicaid costs borne by the federal budget ranges from a minimum of 50 percent in states with high per-capita incomes (for example, Alaska, California, Connecticut, Delaware, Nevada, and New Jersey), to a theoretical maximum of 77.4 percent in low-income states (Mississippi).[8]

Medicaid law mandates that states provide medical services to all those receiving assistance under Aid to Families with Dependent Children programs and, in general, to those eligible for Supplemental Security Income (SSI). (SSI is discussed further later.) Beyond these "categorically needy" persons, states have the flexibility to provide services for additional categorically related groups—for example, children in foster care.

The states also have a great range of choice as to the Medicaid benefits they offer. In relation to the aged, Medicaid's main focus is on institutions, largely nursing homes. Other optional Medicaid-funded programs are designed to help those not enrolled in the categorical programs just cited. These people, termed medically needy, are deemed to have insufficient income to pay for health care. The services include (depending on the state) home health services (see chapter 6), physical therapy and other therapies, personal care services in the home, and adult day care.

People in the medically needy category can be covered by Medicaid if their medical expenses bring net income to below standard eligibility limits. As noted, the phenomenon through which medical costs are deducted from income is termed spend down. It is sometimes by this means, for instance, that Medicaid pays for long term institutional care. Most states, however, determine eligibility for long term institutional care through establishment of a special income standard. At each state's discretion, this can be set as high as 300 percent of the SSI national standard.

For all but the most wealthy, entry into a nursing home depletes personal assets quickly. A study in Massachusetts revealed that for about two-thirds of people this process took approximately thirteen weeks.[9] After virtually all of the individual's money is spent, Medicaid picks up payment to the institution. According to a General Accounting Office report,[10] up to two-thirds of Medicaid-supported nursing home residents originally entered as self-payers. It appears illogical and budgetarily unwise, and pernicious to older individuals, that Medicaid thrusts people into institutions and then must pay for them. The explanation for why this happens may lie in the sense of bureaucratic ease that is achieved. Institutional placement, as opposed to payment for care in community settings, permits the states to have more accurate authority over budgets. By paying only for long term care in institutions, states control total costs by not building new beds. Thus no open-ended expenditure source can develop. In any case, Medicaid's eligibility standards tend to allow relatively easy access to nursing home care (see chapter 11). There is little Medicaid support for other forms of community-based long term care.

THE PRO-INSTITUTIONAL BIAS

The pro-institutional bias is evident: of Medicaid funds spent on long term care, 94 percent are for institutional services (hospitals and nursing homes), in comparison to 6 percent for other long term care options.[11]

In the states that do not have spend-down provisions, the income cut-off point for Medicaid eligibility is higher if one enters a nursing home than if one does not.[12] That is, the state will apply more liberal rules to pay the cost of institutional care than it will to pay for home care. Because in many states the income cut-off for Medicaid eligibility is below federal poverty standards, very poor people are even more likely to be compelled to accept life in a nursing home. When aged Medicaid patients share a home with family members, those relatives are frequently held responsible for the older person's support. Financial relief from medical, pharmaceutical, and supply costs is available only if the frail older person is institutionalized. Thus families may actually be penalized financially for failing to institutionalize.

MEDICAID'S IMPACT ON THE DISTRIBUTION OF PATIENTS

The most disabled older people are unattractive to nursing homes. Chronic care institutions can often choose whom to admit, and when given the choice between accepting a patient who requires large amounts of service and attention and one whose needs are minimal, they will be strongly tempted to opt for the latter.

Furthermore, private-pay patients, because they generally pay more money more quickly, are usually more attractive to nursing home operators than are those whose bills are paid by Medicaid. Again, those who are the sickest, poorest, and least able to find their way through the thicket of rules and regulations are hurt the most by our failure to establish a spectrum of services.

Nursing home administrators have adapted to the various fiscal pressures upon them by resisting admission of Medicaid-eligible patients; discharging self-pay patients who use up their money and must depend on Medicaid to reimburse the institution; striving to minimize the number of beds certified for Medicaid use; placing financial demands on patients and families; and filling beds of undesirable Medicaid patients who become hospitalized with more attractive self-pay patients.[13]

Nursing home proprietors have zigzagged through the maze of state and federal regulations, interpreting them as best they can to turn a profit. No sooner is a law passed than they jump to use every possible loophole. For example, New Jersey developed Medicaid regulations requiring all nursing homes to make available a reasonable number of beds for indigent patients. In response, some smaller facilities began accepting a few poor patients without charge, thereby fulfilling the state regulation, in order to avoid participating in the state Medicaid program.[14] In 1978, Minnesota ruled that all patients—private-pay and Medicaid-supported—must be charged at the same rate in any given nursing home. A court challenge by the nursing home industry failed, but administrators still charge more for private patients, holding the difference in escrow. In this case, the sense that Medicaid patients are less attractive has not diminished and will persist, certainly at least until all appeals are settled. State and federal regulations that protect Medicaid patients from discrimination on the basis of their financial status or degree of disability abound. In some states, to implement the regulations, preadmission screening programs have been devised to discourage nursing homes from accepting only the least disabled Medicaid-eligible patients. There are no restrictions on the admission of private patients, however, and if the institution is full of these more desirable clients, the antidiscrimination rules become moot.

The lack of a spectrum of long term care services for the frail aged has resulted in packed nursing homes. As David Schimel, Director of the New York [Manhattan] County Health Services Review Organization, points out, "There is a perverse financial disincentive at work here. Since nursing home operators receive no additional payment for accepting difficult-care patients . . . admitting such patients can only increase nursing home operating expenses."[15] Administrators favor those patients who are easiest and cheapest to handle, a design that may require modification if application of resource utilization groups (RUGS)—discussed later—becomes a nationwide standard. An odd consequence of the conflict between demand and cost is the development of moratoria in a number of states on new nursing home construction. Development is controlled through refusal to issue Certificates of Need.[16]

MEDICAID: FIFTY DIFFERENT PROGRAMS

In attempting to unravel the strands that make up Medicaid, it is first necessary to recognize that it consists of fifty different programs, one for each state.[17] The matter of Medicaid eligibility is a prime example. The states have discretion about the degree of poverty, income standards, and coverage for varying groups of people. In 1982 the ratio of Medicaid recipients to the number of people in poverty ranged from highs of 104 (Hawaii), 83 (California), and 77 (Rhode Island) to lows of 20 (Texas and Wyoming), 18 (Idaho), and 17 (South Dakota).

Costs of paying for long term care institutions are the largest single component of Medicaid expenditures.[18] In 1984, 49 percent of Medicaid funds were so spent, if psychiatric facilities are included, and 44 percent were specifically used to house older people in chronic care beds, at a cost of $14.8 billion.[19] This stands in contrast to the $765 million (2.3 percent of Medicaid total) spent on home care services.*[,20]

Despite the substantial sum spent on nursing homes, the increase in numbers of Medicaid-covered elderly people so placed is smaller than the overall population growth of the aged. From 1975 to 1982 the nursing home Medicaid population grew 11 percent, while the demographic growth in the elderly as a whole was about 20 percent.[21] Here we see evidence that the elderly poor are in double jeopardy. First, as we have discussed, Medicaid is institutionally biased. Monies can be spent for nursing homes that cannot be used for other elements of the long term care spectrum.

Second, for those aged people who genuinely need nursing home placement, barriers are raised by the industry itself or by government. When a crisis occurs, Medicaid patients are the first victims. For example, as reported in the *New York Times* on November 12, 1986, the state of Louisiana faced a 1986 budget shortfall caused by depressed oil prices. The governor proposed to reduce the deficit in part by evicting about one thousand indigent elderly patients from nursing homes, to save $81 million. The issue remains unresolved at this writing because of a stay of action consequent to the filing of a lawsuit.

THE OMNIBUS BUDGET RECONCILIATION ACT OF 1981

A major development in Medicaid law took place in 1981 through the Omnibus Budget Reconciliation Act (Public Law 97-35). Section 2176 of

---

*George Greenberg, Ph.D., personal communication, October 10, 1986. Compiled from unpublished program data from the U.S. Department of Health and Human Services.

the act granted the states authority to receive certain waivers that liberalized regulations for people at risk of institutional placement. These "2176 waivers" permit payment for social services, chores, adult day care, respite services, and homemakers as well as medical care; allow certain subgroups of the population to achieve eligibility, rather than demanding wholesale coverage, thus helping blind, retarded, and emotionally ill people; and allow the states to designate certain geographical areas with large numbers of elderly or poor persons as eligible zones.

Through concerns about costs, however, the flexibility Congress had given to the states was partially withdrawn. In order to have waivers approved, the applicant state was required to show that community-based programs' expense to Medicaid was not greater than that of institutional care. On balance, the revised legislation has been well received. By mid-1986, some form of 2176 waiver was functional in forty-four states.

MEDICAID: A SUMMARY

In 1986 almost 4 million individuals aged sixty-five and older were enrolled in Medicaid.* The program serves as the largest single payer of long term care costs for the elderly. A substantial portion of Medicaid expenditures is used to pay nursing homes. These fees totaled $14.8 billion in 1984, or 44 percent of all Medicaid expenses. In contrast, Medicaid spent 2.3 percent of its resources, or $765 million, on home care services.† The costs of acute hospital care for the elderly poor, those covered by both Medicaid and Medicare, are borne largely by the latter program.[22]

There is growing concern that state Medicaid programs will not be able to bear the further growth in long term care institutional costs implied by the demographic imperative. In 1986, for instance, in New York State and Minnesota, a new method of reimbursement for nursing homes went into effect, based on earlier work done in Maryland. The approach uses what are called resource utilization groups (RUGS) through which patients are classified according to the degree of service required for care. RUGS defines groups of patients according to similar clinical characteristics and consequent use of resources in a manner designed to be statistically sound. The ultimate goal of RUGS is to create a tool that is simple, flexible, and that can be used for reimbursement purposes, quality of care assessment, design of staffing levels, and utilization review.[23]

Each nursing home resident will be evaluated twice per year. The rate paid to the institution will be based on a measurement of the resources necessary to care for that patient. Facilities whose residents require rela-

*George Greenberg, personal communication.
†Ibid.

tively more expensive care—those who need more staff time, for instance—will receive higher rates. A tendency might develop for such institutions to admit sicker people, for whom they will be paid more. At the
same time, the temptation will grow to give the least possible service
permitted by regulation and surveillance.

Even though Medicaid is protected from cuts under the Gramm-Rudman-Hollings Act, there exists an evident overall design to reduce federal
costs to the program. The stresses that develop from this situation may
ultimately mold Medicaid into a structure more compatible with a spectrum of long term care services. However, the fact that each state may
develop its own Medicaid program limits severely the possibility of coherent planning for care of those frail elderly who are poor. While increasing
numbers of older people in need of help make the case at each state capital
for larger Medicaid programs, the potential for a smaller federal share
places greater financial demand on each state budget.

The states have responded characteristically to the threat of federal
budget cuts by reducing services to Medicaid patients.[24] It may be an
interesting by-product of the 1981 act and its 2176 waivers that states will
encourage provision of long term care services in noninstitutional sites.
Medicaid is the largest payer of nursing home costs, and any reductions
can save money.

The potential decrease in federal Medicaid sharing also makes states
look increasingly to patients and families to share the costs of nursing
home care.[25] To the degree that this effort is pressed by government, there
will be corresponding reluctance from potential patients and families to
accept nursing home placement.

Concern about future costs is ameliorated to a degree by the recognition
that older people in general are more secure financially than were prior
generations. They can, in this view, be expected to bear a greater share of
long term care costs with their own funds, and depend less on government
programs such as Medicaid. In fact, however, improvement in financial
status is concentrated among the relatively young elderly, those in the
sixty-five to eighty-four age group. However, the next thirty years will
bring about a most striking demographic growth in those who are eighty-
five and older, the cohort of people who now make up most of the aged
below the poverty line and who depend on Medicaid.[26]

Therefore, how secure later cohorts of the very old will be is hard to
guess. The analysis must include demographic factors, general economic
conditions, medical advances and the costs of high technology, levels of
Social Security, and pension income. During the next half century, the
pressure of these forces may alter Medicaid considerably.

MEDICARE

Medicare is a health insurance program, primarily for people aged sixty-five and older, established in 1965 as Title XVIII of the Social Security Act. Medicare has uniform eligibility standards throughout the United States, and its covered services apply equally to all beneficiaries. The program, as it stands today, has no means test for entry. It covers people entitled to Social Security benefits, others under age sixty-five who are disabled (under certain definitions), and some people with end-stage kidney disease.

Medicare is by nature and origin focused on the acute health care needs of the elderly. Wilbur J. Cohen, a principal theoretician of this legislation, has summarized the forces that created the program.[27] The first glimmer dates back to the 1930s, and the players include the American Medical Association; legislators of skill and weight such as Wilbur Mills, chairman of the House Ways and Means Committee in the crucial year 1965; and President Lyndon Johnson, who pressed for both Medicare and Medicaid as major elements in his image of a Great Society. Some perceived and feared Medicare as the opening toward national health insurance. Others felt that the program was a deserved tribute to the elderly, a reward of sorts to provide protection from unaffordable health costs.

In 1965, through Medicare, the federal government introduced the concept of entitled benefits on the basis of age alone rather than on ability to pay:

> Many senior citizens who would have experienced no financial hardships in purchasing health insurance, if it had been made *available* before 1965, now have that availability, but they also have their care paid for by younger generations who are still working. A political gift has been made to both the needy and the self-sufficient, and I feel we have crossed a threshold over which there is no easy retreat.[28]

Medicare was in part a product of political expediency, and thus was inevitably born flawed. Chronic health care services were largely omitted from theory, planning, legislation, and regulation, and remain so to this day. Instead, all development was concerned with treatment of *immediate* health care needs. Political judgment supported this viewpoint, and political tactics were applied to give it a successful birth. The following recollection from Cohen is telling:

> One feature that I built into the legislation was making the effective date July 1, 1966. Respiratory diseases have a low incidence in summer, and elective surgery

is at a low ebb immediately before the July 4th holiday period. . . . I think initiating the law during a low-admission period in the summer substantially helped.[29]

Twenty years later the country, and particularly the elderly, pay a heavy price for the omission of chronic health care services from Medicare coverage.

MEDICARE AND LONG TERM CARE

Medicare, now in its third decade, is still virtually intact as an insurance program covering acute illness only, despite the fact that both the overt needs and the perceptions and desires of older people have changed. Medicare pays less than 5 percent of the country's nursing home bill, compared to Medicaid's 41 percent; and the Medicare payments are for those short periods of time when the patient is deemed to require *skilled* nursing services.

The critical legislative concepts that deny significant home care services to Medicare recipients are contained within the definitions of service on an intermittent basis and on the skilled nursing requirement. Current guidelines to fiscal intermediaries for applying the intermittent care requirement affirm that Medicare will pay only for part-time, medically reasonable and necessary skilled nursing care, for a *short* period of time, usually about two to three weeks. Additional service can be considered, based on a physician's documentation of a further, time-limited need, but care of an indefinite duration will not be allowed and is not covered.

The writers of regulations within the Health Care Financing Administration deem the skilled nursing requirement to be consistent with the original concept of Medicare as an acute care insurance program. Thus home care benefits are perceived as simply a continuation of services needed following an acute illness. As a consequence, Medicare entitlements are limited to payment for conditions that are so severe that the individuals must be under a physician's care, homebound, and in need of skilled nursing services. Payment for services is denied when the nature of nursing care required is no longer *skilled*. Assistance to those who are chronically but not acutely ill is barred. Chronically disabled Medicare recipients must then fend for themselves in the health care system, unless poor enough to be eligible for Medicaid.

Numerous attempts have been made to alter the basic nature of Medicare, or to modify it significantly toward support of long term care services. (For examples, see chapter 12.) The changes promulgated since 1965 that appear to bend toward long term care benefits include:

1. Coverage of up to one hundred days of skilled nursing facility (nursing home) care following a hospital stay of at least three consecutive days. This provision was amended by the Omnibus Reconciliation Act of 1980. The three-day prior hospitalization requirement was eliminated, as was the previously established one hundred-visit limit on home care services. These developments suggested a liberalization in the Medicare design toward nursing homes and home care. However, to be eligible the patient, as before, must require *skilled* nursing care. This terminology continues to be used to deny chronic care services for people who hold Medicare entitlements.

2. Home health services as part of the treatment plan for an acute illness, including, by various definitions, part-time nursing care; physical, occupational, and/or speech therapy; services of a social worker; medical supplies, but not drugs; and part-time help·from a home health aide. To be eligible, the patient must, once again, require skilled nursing care. Services must be provided under a care plan authorized by a physician.

3. Hospice benefits. This program has been in place since November 1983 as a provision of the Tax Equity and Fiscal Responsibility Act of 1982 (TEFRA). Medicare hospice offers benefits to people with a life expectancy of less than six months. If patients are terminally ill, they are eligible to receive nursing and various therapy services, the help of physicians and social workers, counseling, and limited inpatient care. Because of the low payment rates of $53.17 per patient day, as established in November 1984, relatively few agencies have developed hospice programs under TEFRA provisions. Modest increases in the daily reimbursement rate may be anticipated in the next several years.

While each of these developments appears to offer genuine long term care benefits, in reality they are illusions. For the first two benefits cited, eligibility requires that the patient need skilled nursing services, defined in a manner that frustrates provision of services to any older person with a chronic disability. To fulfill all the requisites of the third benefit, the patient must die.

In summary, Medicare remains an acute health care insurance program for the elderly and disabled. "To the extent that it provides coverage for certain long term care services, it does so with the intent of reducing the need for more intensive and expensive acute care services; the program was not designed to respond specifically to chronic care needs of the elderly over a sustained period of time."[30]

THE IMPACT OF DRGs ON LONG TERM CARE

The Omnibus Reconciliation Act of 1980 and the TEFRA legislation of 1982 have had a more substantial effect on long term care other than through direct amendment of Medicare long term care provisions. There has been a mandate for the development of a case-based Medicare reimbursement system for acute care hospitals that derives from provisions within these laws. This new method of payment, termed the Prospective Payment System (PPS), is based on Diagnosis-Related Groups (DRGs), and was put into its present legal form as Title VI of the Social Security Amendments of 1983.[31] Political hyperbole is flowing; consider the remarks of Senator John Heinz (R-PA) at a hearing of the Senate Special Committee on Aging: "Built into the DRGs are incentives to compromise high quality care to maximize profits. Second, symptoms of program abuse riddle every level of care, from hospital to nursing home to home health. And finally, the watchdog Peer Review Organizations feel hamstrung to identify and sanction the worst offenders."[32]

In fact, it is broadly recognized that DRGs have markedly altered the approach to payment for hospital services. Such reimbursement is now based on an average predetermined length of stay for Medicare patients, depending on their diagnosis. Discussion is taking place on whether DRGs lead to decreased quality of care, develop pressures that cause elderly patients to be released from hospitals into their homes more quickly than in the past while they are in a sicker state, and result in a higher readmission rate. While a mechanism is available to appeal a hospital discharge date a Medicare patient feels is too early, whether a sick old person will have the ability to appeal is questionable:[33]

Basing payment for Medicare patients on an average length of stay assumes that some portion of patients in any disease group will require longer than the average recovery time. If payment is restricted for those additional days, the only alternative for patients unable to pay the difference is either placement in a nursing home or the provision of highly technical care at home. . . . These conditions lead directly to an increase in the over-65 patient population requiring home care services.[34]

A further potential impact of the Medicare amendments that incorporate the PPSystem and DRGs is the model that they offer for control of other aspects of health care payment. Today in acute care hospitals the emphasis is on efficiency and productivity. Studies are already underway that may extend these or similar payment mechanisms to home care, nursing homes, doctors' private offices, and outpatient departments.[35]

Hospitals were first in line for cost control because their costs appeared to have grown the most and to be most responsible for inflation in medical care. What may follow, however, is a version of the domino theory. As hospitals are forced to discharge older people in a more disabled condition, the pressures will build on other components in the spectrum of care to pick up a greater share of service. A logical consequence will be further demands on nursing homes and their tendency to take sicker patients who can pay the most or for whom RUGS pay well. People who are chronically disabled but with low RUGS scores, and/or paid for by Medicaid, will be less welcome. These individuals will be found increasingly in the community, ill and disabled, unable to receive institutional services.

It is reasonable to imagine that payments for the nation's nursing home and home care bill soon will begin to grow, followed by public outcry and then a governmental response requiring cost controls. In addition, it is inevitable that within the next several years some form of financial or service scandal will occur. The combination of these phenomena will result in ever tighter government control over eligibility for service under long term care programs. A larger bureaucracy will be established to scrutinize admissions to programs; spending caps for people's lifetimes will probably be created; some money will be saved; and a growing proportion of frail, old, chronically disabled people will find themselves ineligible for help.

HOME CARE UNDER MEDICARE

In the home health services, this process is already underway.[36] In 1974 home health care accounted for 1.2 percent of Medicare expenditures, equaling $144 million. By 1984 this figure had grown to 3.1 percent, or $1.9 billion. Thus even though Medicare fills a relatively small portion of the need for home health care—limited by the intermittent care and skilled nursing requirements—costs have grown substantially. The average number of health workers' visits to the home, per *one thousand enrollees,* grew from about 340 to 1,044; and total home visits grew from 8.2 million to 36.7 million. The average number of visits to each individual user has grown more slowly, from 20.6 to 26.3.[37]

While home care costs were only 3.1 percent of Medicare expenditures in 1984, we should remember that this was more than a doubling in percent over a decade: in that period, actual dollars spent increased at a rate of about 29 percent each year, and reached the noteworthy figure of $1.9 billion; the demographic imperative is at work, and increasingly large numbers of disabled old people will need help; and the help needed will be progressively less available from acute care hospitals and nursing homes.

In 1986 researchers Christine Bishop and Margaret Stassen produced a thoughtful, comprehensive analysis of this material, and came to useful conclusions. In their view, the largest factor in the cost increase is the growth in total number of home care visits. This growth can be attributed either to a burgeoning in the raw numbers of people served or to a change in the number of visits per case. Both are clearly responsible:

> We can see that the number of persons served increased dramatically, almost tripling [between 1974 and 1983]; the annual rate of growth for this component of total expense was almost 15 percent. Some of this is to be expected due to the growth in Medicare enrollment. But more important than this is the increased use of home health services by Medicare enrollees: utilization increased from about 17 users per 1000 enrollees in 1984 to almost 40 users per thousand in 1982.[38]

Increase in utilization, according to Bishop and Stassen, was thus the prime source of growth in Medicare expenditures for home care services between 1974 and 1983. They emphasize that attempts to control Medicare cost growth by limiting reimbursement per visit or per individual case therefore would be relatively ineffective. Only by making eligibility for care difficult and restrictive would the major growth factor be controlled.

What can we predict for people who need Medicare-covered home care services during the next twenty years? There will be an increasing concern about costs. This will be followed by development of payment systems that emphasize at-home care for people whose health care needs are increasingly complex. Hospitals and nursing homes will be required by policy to exclude such patients. Highly technical and expensive home care services will be increasingly available, and will be paid for by Medicare because they are seen as less expensive than institutional care. Although some form of payment cap will develop, the bulk of available dollars will be devoted to home care patients who are acutely ill. The problem of chronically disabled frail old people will, as it is today, continue to be pushed aside until they become critically ill and eligible for services, or until they die.

OTHER SOURCES
OF GOVERNMENT FUNDS

SUPPLEMENTAL SECURITY INCOME

Supplemental Security Income (SSI) is an income assistance program administered by the federal government through the states. In its basic form, SSI gives cash, not services. It came into being in 1974, as Title XVI of the Social Security Act amendments of 1972. It was designed to provide some equity across the states in terms of benefits offered to the aged, blind, and/or disabled poor, and to simplify previous variegated state benefits for people so categorized.

The federal government has established uniform national eligibility standards, including those for income and assets. In recent years this standard has been in the range of about 70 percent of the federal poverty level. Thus SSI eligibility is distinguished from that of Medicaid, where fifty different state standards may exist. Nevertheless, it is generally true that SSI recipients are also Medicaid-eligible.[39] The fact that federal standards apply offers those seeking SSI benefits a degree of protection from arbitrary state cutbacks in Medicaid designed to balance budgets. Federal SSI is not at risk during the current budgeting process in Washington because it is protected from any funding cuts under provisions of the Gramm-Rudman-Hollings Act, as it now stands. SSI is perceived as part of the safety net designed to protect the most vulnerable. Social Security benefits and Medicaid are equally protected.

In 1985 about 4 million people received cash from this program. Of these, 1.5 million were aged; the remainder were blind or disabled.[40] Federal SSI was set at $325 per month for an individual and $488 for a couple with no other income and living outside of institutions. The SSI program permits states to supplement the income of federally eligible recipients with additional local funds. With state supplementation, the highest rates for elderly people reached $566 for individuals (in Alaska) and $900 for couples (in Ohio).[41] In 1985 all but seven states took the option of supplemental SSI. For recipients who live in nursing homes, the SSI benefit is reduced to about $25 per month to provide pocket money in a setting where basic living costs are covered.

State eligibility rules vary. In some instances all SSI recipients are permitted to obtain the additional benefits. Other states limit eligibility and have chosen to use some of the available funds to support certain community-based long term care programs such as protective housing or adult foster homes, or the salaries of paraprofessional workers in home care programs.[42] It is in part through these optional state programs that SSI can be understood as helping to pay part of long term care costs. In addition, an estimated $370 million is paid directly to nursing homes through SSI.[43]

The future of SSI, its dollar cost to the federal and various state budgets, depends in part on the fiscal health of the country at large. If we assume that the income standards for entry of older people into the program remain roughly the same, then the major variable will be the number of older people who are poor. As the number of very old people increases, and with their associated likelihood of poverty, demands on the SSI program will grow.

THE OLDER AMERICANS ACT

The intent of the Older Americans Act (OAA) was made clear in the original 1965 legislation: to develop a comprehensive, coordinated system of service for older people. OAA is an umbrella of legislation that is concerned with the needs of the elderly in the areas of income, mental and physical health, housing, jobs, social services, and recreation. The impact of this act is sharply limited by the modest levels of funds made available in the federal budget. For obvious reasons related to budget deficits, the future of OAA is clouded.

The section of the OAA relevant to long term care is Title III. This title is designed to foster the development of a comprehensive and coordinated system of services for the aged, with the goals of securing and maintaining the maximum possible independence for older people in their own homes; removing barriers to economic and personal independence for the elderly; and providing a continuum of services for those who are vulnerable or frail.

Under Title III, the federal government distributes funds to state Agencies on Aging. These extend awards to the 664 local Agencies on Aging. In fiscal year 1985, Title III appropriations were $666 million. Half of this amount was used for nutrition services, such as serving lunches at senior citizen's centers. About 10 percent, or $68 million, was designed for home-delivered meals (Meals-on-Wheels) and 40 percent, or $265 million, for supportive services.

The OAA makes perhaps its most striking impact on the lives of the elderly in the area of supportive services. These OAA dollars are available to local aging agencies with minimal restrictions. Among these few restrictions are that a specific portion of the funds be used to provide transportation, outreach, information, and referral services; legal and other forms of counseling; and in-home care.[44]

The money can be used to fill in where Medicaid and Medicare fail. To receive help, people are not required to pass a means test. The nature of services need not fit Medicare restrictions. Agencies have often chosen to use the supportive services money to increase their in-home meals programs. Some have opted to put funds into housekeeping, personal care, and chore services for the homebound:

Many state and area agencies have made strides to improve long-term care services through coordination [sic] activities with health and other social service agencies, and through the development of a social service infrastructure for the elderly at the local level. Some State agencies on aging have also acted as catalysts to reorganize community-based health and social services systems at the State and local levels so as to serve more effectively the long-term care population. For example, State agencies have developed case management and assessment systems through area agencies on aging and have supported services otherwise unavailable to the frail population.[45]

Title III also mandates that ombudsman programs be conducted at the state level. These programs have direct relevance to the long term care system. The state ombudsman has the authority to investigate and resolve complaints about institutional and boarding home care of the elderly and to monitor compliance with all relevant laws and regulations. In fiscal year 1983 about $12 million of OAA funds was so spent.[46]

SOCIAL SERVICES BLOCK GRANT

The Social Services Block Grant (SSBG) program was passed into law in January 1974 as Title XX of the Social Security Act. It was amended in 1981 through the Omnibus Budget Reconciliation Act to remove the requirement for state matching of funds. SSBG authorizes block grants to the states to assist elderly people, the disabled, and children through reducing or eliminating dependency by improving elderly people's economic status; helping them to maintain self-sufficiency; preventing or correcting neglect, abuse, or exploitation of people unable to protect their own interests; preventing or reducing inappropriate institutional care by providing community-based services; and arranging for institutional placement when appropriate.

In summary, SSBG is a social service program. It is jointly funded by the federal and state governments; administered, defined, and implemented by the states; and focuses on community-based services. SSBG does not support institutional care, nor any service covered by Medicare or Medicaid; and it pays for health services only when such care is integral but subordinate to social services. Eligibility is not limited by any provision of federal statute. However, individual states may establish such standards, including means tests.[47]

The states have substantial leeway in determining the use of SSBG funds, as long as the program's basic goals are met. Monies are allotted to the states on the basis of population size and an approved service program plan, within a ceiling of total expenditures established through the federal budget process. In fiscal years 1983 through 1985 the federal appropriation and the expenditure ceiling were both set at $2.6 billion; and in 1986, at $2.7 billion. In 1981 the expenditure ceiling was $2.9 billion; in 1982, $3.3 billion.[48]

The Omnibus Budget Reconciliation Act of 1981 significantly altered the provisions of SSBG. The preexisting limitations on the population to be served, such as the poor, and of available services were voided. According to the most recent information, SSBG funds can be used for: homemaker, chore, and home management assistance for eligible individuals and families in almost all states; adult day care (available in twenty-six states); and adult foster care (offered in sixteen states).[49]

In 1983 services in the home were given to about 300,000 people under SSBG, or about 11 percent of all Title XX recipients. It is not possible to determine how many of these recipients were elderly; nor is it possible to measure the number of dollars used to support elements on the long term care spectrum for the aged. The reason for the paucity of information is a further condition of the Omnibus Budget Reconciliation Act of 1981, which eliminated state reporting requirements. Therefore we are unable to evaluate the importance of Title XX to the frail elderly.

SSBG is a complex program because it offers services to widely diverse populations, has fifty different sets of state standards, and results in varying groups with differing demands competing for limited funds. Based on the information available, it seems reasonably clear that SSBG gives support to long term care services for the aged at a relatively modest level. As O'Shaughnessy and her associates point out:

> Community care programs such as those supported by Title XX are minimal when compared to programs which support institutional care. For example, Federal funds available for all Title XX activities in 1983 ($2.6 billion) were approximately one-third the total Federal nursing home expenditures in that year ($8.1 billion).[50]

VETERANS ADMINISTRATION PROGRAMS

The demographic imperative applies more strongly to elderly veterans than it does to the U.S. population as a whole. In 1983 there existed 3.5 million veterans age sixty-five or more, who made up slightly more than 12 percent of the total pool of 28 million elderly. By 1990, because of the bulge caused by wartime service, particularly in World War II,[51] the number of older veterans will grow to 9 million; and by the year 2000 the numbers of those aged seventy-five or older will reach 4 million.[52] To meet the consequences of demographic change, the Veterans Administration (VA) will need to enlarge its programs for elderly veterans. A more aged clientele will have greater need.[53]

Eligibility for VA care is based on three criteria, enforced variably by the agency: veteran status, degree of disability, and service-connection of the disability. Access to care was made easier for veterans aged sixty-five and over in 1970, through passage of Public Law 91-500. Since then, older veterans are deemed eligible for service in VA hospitals, nursing homes, and the domiciliary care program for disabilities that may not necessarily be connected with service duty, and regardless of ability to pay.[54]

Currently the VA already offers significant long term care service programs. These include nursing home care, outpatient visits, placement in special housing, personal care, adult day health services, and hospice.

The VA owns more than nine thousand nursing home beds across the country and controls another sixteen thousand in proprietary institutions. About 60 percent of veterans in these homes are aged sixty-five or older.[55] In 1985 the VA spent $708 million for all of these various long term care services.

Three particularly innovative VA programs serve the elderly. The VA has been a leader in establishing *geriatric evaluation units* at its hospitals. Fifteen such programs are now in existence, using a team approach to assess and identify medical and social problems of older veterans and to reduce rehospitalization and nursing home placement. The VA has also established eight *geriatric research, education and clinical centers, or GRECS.* These are designed to be centers of excellence, through which careful study of and research efforts about the elderly will enhance their care. *Hospital-based home care (HBHC)* programs are now in operation at more than seventy major VA medical centers. These programs provide hospital staff members, including physicians from the departments of medicine and surgery, to make home visits as part of interdisciplinary teams. Their geographic base may extend as far as thirty miles from the hospital.[56]

PRIVATE SOURCES
OF LONG TERM CARE FUNDS

Today older people and their families pay for more than half of long term care costs: 50 percent of nursing home fees and 80 percent or more of home care costs are paid with personal dollars.[57] Private support for long term care can take the form of direct payment by or for the person in need of service, or can come from an insurance program. Although, as we shall see, commercial companies are becoming interested in providing insurance coverage in this field, up to now almost all nongovernmental payments for long term care services come from the wallets or purses of individuals. It is essential to identify the people most likely to be faced with these personal expenses. As Dr. Stanley Wallack, policy analyst at Brandeis University, indicates: "It is not the 65-year-old, and it probably is not the 75-year-old; more and more often it is an 80- to 85-year-old woman, who is single, widowed, or divorced."[58]

In general, the older people are, the smaller their financial resources.[59] The 1980 census revealed that married couples with a head of household aged sixty-five to sixty-nine had a median income of $18,400. For those aged eighty-five and over the figure was $11,200. The comparable incomes for single women were $6,800 and $5,200, respectively.[60]

Beyond Social Security, the major sources of income for people aged sixty-five and over are dollars from interest and dividends, public assistance payments for those who can pass a means test and are willing to do so, and pensions. Salaries account for about one-fifth of their income.[61]

Pensions will probably cover an increasing share of long term care costs paid by individuals. People employed now have far greater protection of their pension rights than did retirees of fifteen years ago. The Employee Retirement Income Security Act of 1974 (ERISA) broadened and assured eligibility. Prior to this, substantial numbers of people failed to find the expected income benefits available at retirement.[62]

Thus a primary cause of age-related income differences is the smaller level of pensions received by people who retired from employment in earlier years. Further, Social Security payments are directly related to wages earned. Therefore, the monthly check is progressively smaller for people in each older age group.

Poverty is also more evident among those of greatly advanced age. In general, older people have developed an improved level of economic standing in recent decades. The poverty rate for people over age sixty-four was 35.2 percent in 1959. By 1984 this figure had fallen to 12.4 percent. However, these data tend to obscure the fact that significant subgroups of the old are destitute. To illustrate, using 1980 figures, the poverty rate for people aged sixty-five to sixty-nine was 13.6 percent; and for those eighty-five and over, 27.3 percent.[63] Of people aged sixty-five and over, 39 percent of blacks and 26 percent of Hispanics, compared to 13 percent of whites, were below the poverty line in 1981. Older people, and especially older women, who live alone are more likely to be poor than are those who live with others. This suggests a future problem. Poverty rates may increase as divorced individuals, a group that increased in this era, and members of minority groups, make up larger proportions of the elderly.[64] In addition, aggregate statistics mask the fact that while a large number of the elderly are not formally below the poverty line, their incomes are just above it. For these individuals, modest medical costs will reduce their disposable incomes below the poverty line.

We are faced with a problem: those people most likely to need long term care services are very old women living alone; and it is these individuals who are most likely to be impoverished and unable to share costs for their care from current income.

In order for poor elderly people to be able to pay for long term care services, either their income levels must be increased or methods must be developed that will allow them to tap their noncash assets.

Analysis of private payments made by older people for health care services emphasizes this point. In 1984 about 30 percent of *all* health care costs for those aged sixty-five and more were paid for by the individuals involved. Hospital expenses were dealt with largely by Medicare and Medicaid. Only 3.1 percent were paid for privately. On the other hand, for nursing home care, the most expensive element on the long term care spectrum, Medicare paid 2.1 percent, Medicaid 41.5 percent (this figure includes all nursing home costs, for people of all ages who are so incarcerated), and private monies paid 50.1 percent.[65] Further, as a percentage of income, the elderly who are poor and near poor bear a greater personal burden of health care expenses than do those who are better off financially.[66]

HOME EQUITY CONVERSION

Poor old people will continue to need help from government to sustain their long term care needs. However, if their wealth were to be defined in terms of total assets, the majority of the elderly are not impoverished. If they are in difficulty, it is because they cannot use their assets to pay for current services in cash. Their wealth is not in liquid form. The most prominent asset of older people is equity in a home. For those aged fifty-five to sixty-four, about 40 percent of assets are locked up in their houses.[67]

About 75 percent of people aged sixty-five and over are homeowners.[68] Of these homes, 84 percent are free of debt or mortgage. The total equity value of these real estate holdings is about $550 billion:[69]

Relatively few older homeowners ever use this major asset as a source of income. The vast majority choose to remain in their own homes as long as they can. As a result, most of their financial resources remain tied up in that home. Compared to others, therefore, many older homeowners are asset-rich and income-poor.[70]

Logic suggests that good use can be made of this asset to pay for necessary long term care requirements. One option is home equity conversion. Another allows the use of assets from the sale of a house for purchase of entry into a life care community (see chapter 10).

The potential for using the value of the home for dollars to pay for long term care is significant.[71] One clear goal is to allow elderly homeowners to occupy their own homes while turning a portion of their equity into cash income. Home equity conversions have an additional benefit. They may produce funds to allow older people to purchase long term care insurance policies. Major insurance companies will be looking closely at this rather new form of real estate investment over the next several years. If Metropolitan, Prudential, Equitable, and other behemoths enter the field, both home equity conversion and commercial insurance will become substantial forces in long term care financing.

At this time, there is little experience in the field of home equity conversion. Although considerable discussion of the concept has taken place, only about eight hundred such contracts have been closed throughout the country.* ,[72] Other negatives include homeowners' reluctance to cannibalize an asset that they had hoped to leave to their children, and the possibility that the cash flowing from the transaction might be misused.[73]

Two types of home equity conversion exist, loan plans and sale plans. Under a loan plan, or *reverse mortgage,* the elderly homeowner makes a loan agreement with a lending institution. Through this contract a monthly payment is provided to the borrower. Repayment of principal and interest is deferred until the end of the loan term, which may be as long as forty years, or until the death of the borrower or sale of the house.[74] Under a loan plan the mortgagee retains ownership rights to the home. When the loan comes due, the owner can convert the debt into a regular mortgage, sell the property to settle the debt, or obtain a new reverse mortgage.[75]

Examination of a particular reverse mortgage plan shows what imagination and the entrepreneurial spirit can do. The individual retirement mortgage account (IRMA), now being promoted as an innovative real estate business venture,[76] operates through a long term reverse-shared appreciation mortgage. While other reverse mortgage plans are time-limited, IRMA is for life.[77] Under this plan anyone sixty-two years of age and older who owns a home in good condition and free of debt is eligible, if the home is the principal residence:

> Homeowners receive monthly tax-free loan advances as high as $700 a month for as long as they continue to live in the home [subject to the original terms of the loan]. In return they give up a first-mortgage interest in the home. Borrowers keep title of the home throughout the loan term. . . . Since the payments made to borrowers are installments on a loan, this monthly income is not subject to income tax.[78]

Interest is charged on the loan, but repayment of both interest and principal is deferred until maturity. Under IRMA, loans are not due until the borrower sells the home, moves out, dies, or reaches age one hundred.

At age one hundred borrowers have the option to extend the program for the duration of their lives. If one spouse dies, payments continue without reduction for the life of the survivor.

The monthly income available under IRMA depends on the age of the borrower, the value of the home, the rate of loan interest, and the portion of the home's value committed to the program. The older the borrower and the more valuable the home, the greater the possible monthly payment. In financial counselor Peter Wessel's analysis: "A 70-year-old homeowner

---

*K. Scholen and R. J. Arbogast, personal communications, March 1986 and April 1987.

with a $90,000 home would receive $350 per month. A person 82 years of age with a home valued at the same price would receive twice as much. . . . If the 70-year-old had a home worth $130,000 instead of $90,000, the payment would be $525 per month."[79]

As matters stand today, about forty-four reverse mortgage participants have become associated with IRMA*—a minute number, considering the potential. However, IRMA has grown in availability over the past several years, is now available in five states, and appears to offer a significant prospect of tapping into the massive quantity of frozen funds available to older people through the real estate values of their homes. Through this kind of enterprise, reverse mortgages may become a realistic means of supporting the highly expensive long term care services for the aged that will be necessary over the next half century.

LONG TERM CARE INSURANCE

Health care analyst Laurence F. Lane points out:

> Long term care policy planners—reinforced by consumer naiveté, provider apathy, and insurer indifference—traditionally have relied on government as the primary payer. Therefore the public responsibility model has dominated social planners' quest for the elusive consolidated long term care delivery system. With reductions in public domestic expenditures, however, planners finally are exploring private financing options, one of the most promising of which is insurance for long term care.[80]

The current federal budget deficit makes obvious the need to establish private sources of long term care funds. For the present, Medicare will remain an insurance program covering acute illness; and Medicaid, which pays considerable funds for nursing home care, will continue to be a means-tested program.

Medicare Supplemental Insurance, or so-called Medi-gap policies, do not fill the need for long term care payments. This form of insurance, for years misrepresented as a source of coverage for diverse services needed by the elderly, is now basically an honest venture. The provisions of Medi-gap policies are controlled by the Baucas Amendment of 1980 (PL 96-265) and regulated by the states. However, sellers have finely tuned these policies so that payments are restricted only to those services approved under Medicare. Thus Medi-gap insurance may pay for Medicare deductibles but not for long term care.[81]

Private, or commercial, long term care insurance may develop into such

*R. J. Arbogast, personal communication, March 1986.

a source. As mentioned, paying for long term care places tremendous strain on all concerned: the various levels of government, the individual in need, the family. Insuring against risk makes sense, and long term care insurance may be a logical purchase.[82] Cash to purchase policies may be available. A 1983 study conducted for the Department of Health and Human Services estimated that, based on future income levels and pension growth, about 93 percent of married couples at age sixty-five will be able to purchase long term care insurance policies with less than 5 percent of their cash income by the year 2005. For single persons at age sixty-five, the figure is 60 percent.[83] Unfortunately, this study may be overly optimistic, because of insufficient consideration given to inflation and future long term care costs.*

Tapping into the pool of personal funds available to individuals with reasonable assets will enable available government funds to be used for the poor. In addition, as Lane indicates, private long term care insurance permits people to have money available for higher quality care; gives greater opportunity for individual choice in type of care; benefits people who have prudently saved money for their care in later years; and serves as an alternative to reliance on public support.[84]

Until recently, this form of insurance had not been perceived as viable; and even at this writing a mere 75,000 to 100,000 people in the United States are covered by individual long term care policies. Those policies available up to now, furthermore, have been limited in scope. They pay part of nursing home costs through a form of indemnity benefit and offer minimal genuine coverage of in-home services.[85]

Lane has summarized the key features of long term care insurance. Many policies now being developed: cover professional long term care services for longer than six months; do not use the restrictions for care inherent to Medicare law and regulation as policy criteria; and are based on indemnity payouts—that is, a flat payment is offered for each day of care.[86]

Most such policies also restrict payment largely for institutional placement and limit benefits to three or four years. Cost of premiums is age-rated, and careful underwriting and utilization controls are exercised by insurance companies. Up to this point they remain understandably concerned that these policies may lose money.

Developing a Market

The forces propelling the development of long term care insurance are the need for financial coverage that cannot and will not be provided for most people by any level of government and the increased financial resources possessed by the elderly in general. At the same time that these

*George Greenberg, Ph.D., personal communication, October 1986.

forces begin to drive the market forward, other factors tend to inhibit its growth. Among these are concerns that insurance companies rely on fine print to avoid payouts; that policies are too expensive and provide insurance companies profits that are unreasonably high; that insurance sales practices are deceptive; and that benefits are concentrated excessively on payment for institutional care.

A further concern is the degree to which potential purchasers are uninformed about the need. There remains a widespread misapprehension that Medicare pays for long term care services. In a Gallup survey conducted for the American Association of Retired Persons (AARP) in 1983, the vast majority of respondents indicated their belief that Medicare would be the primary source of payment for such care.[87] Following this survey, the AARP began a process of education for its members and developed a model long term care insurance policy in association with Prudential Insurance Company of America. In October 1985 AARP mailed 215,000 solicitations for its new policy to randomly selected households. The response was considered poor; negative criticism focused particularly on inadequacies in coverage and excessive costs.[88] Details of this policy in comparison with others are summarized in the next section, but it is noteworthy that even when offered under good auspices, such as by the AARP, this form of insurance has yet to prove itself in the marketplace.

Therefore, in order for the insurance industry to accept what it perceives to be a substantial sales gamble, a wider market must be opened. More people, preferably in groups as opposed to individual purchasers, must want a policy that will cover the cost of future long term care. An essential prerequisite to this growth is education of the general populace to the gaps in Medicare coverage. For this, efforts such as that put forth by the AARP must be repeated and expanded.

Further, the information base to support development of logical insurance policy design and pricing remains inadequate. A better understanding of demographic information will help. Also, as the fate of people enrolled in nontraditional insurance programs for the elderly such as Social/Health Maintenance Organizations (SHMOs) and life care retirement centers (see chapter 10) is known, actuarial analysis will become more reliable. These programs can be understood as forms of managed care for the elderly, paid for in a broad sense by capitation. As such, they offer the opportunity to insure for the risks of long term care.[89]

As insurance companies become more comfortable in development and sales of these policies, competition should produce ones that are more appropriate and desirable, and at better prices. Consumer advocacy organizations for the aged, such as the AARP and the Section for Aging and Long Term Care Services of the American Hospital Association, can be relied upon to conduct impartial assessment of policies in the interest of potential purchasers.

The Current Market

Competition in the marketing of policies is developing. As recently as 1982, a year in which less than 1 percent of nursing home costs were covered by private insurance,[90] Art Lifson, an insurance company spokesman, stated that long term care insurance "is a risky venture" and that "demand for a long term care policy is not certain at this time." Lifson predicted that in the next five to ten years, there would be increased private activity, but not in traditional insurance plan settings.[91]

The pace of development of these policies has been considerably faster. At this writing more than sixty companies are reported to offer insurance coverage for long term care, and four to five additional companies enter the field each month. An important caveat: Any potential purchaser must take care when evaluating the coverage offered. Many of the policies now being offered do not provide adequate long term care protection.

It would not be feasible to attempt to compare the various policies here. The variables are uncountable and the details a swamp. However, a summary of the policies offered by several well-known carriers is in order:

AARP/Prudential pays, in a typical policy (several are available), $40 per day for long term institutional care up to a maximum of three years during a lifetime, after a thirty-day waiting period, but only following a hospitalization of at least three days; pays $25 per day for home health services, up to a limit of 365 visits, and service must begin within two weeks of a hospital stay of at least three days, or of discharge from a nursing home; and pays $40 per day for skilled nursing care (note the word skilled) for up to three years with similar hospital stay requirements. Premium varies with age, and ranges from $14.95 per month between ages fifty and fifty-nine, to $94.95 per month for persons in the seventy-five- to seventy-nine-year age group.

Aetna pays $40 per day for skilled nursing care and for long term institutional care, both of which must be in a skilled nursing facility for four years total in a lifetime, within thirty days of a hospitalization of at least three days. For home health care, it pays $20 per day for up to two years. Service begins after a stay of at least 120 days in an skilled nursing facility. Premiums range from $15 to $83 per month, depending on age. As of October 1986 Aetna's policies were available in ten states.

Blue Cross of North America pays $35 per day for skilled nursing care for up to 630 days; and pays $30 per day for intermediate level institutional care, also for up to 630 days. No custodial care or home health benefits are included. Premiums are based on age, and range from $40 to $76 per month.

The details of these and other policies require the closest possible analysis before purchase, and these examples are cited merely to give a sense of the range of available benefits and prices.

Government Responsibilities for Long Term Care Insurance

The federal government has been preoccupied with control of acute care costs. The revolution in fiscal control of hospitals manifested by the Diagnosis-related group legislation is an example. Attention to issues of long term care, however, has been modest, and at this time a perception that inadequate financial resources are available inhibits new government programs. The response of the executive branch in Washington, as expressed by C. M. Haddow, previously of the Health Care Financing Administration (HCFA), is that government must encourage the development of private long term care insurance. HCFA supports legislation that will give greater flexibility to the states "to require middle class families to help bear the cost of maintaining family members in institutions."[92]

Attempts to establish government controls are being developed. In Washington, the Long Term Care Insurance Promotion and Protection Act[93] was introduced as part of the Consolidated Omnibus Reconciliation Act of 1985. No action has been taken yet. This bill includes guidelines for what should be covered under such policies; offers federal certification to those companies which comply; and establishes a federal Task Force on Long Term Care health policies to make recommendations on long term care insurance.

On the state level, at this writing twenty-eight governments have started some form of study to explore their proper role in the field of long term care insurance. The activities range from establishment of study commissions, through reform of insurance regulations and consumer protection standards, to control over recently promulgated insurance policies.

SOLUTIONS: APPROACHES
TO FINANCING LONG TERM CARE

The history of social planning in our country suggests that no overall integrated scheme of financing will take place. Developing an armchair strategy for comprehensive reform may be a pleasant entertainment, and may in fact produce highly worthwhile concepts. However, we must devote the bulk of our planning energies to the hard work of incremental change to meet the need, to the degree that political and financial pressures will give us the leverage. Karen Davis and Diane Rowland, chairman and research associate, respectively, of the Department of Health Policy and Management at Johns Hopkins University, ask the key questions:

What share of the financing should be borne directly by the individual receiving services or by the family? To what extent should care be provided and financed by the public sector? Underlying these questions are issues related to whether eligibility for publicly financed care should be based on income and how to avoid buying much of the care that is now provided free.[94]

CHANGES IN GOVERNMENT FINANCING

Medicare reform is the basic prerequisite for the development of long term care financing. Almost all older people have entitlements under this program, and it is widely accepted as a reliable and effective insurance vehicle for care of the elderly. The major gap is in the area of long term care. Therefore why shouldn't Medicare be changed to fill the gap? The answer is, primarily, lack of money, political desire, and consensus among the various forces that could strive for this result. Medicare is a federal program. Current budget problems inhibit the development of changes in Medicare that might add to costs.

Davis and Rowland[95] have developed a three-pronged theoretical structure for Medicare reform. The components are consumer incentives, provider incentives, and increased revenues:

1. *Consumer incentives to control costs.* Enrollees are given greater responsibility for payment of their own health care expenses. The aim here is to lead to more prudent use of resources and a reduction of the share that younger and less populous generations must pay toward the overall Medicare costs. The means for developing consumer incentives include further increases in the present co-insurance and deductible amounts and creation of a voucher system.

2. *Provider incentives to control costs.* A major first step has been taken with the establishment of PPS and DRGs. Hospitals, the most expensive part of Medicare, are placed under fiscal constraint. Attempts to control other elements of care, such as physicians' fees and nursing home/home care costs, to the extent that they are covered by Medicare, would follow.

3. *Increasing revenues to Medicare.* Among suggested sources of additional money are increases in the payroll tax for employers and employees, use of general tax revenues, and application of specific taxes, including those on alcohol and tobacco. These seem particularly appropriate to use for funding health services.

Beyond these three points, Medicare financing opportunities for consideration include changing the age of eligibility upward; offering a varied program of benefits for different age cohorts under Medicare so that those more elderly would have access to more long term care services; and requiring people of greater means to pay a larger share of costs.[96]

Changes in Medicaid and SSI that might improve financing of the long term care spectrum include: *preservation of income* and requiring that Medicaid's pro-institutional bias be eliminated. In order to permit Medicaid patients to retain their own homes or apartments while in nursing homes, and make it possible for some to return home, they would be allowed to keep their regular sources of income, such as SSI, for a limited period of time, perhaps three months. By eliminating Medicaid's pro-institutional bias, funds would flow as easily for home care as for nursing home placement. Perhaps home care should be the *beneficiary* of bias.[97]

CHANGES IN PRIVATE FINANCING

Change in tax and Social Security law and regulation would help free personal funds, which could be used for long term care of older people. Innovative forms of insurance, reverse mortgages, S/HMOs, and life care communities are some ways of dealing with the problem. Other methods include:

1. *Tax deductions for in-home services.* Amend the tax law to permit families to obtain tax credit for the expenses of caring for an aged relative at home. This development seems preordained by a similar credit already in existence for expenses of the care of a dependent child. This amendment would tend to support care at home as opposed to institutional placement. Negatives include loss of tax revenue, and thus the creation of federal support for services previously given free by the family.

2. *Employee fringe benefits.* Consideration should be given to conversion of benefits in place during working years, such as life insurance policies, into annuities at the time of retirement. Through this means the monies that would be paid off after death could be used instead during life to pay for needed services.[98]

3. *Individual Retirement Accounts (IRAs).* A form of IRA could be developed that was reserved for use in paying long term care costs. The tax deferral value of the IRA concept would be preserved, and thus people could be encouraged to save for their future independence at home, avoid nursing home placement if possible, and in the worst case perhaps have more choice of institutions, and more amenities, than if they became wards of Medicaid.[99]

4. *Social Security Payment Adjustment.* Social Security payments might be made more available to support each beneficiary's long term care needs if the payment schedule allowed increases with age. There is inherent logic to the idea that, as need and expense increase, income should grow in parallel. The idea that as cumbersome a process as Social Security might be made this flexible seems quixotic. However, as pressures grow in the next twenty years for solutions to the long term care payment dilemma, this suggestion, put forth by Dr. Wallack, may become realistic.[100]

Vladeck has summarized the situation:

> If we start by asking ourselves how we can best provide services to frail elderly persons who most need them, we can only conclude that more effective and integrated mechanisms of financing are necessary. . . . Given demographic trends, none of the major sources of financing for long term care are ever going to spend any less than they are now spending. Whether they are prepared to enter into the necessary arrangements to develop effective systems of care while limiting their future liabilities is fundamentally a political question.[101]

Regulations covering long term care services will be altered when the climate is favorable. At that time, logic says, money from payroll taxes, general revenues of the government, and premium contributions to Medicare will be combined with an array of funds generated from the private sector effectively to finance long term care services for the elderly.

PART TWO

CLINICAL
CONCERNS

Chapter 3

Health, Disease, and Functional Ability

Knowledge in the fields of geriatrics and gerontology has begun to approach that of other medical and social science disciplines in complexity and scholarship. Substantial information is available in the areas of cellular aging, metabolism, and neurobiology. In other aspects, such as the practice of medicine in the nursing home, growth has been erratic. In any case, these advances lack immediate practical value unless responsible clinicians can use the data effectively to benefit individual older persons.

Only a sensitive and integrated approach to health care services for the elderly should be acceptable. Their needs are dynamic—subject to change—as is the environment in which health care is given. A balance must exist between prudent use of fiscal resources and sound, comprehensive medical care. The current national concern with economy in the use of health personnel, equipment, and institutional resources has caused realistic restrictions in what care can be offered. Will the demand for cost efficiency yield to crude expediency, such as the denial of renal dialysis to persons over age fifty-five? Or, through diligent research and analysis, will we find the techniques to offer pertinent forms of health care to all who can benefit, without excessive and too-burdensome cost?

Various attempts have been made to integrate physical, psychological, and social factors that affect human health.[1] This chapter is based on a model that integrates these elements. Factors intrinsic and extrinsic to each older individual are considered, but it is understood that in real life boundaries are not always easily distinguished. Further, it is essential to understand that in the long term care spectrum all the biological and environmental stresses that relate to the welfare of each person are in flux.

This analysis also suggests possible compensatory mechanisms people may use to preserve basic and valued functions and needs. As an example, for some, loss of a physical ability, such as walking, can lead to development of creative psychological adaptations and compensations.

The forces that influence the fate of the aged in their relationship to long term care are innumerable. While we discuss a particular set of factors of clear significance, it should be understood that many additional influences could well be included.

INTRINSIC FACTORS: PHYSICAL AND PSYCHOLOGICAL CHARACTERISTICS

THE BODY

The rate at which people age is associated with a myriad of factors unique to each individual's own body. Despite this, efforts to develop a general understanding of the causes of aging through studies of human tissue at subcellular and cellular levels are critically important. Only by comprehending the effects of normal aging on tissue can we expect to understand the results of disease and thus to distinguish between normal senescence and morbid states.

For example, fibroblasts are primitive cells often used as markers in aging research. It is now known that fibroblasts derived from patients with diseases that in some ways mimic advanced aging, in rare conditions such as Werner's syndrome and progeria, and in diabetes mellitus, have shorter life-spans in tissue culture than do those cells from age-matched controls.[2] This suggests strongly that even in the absence of identifiable disease, each person's cells age at a pace preordained by that individual's genetic structure. Through this kind of study it becomes possible to explain differences in bodily function and ability among people of the same chronological age and, by extension, the differences in their relative abilities to remain independent as they grow older.

DISEASE

Disease is a process that produces dysfunction of the body and meets definable clinical criteria. It is an abnormal state that must be distinguished from aging as such. In a simplistic categorization, diseases in older people can be divided into two groups: conditions particularly common to the elderly, such as osteoporosis, and those that may occur at any age, such as pneumonia. Geriatricians have learned that, while the underlying conditions may be common, the second group of disorders can present aberrantly in people of advanced age and thus not be easily recognized. Examples include depression, thyroid disease, pneumonia, and myocardial infarction.[3]

A paradoxical result of medical progress is the survival of more people with chronic disease. This phenomenon is particularly evident in the fifth through the tenth decades of life, a consequence of the fact that many acute conditions that were killers of the elderly in prior decades, such as bacterial pneumonia, are now treatable or curable. Today older people are subject to long term illness or disability that in the past they would not have survived to face.[4] Further, the mix of clinical disorders among the very old has changed. The ability of physicians to treat high blood pressure, for instance, has caused a significant reduction in the incidence of strokes.[5]

NUTRITION

Nutritional considerations for the elderly vary widely with their health status and living situation, because the process of aging causes in most physiologic measurements to be increasingly heterogeneous.[6] While the past scientific understanding of diet-related health problems was modest, today a broad knowledge exists.[7] However, the abundant medical literature that describes essential nutrients, anthropomorphic indices (measures of body composition), and recommended dietary allowances for human beings in general is markedly inadequate for people over age seventy-five.[8] While many basic nutritional principles probably can be applied broadly across all ages as long as the people under study are vigorous and healthy,[9] nutritional concerns change radically as people grow more frail and thus require higher levels of care.[10] For instance, the side effects of therapeutic drugs and chronic diseases such as depression and malignancy may cause anorexia and lead to a poor state of nutrition. Aging itself, which has certain effects on the cells of the gut and thus on the absorption of nutrients, may do so as well.

Many older people, particularly those whose lives are physically restricted and who are inactive, need less nutrients. Nursing home dietary departments must concentrate planning on the correct mix of foods rather than assuming that more calories are better.

As people reach advanced degrees of disability—for instance, when they have lost the gag reflex or require feeding through a nasogastric tube—

nutritional issues become further complicated. In this case food consistency and mode of ingestion are a concern in order to avoid aspiration into the lungs, with consequent pneumonia.

FITNESS

We use the term fitness to refer to the degree to which the body's ability to resist fatigue has been developed. Body function, in a simplified way, can be explained through this term. Each organ may be free of disease and may have escaped the negative effects of accelerated aging, but may fall below functional potential because of poor fitness. In the presence of disease, the question of bodily fitness becomes of greater importance. For instance, an older person with a fractured hip is more likely to recover fully if she walked three miles a day regularly before the injury than if she had led a sedentary life.[11]

The concept of fitness as interpreted by investigators in the field of rehabilitation medicine is quite specific and can be measured objectively. It is possible to determine, for example, the specific effects of fitness on certain bone, muscle, and nerve cells. In muscle, distinctions can be made between various types of fibers, based on the amount of activity of certain enzymes. Specifically, the types of fibers in a bundle of striated muscle can be distinguished by the level and proportion of myosin-adenosinetriphosphatase activity and oxidative capacity. Certain fibers have been shown to remain constant in number with age. Others decline markedly, a fact that may relate to the loss of strength and agility experienced by older people in general.[12]

The practical effects of fitness on functional ability are noteworthy. In an older person with physical reserves reduced by normal senescence, effective conditioning may alter the balance at a critical moment in favor of independence rather than another option on the long term care spectrum. A person less fit, and thus less able to engage in self-care, may require institutional placement.

PSYCHOLOGICAL STRENGTH

The psychological makeup of each person includes intellectual function, organization of the personality, and psychodynamics. While these factors interact, each has distinct and identifiable qualities of its own. For example, a cognitive function such as memory can be measured through reproducible tests. An intact short term memory suggests that the person has a relatively good likelihood of maintaining a safe life in the home. Short term memory difficulties may be manifested by risks such as leaving on the gas, forgetting to turn off the tap, or getting lost on familiar streets. The relationship of short term memory to the long term care spectrum is evident.

If a person is psychiatrically ill, symptoms are likely to interfere with functioning, have a significant impact on ability to handle problems, and also relate to the individual's placement on the spectrum. Depression and suicide are relatively common in the elderly. If the patient is seriously depressed, the total approach to a plan of long term care will be affected. It may be especially difficult for hypochondrical patients to adjust to the characteristics of normal aging.

It is helpful to emphasize nurturing the psychological strengths of each older person rather than dwelling on frailty. Family and friends, for instance, or the concerned physician, may opt to confine the older person once forgetfulness becomes evident. The temptation to do so ignores residual psychological forces in the individual that may be ample to handle a life of reasonable independence, if some help is provided. Friendly visits, Meals-on-Wheels, telephone reassurance and/or telephone buddy systems, part-time paraprofessional service, and careful use of psychotropic medications all may serve to strengthen and validate the patient's remaining resources of psychological strength.

Some people have psychological qualities that endear them to others. Their natures seem to engender loving, nurturing behavior from caregivers, friends, and family members, an empathic response that well serves the person in need. A cheerful disposition may preserve independence, and grumpiness may cause alienation, isolation, and danger. On the other hand, sweetness must not be equated with passivity. Therein lies risk. Sometimes it is healthy to be unpleasant.

COPING SKILLS

Each individual has a certain innate capacity to handle pain, anxiety, loneliness, helplessness, and other stresses. Gerontologists and psychologists are studying these capacities, or coping skills, which influence an older person's ability to retain independence.

An early focus of interest has been the ability of older people to cope with relocation from a familiar setting. One study describes three components of a coping strategy: the degree of coping effort, the level of ability to integrate (also called cognitive restructuring), and the person's perceived degree of mastery over the relocation process and over the new situation.[13] In this study, the individual's abilities to handle the challenge (termed management strategies) were measured against the degree of depression shortly after the relocation and also with long term outcomes. Those people with high degrees of mastery and control (that is, those with better coping skills) had lower levels of postmove depression and better long term results. This analysis proved again the validity of the truism: passivity is dangerous. It is healthy for all persons, specifically including the elderly, to remain in control of major life decisions. Sometimes the frail older person, always at risk of manipulation by others, must be devious and crafty, when common sense and sweet reason are insufficient.[14]

A good ability to cope, to accept and work through life's challenges with equanimity, seems to serve people well. This point is supported by interviews with twelve hundred centenarians conducted by the Social Security Administration.[15] Enjoyment of work and a strong will to live emerged as the dominant common themes. Most of the people interviewed had lived quiet, circumscribed, independent lives; were content with their lot; ate a balanced diet; were devoted to family and religion; and worked hard and enjoyed it. In general, they did not have high ambitions and lacked regrets, self-pity, and combativeness.

In crises, an individual's coping strategies are formed from initial interpretation of the stressful event, a process that requires cognitive ability. If cognitive function is diminished by disease or otherwise, coping ability is reduced. This fact has direct impact on the placement of a person on the long term care spectrum. To illustrate, if an elderly man living at home successfully with a part-time homemaker becomes ill, his cognitive ability may become temporarily impaired. His ability to cope with the environment is reduced, and feelings of depression rise. His appetite worsens, and the reduction in caloric intake impedes recovery from the illness. The downhill spiral of system failure proceeds, with the ultimate conclusion of nursing home placement or death.

EXTRINSIC FACTORS: THE ENVIRONMENT, PEOPLE WHO HELP, AND COMMUNITY RESOURCES

LIVING SPACE

For a frail older person, the area in which the activities of daily living take place may range from a bed to an entire house. If living space is reduced to a bed, the focus of major attention will be on such matters as whether the risk of decubitus ulcer formation by the pressure of the bedding is controlled; or it may become critical to know whether the bed is near the bathroom, if the patient is able to walk a few unassisted steps. This simple ability may prevent the patient from developing functional urinary incontinence caused by failure to reach the toilet in time.

The discussion of living space may be extended to include the workplace of the employed older person. If the room is polluted with fumes from industry or tobacco, the employee with lung disease and borderline bronchial airway obstruction may become unable to work. Since older people are more likely to have lost functional physical reserve than those who are younger,[16] they may be tipped into a symptomatic state and disability.

Falls, a relatively common problem in the elderly, produce substantial morbidity and mortality.[17] Intensive studies done in institutions[18] have shown that the living space is responsible for about 40 percent of falls by older people. This is a pertinent illustration of how extrinsic factors affect health.

CLIMATE

Factors such as altitude, sunlight, and ambient temperature influence health status. For instance, the Hunzas,[19] a people who live at an altitude of eight thousand feet and who walk great distances, are extremely long-lived, relatively free of cardiovascular disease, and thus stand in contrast to people living near sea level and in smog.

The importance of climatological influences changes as the older person moves from place to place on the spectrum of care. For example, the climate in a nursing home is probably fairly well controlled. Yet it can be influenced by extremes of heat and cold. The nursing home resident, unable to alter the environment, may suffer inadvertent hyper- or hypothermia. Cases of dehydration among frail residents of institutions are relatively common in hot summer months, a problem caused largely by the elderly's decreased homeostatic ability.[20] During long periods of cold, nursing homes must remain relatively sealed, a factor that encourages the spread of infections within the environment.

During the last several decades, climate has been responsible for the migration of many older people to the sunbelt of the United States. As a result, these individuals have become separated from friends and family, with the inevitable loss of normal natural supporters who might have helped during times of illness or disability. As these immigrants become the old-old, the local cities and counties have been hard-pressed to meet the need for institutional beds and community home care services. Because of the lack of available services, a small reverse migration to the north has occurred.

SUPPORT PERSONS

At every point on the long term care spectrum, older people need the help of others. These range from highly skilled professionals, through salaried homemakers and aides, to friends and family members (see chapters 7 and 8). The timely availability of support persons is a critical factor in the preservation of independence for frail older people. If an elderly individual living alone and in control of his or her life suddenly becomes unable to walk, who will help? Can technical assistance be found? Will helpers be trained, consistent, resourceful? If the person becomes more dependent, will they be able to step up the effort?

FINANCE

The financial factors that influence the fate of older people can be considered on individual, family, community, state, and national levels. As the dollar costs of services on the long term care spectrum rise, personal wealth is placed increasingly at risk. It has already been noted that Medicaid, a means-tested government health insurance program, will pay nursing home and other costs only if the person in need is virtually impoverished. Because of this, occasionally an older person's wealth has been transferred to other family members, sometimes illegally; or he or she has been divorced in order to obtain benefits. Given the harsh choices imposed by the cost of long term care, some older people have preferred to leave a legacy of money or property to their kin rather than exhaust their funds in order to add a few more months or years of totally dependent life. Some have committed suicide. Sometimes, when family members are in control, they will opt to preserve money for themselves rather than preserve life.

DR, a man in his eighties, lived in a skilled nursing facility for three years as a self-pay resident. He was vigorous, ambulatory, and seemed to enjoy life, although he could not communicate. He survived frequent episodes of hospitalization for treatment of aspiration pneumonia and infection of a suprapubic tube, but his Medicare allowance for inpatient days became exhausted. He would have to pay himself for any future hospital placement.

Suddenly, at this point the family members decided that the situation was intolerable, further hospitalization was inhumane, the patient "would not want to continue living this way," and "if he knew he would have to accept Medicaid he would kill himself." The next time the patient developed aspiration pneumonia, they insisted that he not be placed in the hospital. The nursing home physician opposed their decision but honored it, and the patient died several days later.

Financial incentives to hospitals under the Diagnosis-Related Group (DRG) system now in place in this country encourage a tendency to discharge older people sooner, and while still in poor health. The assumption has been that less expensive forms of community care would be available to assume responsibility for patients. Yet the presence of such services in the community is, in fact, highly variable. In parts of the country, particularly rural areas, home health care programs, day care, homemakers, and nursing homes are hard to tap or simply nonexistent.[21] Under these circumstances, even for those people who may have ample funds, there is no help. They cannot buy what is not available.

States are seeking methods to reduce their long term care costs further. In New York State, nursing homes now function under a rating system (resource utilization groups, or RUGs)[22] designed to encourage retention of only the sickest people and to discharge others to less intense levels of care. Since the program became effective on January 1, 1986, about 20 percent of nursing home residents have been deemed too physically able, too functionally independent, to warrant full Medicaid reimbursement to the institution. As they no longer generate full Medicaid payment, such people will become unwelcome, because the institution will be placed under fiscal strain for their care. Ultimately, nursing homes will be populated by patients who require highly intense levels of care—those who are sicker, more frail, closer to death, more likely to be hospitalized repeatedly. If the state is to continue to pay the costs, those older people who are not demented, who can walk, eat, and toilet themselves, will be squeezed down to a lower level of care.

ASSESSMENT

A comprehensive evaluation of each older person's situation is essential to the provision of the right services at the right time, when issues of long term care arise. This assessment should concern the individual's state of physical and emotional health, finances, and relations with family and others. More important, the focus should be on the person's own goals and on realistic means for reaching them.

Assessment has been studied as a process in itself, and several health care institutions have created inpatient or clinic units for this purpose. The claim is probably valid that comprehensive assessment techniques have proven useful in improving the outcome for the older people under review.[23] A particularly effective example is the series of geriatric evaluation units (GEUs) established at a number of Veterans Administration Medical

Centers.[24] Through these programs professional staff members complete assessments of older veterans while they are at the hospital and then maintain a long term follow-up relationship with the patients in their own homes.

Institution-based programs are few in number. Therefore, older people largely do without a comprehensive review and suffer an ad hoc fate, or depend on their own physician's experience. In real life most assessments are performed in the offices of private practitioners, who tend to employ an intuitive approach based on knowledge of the patient's personal and family history and observations over time.

Any worthy assessment, whether done over several days in a hospital or alone with a physician in the office, must integrate, insofar as possible, all the factors that relate to a person's health, disease, and functional ability. Each finding of the assessment must be interpreted in the context of the place on the spectrum of care where the patient sits at the time. A judgment then must be made as to the impact of all these points on the patient's ability to function, subject to refinement as time passes and the dynamics of the situation.

MEDICAL CARE

Medical care, as used in this discussion, means all the aspects of long term health care necessary to help an older person maintain the best possible physical, social, and psychological function. Complexity ranges from routine visits to a physician's office by a well elderly person, to hospitalization in an intensive care unit. The term includes diagnosis, prevention, therapy, rehabilitation, support, and maintenance.[25] Medical care must be resourceful and dynamic, available to older people as needed to maximize functioning and to avoid deterioration leading to loss of independence.

The physician is usually responsible for the patient's entry into the long term care spectrum, either through deliberate planning and consultation with the patient, family, and other health workers; or inadvertently, by lack of attention, stereotyping, assumptions of the inevitability of nursing home placement, or diagnosis and treatment inappropriate to a very old patient. There are four specific points that require understanding.

First, the *risk-benefit ratio of medical procedures* must be understood. For instance, the noting of blood in the stool of a frail ninety-year old person with dementia who is known to have hemorrhoids (a common explanation for this finding) does not necessarily demand a sigmoidoscopy and a barium enema. Such studies carry some risk,[26] may cause considerable discomfort, and can lead to findings of abnormalities that the patient and/or family would choose to ignore. If a cancer of the colon were found, the diagnostic effort would be futile if treatment by surgery or other means were to be refused. A clear understanding of the meaning and consequence of each procedure should exist between all parties.

Second, *transportation problems* must be recognized. The moment when the patient cannot get to the physician's office independently because she cannot climb the bus steps or has lost the visual acuity necessary to drive safely is often the time when medical supervision is most needed. The consequence of the new difficulty in mobility may therefore be an undetected but treatable lesion or an insidious weight loss that goes undetected. Unchecked, the disorder may reach a more critical point.

A third point to consider is the *physician's attitude.* Physicians must maintain an attitude toward their older patients that is supportive, understanding, honest, good-humored, and respectful. For instance, when an older patient is in the office with an accompanying relative, the doctor's attention should be directed appropriately. Ignoring the patient and discussing the case instead with the relative is an infantilizing discourtesy. The doctor's conduct should manifest a pledge of assistance and guidance to fellow human beings at this vulnerable time in their lives.

Fourth, *research* must be ongoing. The phenomenon of long term care is now a matter of major national importance. Therefore it has become a fruitful, rewarding subject for analysis. The opportunity to effect change seems substantial. The basic research questions in this field might be: How can appropriate assessment, health care services, and programs for older people be defined and developed?[27] What are the necessary costs, and how can we secure the needed funds?

The national forum of the 1981 White House Conference on Aging set the basic research agenda for the final two decades of the century.[28] Final recommendations included the following points:

1. Research in disease prevention and health promotion should receive the highest priority. The knowledge we already possess must be exploited. New studies are needed to establish improved biological markers of physiological age. Study of the personal motivators for improved health habits is also essential.

2. The Department of Health and Human Services (HHS) should improve its coordination of overall strategy for its research on aging, to insure that high-priority concerns are adequately funded. Duplication of research activities should be avoided.

3. The HHS should meet with private foundations and corporations to coordinate and encourage their involvement in aging research activities.

4. Cooperation and coordination in this field between United States scientists, and with their foreign counterparts, should be fostered, and information disseminated broadly.

As people age, their need for services within the long term care spectrum becomes increasingly likely. Their health and social conditions are dynamic, and thus the intrinsic and extrinsic forces will vary in importance. Even as people advance in chronological age, modification of lifestyle and proper treatment of illness can help maintain the maximum possible degree of physical independence.

In older people, a delicate balance of functions exists. A small gain in strength, agility, or self-confidence can result in major positive effects on an individual's life, just as a minor physical insult may have devastating consequences. For young people, with greater physical reserves, the situation may have a greater amount of forgiveness built in. For example, ingestion of two ounces of alcohol may cause no appreciable physical problem in a twenty-year-old, but it may produce severe disability in an octogenarian (see chapter 5).

Urinary incontinence is a prototypical major concern of older people. The consequences of incontinence depend on the impact of the extrinsic and intrinsic factors. These forces produce a dynamic set of interactions that require responses from the patient, family, friends, and health care personnel.[29] The patient's coping skills are needed to avoid retreat into isolation, but personal attitudes differ. One man's dribbling is another's incontinence. Among the physician's considerations is the disease or dysfunctional process that may underlie the incontinence.[30] The numerous possible etiologies include confusion, dementia and delerium, infection, side effects of drugs such as diuretics and sedatives, psychological disorders, poor mobility that denies the patient adequate speed to reach the toilet, urethritis, and vaginitis. The condition may relate to nutritional considerations such as obesity or vitamin B12 deficiency, or to poorly controlled diabetes mellitus.

The degree of threat imposed by incontinence varies with each person's situation, and the means to control or limit the problem are equally diverse. For the alert older person faced with the loss of Saturday theater matinees because of dribbling, aggressive measures to diagnose, treat and/or absorb the problem are appropriate. On the other hand, for a nursing home patient with Alzheimer's disease and urinary incontinence, development of simple plans for placement of a commode in the patient's room and encouragement of frequent urination may be sufficient.

It is important for patients, family members, and health care workers to understand that numerous forces have an impact on the lives of older people, and that many of these forces can be controlled. Personal interactions and treatment plans should be developed with this view clearly in mind.

INTEGRATING HEALTH, DISEASE, AND FUNCTIONAL ABILITY: CASE EXAMPLES

The hypothetical composite studies that follow illustrate how the numerous intrinsic and extrinsic forces applied to each person can affect major life decisions. They demand recognition that aging is both a psychosocial and a biological process.[31]

RT is a youthful-appearing sixty-six-year-old employed man who hobbles to his physician's office after a two-year absence complaining of exquisite pain in the knee. For several years he has taken a diuretic medication for control of high blood pressure. The only abnormality on the physical examination is a hot, tender, swollen, red knee.

His *body* is in good shape and highly functional. He looks about twenty years younger than his stated age. Nevertheless, normal aging has had a physiologic impact on the joints. Cartilage begins to undergo degeneration after about age thirty. Because he is a man in his seventh decade, the diagnostic considerations for his knee *disease* differ from those of a younger person or from a contemporary who is bed-bound in a nursing home. Here, gout is the prime candidate. RT's doctor must be aware, however, that pseudogout is also a disorder with a high prevalence in the elderly. There may, in addition, be a coexisting condition, such as osteoarthritis, which is likely to be present in people of this age group. Establishing the proper diagnosis is complicated because laboratory values for elderly persons differ quantitatively from those of younger people.[32] Thus physicians must expand their fund of knowledge in order to treat the elderly.

RT's *nutritional status* requires attention. He appears youthful, but his body is not metabolizing food as it did decades earlier. His ability to control the metabolism of uric acid may have altered as well and this, combined with gout-inducing side effects of his diuretic, may have been the precipitating cause of his illness. Furthermore, his home circumstances may have changed—the death of a spouse, the marriage of a child, or other events may have resulted in changes in his habitual diet. He may now be eating large quantities of anchovies and organ meats, such as liver and sweetbreads, all gout-inducing foods, rather than his wife's careful, prudent cooking.

RT's *psychological strengths* are relevant to the outcome of his ailment. His cognitive skills will be called upon to understand the doctor's explanation of his disease, the therapeutic regime, and methods of functioning with a game leg. His personality and character will sustain him through treatment, allow him to be overwhelmed with anxiety ("Is the doctor telling me the truth? Do I really have cancer?"), or cause him to deny the condition and impair its healing. The ultimate result of this event—full recovery and return to work versus the possibility of a collapse into a dependent state—will be determined in large part by the patient's *coping skills.* How will RT adapt? He has shown vigor and strength through the fact that he is still working and is in a healthy state in general, despite long gaps between doctor visits. New challenges to the patient's coping skills have now arisen, however. Is his job secure? An episode of illness may present the excuse the employer was seeking to fire RT. Is he the principle caretaker of an invalid spouse? The attack of gout may necessitate the wife's hospitalization, or outside help may be needed.

The patient's underlying *fitness* is the key to recovery. Considerations during a gout attack include the underlying strength of the leg. The supporting muscles of the knee will weaken through disuse during the illness and recovery periods. Therefore RT's ability to walk with crutches and his later return to full function will depend in part on prior muscle tone. The bone and cartilage of the joint on which this attack is imposed are also affected by previous fitness levels,[33] and their condition will affect the possibility of full recovery.

Prior to this illness RT had good mobility. How can he preserve the maximum possible normal function? Numerous factors in his *living space* at home and worksite are pertinent. Are there stairs to climb? Does he drive a stick-shift car? Mobility is essential to this man's functioning. For example, if the *climate* in his area is snowy when he requires crutches, his difficulties will grow.

Before the illness, RT's need for a network of *support persons* to assist him physically in carrying out normal activities was minimal. This has now changed. Further, the issues of emotional support that surround convalescence will require that he have good relations with others. Many aspects of coping and mental health depend on the intangible qualities of the support network. How well the surrounding persons work with RT in his new state of dependency will affect the long term outcome substantially.

Are RT's finances secure? While the expense of this episode of illness will probably be relatively light, it may still produce hardship. He will have considerable personal costs. He will have to meet the deductible portion of Medicare for payment of his physician's bill. If the cost of medication is not covered by insurance through his job, he will have to pay for drugs. Will he require paraprofessional assistance temporarily? If so, he will have to pay.

This patient arrived in the doctor's office for *medical care* of an acute illness. If the doctor can integrate a response to the multitude of forces that affect RT with good diagnostic, preventive, therapeutic, supportive, rehabilitative, and maintenance measures, he or she will be able to help RT. The doctor's assessment must be comprehensive and must consider illnesses common to people of RT's chronological age. An examination of the necessary thoroughness is perhaps less likely to occur when a patient visits the physician for an isolated complaint, as in this instance, than when the doctor-patient relationship has been stronger.

The risk-benefit ratio of each treatment requires careful thought, because there is a negative side to each decision. Therapy in this case might require the use of drugs such as colchicine, indomethacin, or phenylbutazone. The diarrhea and vomiting sometimes induced by colchicine can cause dehydration or aspiration of vomitus into the lungs. Indomethacin can cause a soporific state, leaving the patient at risk of falls or other consequences of inattention. Phenylbutazone may result in fluid retention and lead to congestive heart failure. An underlying, as yet undetected, cardiac disorder is a realistic possibility in a sixty-six-year-old man. There is a risk that RT might suffer the cascade effect, a series of complications, one leading to the next.[34]

To minimize the risks of treatment, the following principles should be considered by the physician and understood and supported by the patient and available family members:

1. The medical history must be accurate and thorough. It should include family information and prior medical records from other physicians.
2. Findings on the physical examination or from laboratory tests should be interpreted in the light of their predictive value, sensitivity, and specificity, and the prevalence of the conditions under evaluation.
3. Tests should be ordered only if the results will produce a difference in clinical decisions. For example, in the case of a very old person with coronary disease, it is pointless to carry out a coronary arteriogram, with its risks and its implications for heart surgery, if surgery has already been ruled out by other considerations. On the other hand, some risk may be acceptable in testing, and should not be avoided if it is determined that the likelihood of benefit is high.[35]

In RT's case, the consequences of an acute attack of gout will probably not be especially onerous, because it is a self-limited and treatable condition. Still, there are threats to his quality of life, and if the forces that place him at risk are not appreciated his situation could collapse. In the worst case, this man, highly functional in many ways, could be left jobless, friendless, and an institutionalized destitute ward of the state.

The next person under review is at far graver risk of entering the long term care spectrum than is RT. The admixture of chronic illness, poor ego strength, unsafe personal habits, a more advanced chronological and biological age, and poor support from family are the issues here.

JB, a seventy-five-year-old woman, seeks advice from a private physician, an internist, at the urging of her daughter, who has heard that he is "good with the elderly." The patient arrives in the office unaccompanied, and gives a history of feeling weak, poor appetite, chronic constipation, increasing unsteadiness, and numbness in the feet. When pressed for further historical information, she relates that she drinks three martinis per day, has smoked two packs of Camels daily since she was a teenager, and has experienced vague chest discomfort for the last seventy-two hours.

On physical examination she is found to be frail, slightly hypertensive, mildly unsteady, with signs of liver disease. An electrocardiogram shows evidence of both old and acute damage. The physician advises immediate hospitalization, but the patient refuses: "Let me just go home and if I die tonight that'll be all right too." After failing to reach the daughter on the telephone, the doctor coaxes JB into his own car, since she adamantly refuses an ambulance, and takes her to the emergency room of the local hospital. The diagnosis of an acute myocardial infarction is established, and she is admitted.

During the hospital stay, additional information is provided by the daughter. There exists a more substantial history of heavy drinking, and JB had had another heart attack a year earlier but had not followed medical orders since that time. The hospital stay is uneventful, but discharge planning is complicated by JB's resistance to change, the recognition that she cannot happily live with her daughter but that she will be unsafe alone, and her refusal to consider nursing home placement.

JB's *body* has been assaulted by years of alcohol and tobacco abuse. She is significantly depressed as well. Therefore it may be difficult to tease out the basic underlying structural and physiological qualities of her organs, which consist of a mix of diseased and normal cells, all of which are also subject to the consequences of aging. The reserves of functional tissue that to date have permitted her survival are at their limits in the heart and liver. Moreover, the residual functional ability of her other organs will dictate the effectiveness of medications, rehabilitation potential, and the likelihood of other illnesses.

JB is on the downhill slope of increased frailty and dependence because she suffers from *disease* of both heart and liver. The most immediate concern is her cardiac status, with the threat of a further myocardial infarction and death. The physician recognized the significance of JB's complaint of chest pain while she was in his office and dealt vigorously with the need for immediate hospital care. It took good clinical judgment and careful attention to recognize this problem in the confused context of information the patient presented. In the elderly, typical crushing chest pain, so often a sign of heart attack in younger people, is much less a constant.[36] The patient's survival past the immediate postinfarction hours, the period of greatest risk to life, was somewhat in question because of her age.[37] The increased relative risk in older people results from the greater likelihood of preexisting heart disease, with particular reference to disorders of rhythm conduction, and to abnormalities of sodium and potassium metabolism.

The disease of alcoholism is a problem here as well. Alcohol harms many organs and functions, several of which have been cited in JB's history and physical examination. An immediate related problem during the hospital period is the possibility of an alcohol withdrawal syndrome, with rapid heart rate, elevation in blood pressure, and fever. These additional physical stresses would hardly be helpful to a cardiac patient. That JB escaped these problems in this instance may be due to the decreased tolerance for alcohol that gradually occurs in elderly alcoholics (see chapter 5). An additional problem in this case is the possible appearance of an alcohol-related dementia. If this occurs, the end result may be institutionalization in order to cope with the essentials of daily care such as washing, feeding, and toileting. It should also be understood that the patient's alcoholism may be relevant to her refusal to accept nursing home placement or to live with her daughter. In each instance she would recognize the potential loss of access to alcohol.

Since JB survived her heart attack, the generic concerns that can affect her level of placement on the long term care spectrum must be faced. Among these, her *nutritional status* impacts strongly on her ability to recover and on the prevention of a further heart attack. Because she lived alone, she may have eaten largely at fast food restaurants. The consumption of high-fat meals may have contributed to her coronary artery disease. Even at this stage of her life, use of a cardiac-prudent diet[38] might decrease the chance of further heart damage. Nutritional issues relate to the consequences of her alcoholism as well. Because she has in part substituted the calories in alcohol for those in food, she may have a diet low in vitamin B1. Thus she is a candidate for beriberi, a deficiency disease that involves the heart.

JB's level of *psychological strength* is poor. If she were tested, deficiencies of memory, cognition, and personality organization would probably surface. These qualities will harm her ability to recover quickly from the rigors of a heart attack and its explicit threat to life. Further, the patient was overtly depressed on arrival in the doctor's office, a clinical problem that alone will impede vigorous recovery from a major illness.

Her *coping skills* are modest. JB's passive and fatalistic resolve would tend to thwart an assiduous adherence to a complex treatment regimen,[39] particularly one that demands giving up her addictions to alcohol and tobacco. Healthy coping mechanisms require careful appraisal of therapeutic choices, a vigilant approach to recovery, and adequate cognitive skills. They will be undermined by depression.[40]

JB's daughter was her only available *support person*. Unfortunately, the two women had a tense, ambivalent, and conflicted relationship. The daughter tried to be helpful and sought out a physician she thought might be especially appropriate, but she did not come to the appointment with her mother. Although the sharing of living quarters might have been life-saving for the mother, the proposal was unacceptable to the older woman. Later discussion revealed that the daughter held deep-seated resentment because of her mother's lifelong alcohol abuse and JB's inconsistent evidence of affection toward her child, which seemed to deny meaningful maternal support.

JB's *financial status* was unclear because of her confusion and apparent resistance to giving information about access to cash. There was sufficient money in a checking account to deny her eligibility for Medicaid, thereby largely eliminating payment for home care or nursing home services by any level of government. She resisted suggestions to spend down her assets to make herself Medicaid-eligible. Although JB refused to acknowledge the point, it seemed possible that she was striving through these mechanisms to retain control over her own life, including her freedom to drink.

JB's use of *medical care* services seemed imprudent. She sought the doctor's attention only after prodding from her daughter, and in regard to isolated complaints. There existed no effective, ongoing physician-patient relationship, a partnership that might have provided preventive treatment and helped JB avoid the brink of involvement with the long term care spectrum. Indeed, that she resisted medical treatment for several years despite considerable illness and disability emphasizes her need for independence and the strength of her denials. In an ironic defense of her rationale, one that might well be considered maladaptive, it is reasonable to ask how likely it was that JB would find appropriate, sensitive care from a doctor. Many well-trained internists and family physicians lack training in care of older people and of alcoholics.

Assessment of JB's health and social needs while in the hospital was carried out by a staff social worker. This employee faced dual demands on her motivation and skill. She wanted to help the patient achieve a safe and attractive living situation after discharge. She needed time for evaluation of a complex case and for counseling with patient and daughter. She also had to respond to the hospital's need for JB's prompt discharge to the community because of financial concerns imposed by DRG regulations. Hospital peer review mechanisms triggered a speedy release, as soon as JB's medical clearance occurred. These pressures, coupled with the patient's own eagerness to go home and unwillingness to address issues such as her alcoholism, isolation, and poor nutrition, resulted in a hasty discharge. Provision for adequate follow-up was lacking and JB was left at high risk for recurrence of acute illness and hospital readmission. For a reasonable chance of salvage, JB would have required a hospital that maintained a geriatric assessment team and a community-based long term home health care program.[41]

The following situation created the need for consideration of ethical questions. When a very old and frail person seems to be dying, who makes the decisions about treatment? Where lies the balance between aggressive attempts to preserve life at any cost and resignation to fate?

RB was a ninety-five-year old woman, a member of a loving and caring family. She had always been a vibrant person, but made a poor psychological adjustment to the death of her husband three years earlier. Shortly thereafter she developed carcinoma of the breast and underwent a mastectomy. No recurrence had been noted to date. Eight months later she required major surgery for repair of an abdominal aortic aneurysm, and had a lengthy convalescence.

She was admitted to a nursing home because of increasing dementia. She had turned on the stove and forgotten to turn it off; and had been found wandering in the street on three occasions. Her children felt that safety required that she be institutionalized.

RB seemed to adapt well to life in the nursing home. Her entry physical examination and laboratory screening tests proved unremarkable. She became a leader of group book discussions, took care of her personal needs well with some guidance, and developed a flirting interaction with members of the professional staff. As an instance, the following conversation was noted during a visit by a daughter when the home's physician was present:

Daughter: Mother! Cover yourself. You're indecent.

RB: This doctor doesn't even look at me. He's got younger girls to look at.

After three stable months in the nursing home, RB underwent a change. She was less ebullient, lost her appetite, and lost twelve pounds over a ten-week period. Physical examinations, X-rays, and blood tests yielded little explanatory information. She became listless, then semicomatose; spiked a fever to 102.5° F; was unable to drink and became dehydrated.[42] Daily discussion took place between staff of the nursing home and delegated representatives of RB's family. The doctor wanted to place RB in the hospital in order to establish a diagnostic cause for the physical collapse; and he was quite free as well in expressing the fear that he might be open to a malpractice suit by the family if he did not press for the use of all available measures to preserve life. The nursing home administrator seemed to want RB placed in a hospital because the death of a resident in the nursing home might create an unpleasant ambiance for other patients and causes negative responses from state surveyors. The family, on the other hand, realized that RB was dying and wanted the event to take place naturally and without further action, peacefully, and in the nursing home.[43] They recognized that RB would probably undergo aggressive treatment if she was transferred to a hospital. Because a trusting and caring relationship had been established over the six-month period, family wishes were permitted to prevail, and RB died in bed in her final home, without a tube inserted into her body.

RB reached a great age. What were the physical qualities of her *body* that permitted her to be vibrant and agile into her tenth decade? A combination of genetic sturdiness and a prudent style of life with avoidance of risk factors offers the best general explanation available. Senescence of body tissues and organs had proceeded, however, and RB had lost much of her reserve capacity. Any minor change in her physical state put her at risk for death.

RB had, in fact, already been faced with two significant major *diseases:* arteriosclerosis, manifested by an aortic aneurysm,[44] and cancer of the breast.[45] Both of these conditions could recur.

The approach to diagnosis and treatment of disease among very old individuals in institutions differs from that of people living independent lives in the community. The thinking of clinical investigators or nursing home physicians may need modification to accommodate the setting in which the aged live. Nursing home residents have a greater likelihood of dementia and chronic disability. They are therefore less able to exert full control over decisions regarding health care. This power tends to lie in the hands of their children. When no family member exists, the staff physician or administrator may be forced into that role.

RB's *nutritional status* was a concern during her last months of life, because of her noticeable loss of appetite and weight. A question arose as to whether her general body failure was primarily a disease consequent to inadequate nourishment, or whether her inability to eat followed the development of an illness, albeit one as yet not diagnosed. Nutritional deficiencies in the elderly population, although widely reported,[46] are difficult to implicate as causative in RB's complex situation. After all, she had eaten well and with pleasure during her first three months in the nursing home. In this instance, the physician felt the weight loss to be a result of anorexia, a condition probably caused by a preexisting disease. Metastases to other organs from her earlier carcinoma of the breast were suspected. It deserves emphasis that weight loss in an older person is frequently an early sign of impending disease and should always trigger consideration of screening, testing, and nutritional consultation.

The quality of *living space* in this case assumes a substantial importance. Life confined to a nursing home called forth all of RB's *psychological strength* in order to thrive. It takes qualities of vigor and optimism, a humorous and ironic view of life, tolerance and equanimity to accept regimentation and loss of personal control without depression. RB was able to engage with staff and program happily, it seemed, for about three months. Then she began to fail. Had she become depressed? Had her *coping skills* failed her? This aged woman had shown the ability to survive two major illnesses and the associated surgery, but coping with an institutional environment, especially considering her cognitive deficits, perhaps was a greater challenge. The explanation for her illness and death remains elusive, but could the communal nature of nursing home living itself be responsible? It is recognized that institutions, as well as their residents, can be the source of disease spread and transmission. Problems have ranged in severity from lice spread through communal contact, to the wide dispersion of tubercule bacilli through the air vents of the structure and a series of tuberculosis cases.[47]

The most important purposes served here by the *natural support* persons in the institutional setting were stimulation of the patient's interests, monitoring of therapeutic decisions for consistency with her previously expressed wishes and her dignity, and establishing relationships with staff. In nursing homes, it is commonplace for family and friends to be brushed aside and for institutional rather than human goals to rule.[48] Friends and family members may have to be assertive, and even become difficult and unpopular, in order to secure adequate attention for the patient. Sometimes, despite all such efforts, residents are ignored or maltreated. The question of who is in control when major decisions must be made is a critical matter. For instance, what if RB had been found collapsed at 4:00 A.M. by the lone nurse on the night shift who was a new employee and lacked understanding about the case? The hospital ambulance would certainly have been called.

Medical care in the nursing home setting is often provided intuitively, by physicians who are otherwise extremely busy and for whom the work has a low priority.[49] The textbook that details standards for proper care in this setting has yet to be written. The current result is an emphasis, imposed by government regulations, on documentation and monitoring. There is less concern with clinical, decision-making behavior of physicians, the amount of time they actually spend with patients, or the degree of rapport among doctor, patient, and family members. Yet these are the elements that make up the reality of good care.

The cause of RB's illness and death was never determined. Can the physician be criticized for failing to give medical care up to present-day standards? The concerned persons had agreed to allow death to occur. What about the views of RB herself? In her last months she was too obtunded to express her intentions about aggressive life support. However, several years earlier she had completed a Living Will.[50] Her family understood that she was prepared to die.

As yet there exists no consensus regarding whether the quality of ethical decisions so often required in institutional settings should be reviewed.[51] Ethics committees recently established in some nursing homes are barely beginning to learn how to make day-to-day decisions. Basic matters such as the insertion of a nasogastric tube to continue to nourish a patient arise regularly. When such routine subjects are bitterly contested by four philosophers and three physicians testifying as expert witnesses,[52] it is easy to comprehend the perplexity that nursing home staff and concerned family members may face, and their anxiety and self-reproach.

In sum, a multitude of factors, intrinsic and extrinsic, influence the relationship of each older person to the network of services that make up the long term care spectrum, and these factors differ with each case and change over time. If institutions do not recognize their responsibility for the provision of humane, erudite, sensitive care, they will be challenged. If medical schools do not educate students sufficiently in geriatric care, the elderly patients that almost all of the graduates will treat will be deprived.[53]

At the interface of these intrinsic and extrinsic forces lie the ethical and moral issues that abound in the field of care for the aged today. These questions can be scaled down to the level of individuals, or can be as broad as society itself.

Chapter 4

Dementia

Dementia in older persons is a condition of major significance. Misery and anxiety may arise in people who experience memory failure, fear loss of control over their own lives, and grieve and feel shame about their behavior. The effect on family members is often devastating, and the emotional and dollar costs to all involved are beyond counting.

Dementia is defined as a global loss of cognitive function causing evident intellectual impairment without alteration of the state of consciousness. The spectrum of severity is great, and there is ample room for diagnostic confusion. Criteria in the third edition of the *Diagnostic and Statistical Manual of Mental Disorders* (DSM-III)[1] provide a standardized framework for clinicians to establish the diagnosis of dementia. In practice, however, the basis for identifying dementia in a patient often differs among physicians.[2] In some cases a combination of reported and observed impairment in the patient's memory, judgment, and abstract thinking may serve. In other instances it may be wise to employ a formal or informal mental status examination to confirm suspected intellectual deficit.

Studies on the epidemiology of dementia in various population groups have shown prevalence rates of from 3 to 20 percent in people aged sixty-five and over who are living in the community.[3] The incidence in those who are institutionalized is considerably higher.[4] It is a reasonable estimate that in the year 2000 there may be 4 million persons with Alzheimer's disease, the commonest dementia, in the United States.[5] Concern about dementia is therefore clearly a legitimate issue when matters of public health and monies are under discussion. Generalizations are risky, however, when individuals and their mental status are being considered. It is essential to recognize, for instance, that minor changes in memory capacity are common among older people and do not by any means suggest that progressive deterioration will follow.

From health workers' viewpoints, failure to identify dementia as a problem and to pursue possible treatable causes of the disorder are the two major obstacles to proper care. In older people dementia of modest to formidable degree has many etiologies. A number of these conditions, such as Alzheimer's disease and multi-infarct dementia, are caused by changes in brain cells, or loss of brain tissue, that are essentially irreversible. However, there are many other disease states, and numerous drugs, that through secondary effects can cause confusion, disorientation, and decreased mental function.

Often these other conditions are reversible. Examples include the consequences of acute and chronic alcoholism and the various syndromes of alcohol withdrawal; uncontrolled diabetes mellitus; numerous forms of infection; depletion of body fluids resulting from diseases that produce fever, diarrhea, persistent vomiting, or excessive sweating, or from inappropriate use of diuretic agents; digitalis intoxication; thyroid disease; and abnormal cardiac rate or rhythm.

Psychiatric disorders are as likely to occur in the elderly as in any age group, and depression is relatively more common.[6] States of depression may be reactive to loss of physical ability and threats to independence or may be situational and related, for instance, to poverty and isolation. Whatever the cause, depression can simulate dementia,[7] but may be overlooked or not sought as a cause. Diagnostic confusion results from the fact that symptoms we may perceive as characteristic of depression, such as sad feelings, episodes of crying, or self-denunciation, are relatively infrequent among depressed older people. Rather, somatic signs such as poor appetite, weight loss, constipation, slowness of movement, decreased attention span, and lack of drive or initiative are more likely in the elderly who are depressed. To the inexperienced observer the patient may appear demented. This diagnostic error is significant, because depression is a treatable disease.

Among the most striking correctible causes of dementia is that caused by placement of a frail aged person, previously well connected to reality, into a strange environment. Older people, found confused in a hospital bed, isolated from all the familiar clues that create a daily routine, will often become fully oriented if permitted to return home. Failure to appreciate this point has led to many an inappropriate nursing home placement.

It is unfortunate that on occasion dementia may be attributed to "old age" or "senility"; or evidence for the diagnosis may be glossed over because of the stigma of hopelessness long attached to its symptoms by health professionals and lay persons alike. It is clearly in the interest of every patient presenting with confusion or memory loss for a diagnosis to be properly established. To assume that an older person with symptoms suggesting dementia is permanently disabled, with a grave prognosis, is a conclusion based on inexperience, fatalism, stereotyping, or poor judgment.

DEFINING DEMENTIA

The subject of dementia in older people is bedeviled by difficulties in terminology. The difficulties are caused in part by the great variety of clinical conditions that can produce symptoms of dementia; in part by the overlapping disciplines concerned, including psychiatry, neurology, and internal medicine; and to a major degree by the explosive growth of investigational interest in the field, which itself creates new terminology. The following taxonomy includes definitions in current or frequent use.

1. *Alzheimer's disease (AD):* A condition marked by gradual, significant decline in intellectual function, associated with established pathological changes in the brain. The diagnosis can be established with certainty only by brain biopsy or at autopsy.
2. *Senile dementia:* Dementia that develops in older people (the age range is not precise) that may be produced by a great variety of medical disorders, including AD.
3. *Senile dementia of the Alzheimer's type (SDAT):* A disease that causes characteristic changes in intellect and conduct, comparable to those recognized in patients with proven AD. This term is in regular use and, if based on thorough, careful case analysis, is applicable to those people with apparent AD but for whom tissue diagnosis is not obtainable.
4. *Cortical dementias:* Dementing disorders caused by disease primary within the brain cells of the cortices. AD is the definitive example.
5. *Subcortical dementias:* Conditions with primary cell disorders in subcortical areas of the brain. Huntington's disease and the dementia of Parkinson's disease are examples.

These categories of cortical and subcortical dementia are clinically distinguishable. As neurologist D. F. Benson indicates:

The cortical dementias feature aphasia, amnesia, apraxia, and significant cognitive impairment. . . . In contrast, these functions are only mildly disturbed in the subcortical dementias but speech function . . . gait disturbance, abnormal posture, tremor, or other types of movement disorders [are prominent]. . . . [The latter are characterized by] extreme slowness of movement, comprehension, thinking and verbal response.[8]

THE HISTORICAL BACKGROUND
OF DEMENTIAS

"Dotage has been considered an equivalent of senile dementia" states pathologist Richard M. Torack.[9] During the time the ancient Greek civilization was at its height, the belief that loss of intellectual function accompanies advanced age had already achieved the status of a truism. Solon, the Greek sage and *archon,* or lawgiver (c. 638–c. 558 B.C.), stated that a person's judgment could be harmed by old age. He developed laws that permitted abrogation of a will if old age influenced judgment.[10] The ambiguities that seem always to have been inherent in our attitudes toward the old are pointed up, however, by Solon's view that he himself "each day grew older, and learned something new."[11]

Through the millennia, scientists have attempted to understand the basis of senile dementia, influenced always by the philosophy, standards, and prejudices of the era. As Torack indicates, the first definition of senile dementia consonant with our current views was coined in 1838 by J. E. D. Esquirol, clinician and student of mental disorders: "Senile dementia is established slowly. It commences with enfeeblement of memory, particularly in the memory of recent impressions. The sensations are feeble; the attention, at first fatiguing, at length becomes impossible; the will is uncertain and without impulsion; the movements are slow and impractical."[12]

Esquirol recognized the distinctions between dementias of various origins and attempted to classify dementias into acute, chronic, and senile, the latter caused by advanced age. While we now perceive the clumsiness of this definition, it marked a major step in discriminating causes. According to G. D. Cohen of the National Institute of Mental Health, throughout the nineteenth century, discussions of dementia did not distinguish between those of organic and psychiatric, or "functional," origins.[13]

The ability of scientists, and people in general, to comprehend the bases of this disorder remained confounded by emotional response to the condition, fear, and, above all, lack of knowledge. What we may now call the modern era of investigation began in the late nineteenth century, with an open mind as essential tool, the autopsy as the source of clinical material, and the light microscope as the necessary technical device. Landmarks are the findings of the English pathologist S. Wilks in 1864 that brain atrophy accompanied senile dementia and the description by the German physician Alois Alzheimer in 1907 of a dementing disease in a fifty-one-year-old patient with specific historical and physical findings and pathological brain changes.[14] Twentieth-century studies have shown that certain bacteria— the spirochete that causes syphilis, for instance—can produce clinical syndromes that can be distinguished from other categories of the senile dementias.

The view that aberration of mind in the aged is expected, if not inevitable, is expressed for us most memorably by Shakespeare's seventh age of man in *As You Like It*:

> Last scene of all,
> That ends this strange eventful history,
> Is second childishness and mere oblivion;
> Sans teeth, sans eyes, sans taste, sans everything

and is exemplified in *King Lear.* Was Lear's problem the pseudodementia of reactive depression? Had he taken an overdose of a drug given in his day to the distraught? Might that drug have contained a toxic substance, such as lead or mercury? Did Lear have Parkinson's disease, or had several small strokes occurred? Or did he have SDAT? We might know, were he living in our era and been subjected to investigation that might have included brain biopsy. And he might have been successfully treated for his demented state. But even now, we could not bring back Cordelia.

ALZHEIMER'S DISEASE

The disorder known as Alzheimer's disease is the paradigm of illnesses that produce loss of intelligence. It is the most frequent reason for institutional placement of older people in the United States, and at this time is responsible for the incarceration of more than 1 million individuals in nursing homes and state mental hospitals.[15] Thorough elaboration of available information about this disease is essential for clear understanding and rational development of the long term care spectrum for the aged.

AD, which threatens to become the bogey of the old and has been termed the disease of the century,[16] has drawn the attention of all caring people. After a long period of therapeutic and investigational nihilism, AD is now at the forefront of scientific study. Government and philanthropic funds are available to define the cause of AD, seek therapies, and assist patients and families. These developments are of notable importance and virtue.

PREVALENCE

The number of persons in the United States suffering from dementia is not known. Availability of this demographic information is obscured by definitional problems, as already noted, by the broad range and intermittency of symptoms, and by the feelings of fear and shame that prevent many patients and families from seeking help. General estimates suggest that from 5 to 10 percent of people sixty-five years of age and older have symptoms of dementia to a degree sufficient to be recognizable.[17] Of these patients with dementia, about 50 percent[18] suffer from SDAT. The rest suffer from the other forms of dementia.

Countrywide, approximately 1 to 1.3 million people suffer from dementia to a severe degree, and almost 3 million others have mild to moderate symptoms.[19] One percent or so of people sixty-five and over develop senile dementia each year.[20] In patients so impaired that they lack the ability to care for themselves, institutional placement is frequent. Psychiatrist and geriatrician Barry Reisberg[21] points out that SDAT is the most frequent diagnosis among nursing home patients, and it is also prevalent in populations living in state mental institutions and Veterans Administration hospitals.

We have noted the best estimates of dementia in the large group of people sixty-five and older. This rough assessment requires breakdown into subgroups to improve its significance and value as data. Incidence changes with increasing age,[22] from about 5 percent at sixty-five to 20 percent or more at eighty years plus.[23] An aged and demented man under care in a long term home health care program was, in his own way, correct when he said, "I've got old-timer's disease."[24] While some studies disagree,[25] it is a general consensus that SDAT is more frequent in women. This could be explained by hypothesizing greater susceptibility in women or by the statistical evidence of higher male mortality in these age groups.[26]

SDAT is a frequent cause of death, the result of poor self-care or of stress—following a move, for instance.[27] Pneumonia following aspiration of food or liquid or following inappropriate exposure to the elements is a common consequence of the disease. Despite the increased mortality rate for SDAT patients, however, many may live for several decades after the start of symptoms, and can remain physically robust despite the loss of intellect.[28]

SDAT is a significant public health concern. It has substantial impact on public policy as it relates to health care costs, the nature and development of institutions,[29] the legal rights of mentally disabled people, and the family's way of life. These matters will grow in prominence as the population ages.

DEFINING ALZHEIMER'S DISEASE

Alzheimer's disease is defined by neuropathological changes in brain tissue. In practical terms, since tissue is not available for examination in most cases, it is necessary to define the disorder through its clinical manifestations, or signs and symptoms. When the diagnosis is established through these means, the disorder is termed senile dementia of the Alzheimer type. In recent years careful study of demented patients who died and were subjected to autopsy has permitted physicians to establish standard diagnostic criteria that can be used reliably, permitting individuals with SDAT to be distinguished from patients with other forms of dementia, pseudodementia, and those undergoing normal aging.[30]

SDAT is recognized by its insidious onset and its progressive destruction of the patient's intellect. Memory loss is particularly prominent. Confusion, disorientation, and loss of affect are part of the clinical picture.[31] In many cases, evidence of accompanying physical deterioration is lacking. The advanced stage, called the "dementia phase" by Reisberg,[32] marks the point at which patients must, for survival, be cared for by others. Individuals now cannot carry out their own activities of daily living. Capacity to eat, dress, and bathe is lost. Patients may lose the ability to recognize their caregivers and closest relatives. "Patients forget the name of the spouse upon whom they are entirely dependent for survival and, subsequently, cannot even recognize their own name. In short, all identity is lost."[33]

Many older people have a modest loss of some intellectual functions, particularly memory. Neurologist V. A. Kral[34] has proposed the attractive term benign senescent forgetfulness for this clinical state. Small-scale studies of older people indicate that in most instances these symptoms do not progress to more advanced forms of mental impairment.[35] This is a point worthy of emphasis because of the understandable fear that mild memory loss inevitably leads to conditions like SDAT.

Benign senescent forgetfulness appears to occur in about 80 percent of the elderly, with recent memory loss the most common problem. It has become common knowledge that, while an older person may remember with clarity the details of an event that took place decades past, a routine matter, such as finding the car keys used a few minutes earlier, may become a challenge.

In a small but unknown number of people with mild clinical symptoms, as Reisberg points out, "forgetfulness symptomatology does presage a more overt phase of cognitive deterioration."[36] He has developed the term confusional phase for this development. Surveys reported by neurologist Robert Katzman[37] and neuropathologist Robert Terry[38] indicate that 10 percent or slightly more of people aged sixty-five and older may be so categorized. Older people in this phase of mental impairment lose the capacity to function effectively in common stressful situations. Life in the business world or in the home suffers. Memory loss is more obvious. Ability to recall names at opportune moments fails, an aggravation of the pervasive difficulty that we all note occasionally, especially at critical moments.

The loss of self-confidence that these symptoms may cause is obvious. People will expect and fear failure, and a form of self-fulfilling prophecy develops. Close family members and business associates may not appreciate that the symptoms are manifestations of an illness, and may become angry and critical. In this situation individuals with a clinical disorder causing loss of mental acuity, and who are painfully aware of the problem, are subjected to the negative emotional forces of closest companions and friends, and, in addition, are made to feel guilt.

In order to avoid revealing evidence of symptoms, withdrawal may be the patient's most effective response. Anxiety and depression are additional and understandable results. It is in this situation that supportive efforts, and family involvement in therapeutic programs with the patient, may be most effective.

The likelihood of further intellectual decline for patients in the confusional phase is not known. Studies of small groups of patients suggest, however, that progress to more severe dementia, or SDAT, may occur in about half of the cases.[39]

Proper diagnosis of AD may be a challenge to any clinician. The course of the disorder and the time of onset may be unknown to the physician, unstatable by the patient, and obscured by the doubts or ambivalence of family members. The phases of SDAT just outlined are theoretical only, and hardly form a clear guide for diagnostic judgment. Clarity of the evaluation may be further obscured by the fact that symptoms may be of multiple origin. For instance, a patient with SDAT may, quite appropriately, be significantly depressed; or may be taking substantial doses of a broad range of drugs, some of which are capable of inducing symptoms of dementia.

Doctors working with the elderly have begun to recognize that patients who ultimately are recognized as suffering from SDAT may present atypically. Neurologist E. C. Shuttleworth,[40] in making this point, cites examples: a patient whose first symptom was an inability to calculate but whose memory was preserved; an individual whose symptoms at first were confined to lapses in visual memory but whose verbal memory was preserved; and a patient who apparently had dementia of sudden rather than gradual onset, a consequence, it was ultimately revealed, of relatives having hidden the earlier symptoms.

The differential diagnosis of dementia, including the ability to make a clear case for SDAT, brings the physician back to basics: a thorough history and physical examinations of the patient and careful follow-up to observe the course of symptoms. The doctor must place particular emphasis on obtaining from a reliable observer the following information about the patient: time and character of onset of dementia symptoms, manner of progression, prior intellectual status and physical health, presence and time of onset of mood alteration and change in personality, and degree of impairment of judgment.[41]

The usual clinical course of patients with SDAT is now sufficiently clarified to permit a positive diagnosis, as opposed to assuming SDAT only after excluding all other origins of dementia.

BRAIN ALTERATIONS IN ALZHEIMER'S DISEASE

Changes in Gross Structure

Loss of brain tissue sufficient to cause measurable atrophy occurs in AD patients. These changes are manifested both by shrinkage of the cerebral cortex and by enlargement, or dilatation, of the brain ventricles. Studies using the technique of computed tomography (CT) have been effective in providing visible X-ray evidence of these changes in living subjects; however, the extent of the information obtained through these analyses has also served to confuse matters: It is now clear that similar gross changes in brain size occur in normal aging as well.[42]

In a definitive study of the normal aging process, radiologists Shumpei Takeda and Taiju Matsuzawa[43] carried out brain CT scans on 483 males and 497 females between the ages of ten and eighty-eight years. None had evidence of neurological disease. The extent of brain atrophy development over this age span was analyzed, and "exponential progression of brain atrophy during aging after age thirty in both men and women" was found.

Marked atrophy has been found in the brains of patients with advanced AD who come to autopsy. In extreme cases, as neuropathologist Arne Brun[44] points out, the brain may have lost one-third of its weight, compared to normal age-matched controls. Certain areas of the brain, particularly the temporal lobe and its hippocampus and amygdaloid nucleus, are targets. Further careful use of advanced scanning techniques will, in all likelihood, be useful in distinguishing the atrophy of normal aging from that in AD.

While it is not as yet firmly established that severe brain atrophy is an essential hallmark of AD, there is nevertheless value in understanding the details of the anatomical changes in AD brains. These help point toward the brain areas where loss of tissue is most severe, and thus where changes at the cellular and biochemical levels must be sought. It is through this process of investigation that an understanding of the cause or causes of AD may be found. Only once the cause is established can we expect definitive, nonhazardous diagnostic tests and effective therapy to be developed.

Changes in Microscopic Structure

AD is defined by the presence of characteristic abnormalities in brain tissue observed through microscopic examination.[45] These findings, termed senile plaques and neurofibrillary tangles (NFTs), are "classical and compulsory for the pathologic diagnosis"[46] of this disorder.

Plaques range from 5 to 200 panometers in diameter and are spherical. Electron microscopic study reveals that they are constituted, in part, of distorted and degenerating pieces of brain cells; in part, of normal cells of other types attracted to the damaged area; and last, by amyloid, a protein substance, the origin of which is speculative. Material within the plaques has been identified as derived from the parts of brain cells that synapse, or connect, with other cells. As we will see, this finding is compatible with biochemical abnormalities found in the brains of Alzheimer patients and with the characteristic symptoms of the disease.

NFTs are hairlike strands of protein found within the bodies of neurons, or cells, of the brain. As seen through the electron microscope, NFTs consist of bundles, or pairs, of filaments wrapped about each other in a helical form. Their presence within cells is abnormal, although older people without AD may also harbor small quantities of NFTs in their brain cells. Information about the origin of NFTs remains vague, but it may be a reasonable hypothesis that they derive, in some as yet unexplained manner, from deterioration of the neuron.[47]

In addition to the presence of these specific abnormalities, other major changes occur in the brains of demented patients with AD. The most significant is substantial and progressive deterioration and destruction of the dendrites of the neuronal cells. These extensions of the cell body are the components that connect with other cells and allow for the vast and complex orchestration of intellectual and other bodily activity controlled by the brain. "The result of this process is decreasing synaptic interaction and diminishing computational power."[48] The cause of this dendritic destruction is unknown. Hypothetical explanations, to be detailed, include a destructive effect of the NFTs within the brain cell, interference with axonal transport of neurofilament,[49] the harmful consequences of amyloid within cells or near them, or amyloid interference with the small blood vessels that supply these cells.

Amyloid, as we have noted, is a constituent of senile plaques. It is also found abundantly in and near blood vessels of the brain of patients with

AD. Amyloid may, in fact, infiltrate blood vessel walls to such an extent that blood flow is interfered with or the vessel walls themselves are destroyed. Neuropharmacologist Richard J. Wurtman[50] suggests that the presence of large quantities of amyloid in microscopic examination of the brain is itself almost diagnostic of AD.

Although the presence of these specific lesions is essential for determining whether AD exists, the pathologist's skill and experience remain necessary for the differential diagnosis. Both plaques and NFTs may occur in other neurological disorders, and amyloid, as it is generally defined, is present in many diseases. Moreover, plaques and tangles occasionally may be found in normal brains as well.[51] It is the large quantity of plaques and tangles, and the specificity of the brain areas in which they are concentrated, that distinguish AD from other neurologically abnormal conditions and from normals.[52] Hence a problem arises related to the .use of brain material for pathologic diagnosis: An area selected at random, either at time of biopsy or during autopsy, may not represent accurately the true state of the disease.

Studies of brain tissue, increasingly refined over the past twenty-five years, have consistently shown an age-related decrease in brain cells, or neurons.[53] These cellular losses, however, are not responsible for dementia. As far as AD is concerned, destruction of cells in clearly defined and specific areas of the brain is the basis for the symptoms. Investigators' attention has been drawn to these areas by the presence of large numbers of the pathological markers, NFTs and senile plaques.

In recent years, through extensive studies in animals and humans, the portions of the brain responsible for memory have been mapped with increasing accuracy. It is now generally accepted that portions of the temporal lobes, and the hippocampus[54] and associated structures, are in a sense the seat of memory. These are the precise areas that suffer the greatest cellular destruction and reveal the most prominent presence of the pathological markers in the brains of Alzheimer's patients that have been studied. As Wurtman points out, "the long axon cholinergic neurons to the hippocampus and cerebral cortex [are] particularly vulnerable."[55]

The brain areas that are damaged and show involvement of one or more of the neurotransmitter systems in AD have been refined with remarkable specificity. These involve largely the cerebral cortex and include the basal nucleus and nucleus lócus ceruleus.[56] Researcher Bradley T. Hyman and associates[57] report recent analysis of brain sections from five elderly deceased patients with this disorder. Tissues were studied in detail by microscope and compared to brains of five autopsied patients of comparable ages without AD. There were marked differences between the two groups in portions of the temporal lobes, specifically the subiculum of the hippocampal formation and layers II and IV of the enterohinal cortex. The brains of the AD patients showed a major loss of brain cells in these sites, a finding not matched in the controls. Further, in the AD group, no alterations in brain cell numbers were observed in tissues close to the sections of the temporal lobe just mentioned. The work of these researchers therefore seems to suggest that AD is due at least in part to destruction of cells in a circumscribed area of the brain, that other sections of the brain are spared, and that the portion of the brain afflicted is particularly crucial to the functions that we call memory.

> . . . it is difficult to conceive that the hippocampal formation in the brains of Alzheimer's patients is functionally useful. This isolation of the hippocampal formation may be no less devastating . . . with regard to memory than removal or destruction of the entire structure, and contribute to the contextual memory defect that is a major component of the amnesia in Alzheimer's disease.[58]

The Metabolism of Neurotransmitters

In order for nerve cells to receive and transmit stimuli to and from each other, chemical substances must be available in the proper quantity and location. These agents, called neurotransmitters, are enzymes elaborated inside the nerve cells that circulate within the cells' structure to the juncture points with other cells, where they are active. Maintenance of the normal functional level of neurotransmitter enzymes is sustained by the ability of the nerve cell to synthesize the specific material from building blocks made available through the bloodstream, and by reuse.[59] The exquisite degree of control that characterizes neurotransmission in normal persons can be negatively influenced by disease and, to a degree, by advancing age.

In the brains of AD patients, major deficits in those neurotransmitter systems that involve norepinephrine, serotonin, and acetylcholine have been found. These deficiencies have led many researchers to believe that both the cause of the disease and its possible treatment may be related to neurotransmitters.[60] A flowering of investigational effort has ensued, focused particularly on the acetylcholine system, long known to have a relationship to memory function. Recent work has revealed the striking finding that choline acetyltransferase (CAT), an enzyme that is required for the synthesis of acetylcholine, is markedly reduced in certain areas of the brain in Alzheimer's patients.[61] Among these areas is the hippocampus.

Acceptable evidence allows us to state that transmission of neuronal impulses depends both on intact neuronal cells and their axons and dendrites and on a functioning neurotransmitter enzyme system. We have noted that brain cells critical to the function of memory are damaged in AD, that the dendrites are injured and destroyed as well, and that enzymatic deficits have been found. The latter may theoretically be considered the primary cause of the disease, or damage to the neuronal bodies and synaptic extensions (the axons and dendrites) may interrupt the flow of the enzymatic transmitters to their site of function.[62] Which comes first, damage to the brain cells or destruction of the enzyme system? Does the identification of this specific biochemical abnormality offer the possibility of effective treatment for AD? The answers are not yet known.

The brilliant concept that AD can be treated by providing the patient with missing chemical substrates of neurotransmitters has not to date been realized,[63] but a recent study by psychiatrist William K. Summers and associates shows some promise.[64]

THE CAUSE OF ALZHEIMER'S DISEASE: A MATTER OF SPECULATION

Significant advances have been made in understanding the nature of injury to the brain caused by AD. Data extend to the details of damage within injured cells and to refinements of information about aberrant neurobiochemical states. However, an explanation for the cause or causes of AD remains elusive. Theories abound and are supported by evidence of varying believability. And as is frequently the case when so many avenues of investigation are open, no one is yet established as the road to truth.

Infection

Infection continues to interest investigators as a possible etiology, although no infectious agent has been identified in tissues from the brains of AD patients. Neither has transmissibility to other animal species been established by passage of brain material from AD patients. However, clinical parellels exist between this condition and two other chronic, degenerative diseases of the central nervous system in humans, Creutzfeldt-Jakob disease (CJD) and kuru; and with the disease of animals called scrapie, in which infectivity has been proven.

CJD causes progressive dementia, starting at an age similar to that now typical for Alzheimer's patients.[65] It can usually be distinguished from AD by the symptoms of loss of muscular control, myoclonus (muscular rigidity and spasm), visual disturbances, and specific changes in the electroencephalogram. In most cases of CJD there is a shorter period from the first appearance of symptoms to death, about six to twelve months, compared to several years in Alzheimer's. At autopsy, the two disorders can be distinguished. However, as neurologist Andrés Salazar points out,[66] clinically and even pathologically these two disorders overlap, a fact that suggests that ultimately their cause may be similar. CJD has been transmitted to a variety of other species, including chimpanzees, cats, and mice; in the laboratory it has an incubation period of two to three years in primates.[67]

Kuru, also a chronic degenerative brain disease, is found in a specific tribe in Papua New Guinea that, until recently, had been known to cannibalize the brains of its own tribal members. Symptoms, which do not ordinarily include dementia, are striking ataxia (loss of control over balance), marked tremor, and involuntary movements. Death occurs in two years or less. Pathologic brain changes are similar to those seen in CJD and AD: loss of neurons and presence of amyloid plaques. That kuru is an infectious disorder is satisfactorily proven by the fact that tissue from diseased patients has been transmitted to other species, specifically chimpanzees and the same symptoms, course, and pathological changes have been noted. That kuru was transmitted through cannibalism also seems to be established by the fact that the disorder is dying out. While instances in children were frequent in the past, "the age of onset of new cases has gradually increased over the past 20 years such that only villagers old enough to have participated in the ritual cannibalism (which ceased about 1959) have developed the disease."[68] This point also indicates the long incubation period of kuru and tended to support the view held until recently that its cause, and thus perhaps the cause of CJD and AD as well, was a "slow" virus, one that took years, perhaps decades, to cause evidence of illness.[69]

Scrapie is a fatal disease of the central nervous system that occurs in sheep and goats. Experimental studies have revealed that the disease is transmissible to previously healthy animals of a variety of species and is thus infectious in nature.[70] Study of brains of animals dead of scrapie reveal abnormalities similar to those found in AD, CJD, and kuru: amyloid plaques and deposits and loss of neurons. It has been shown recently[71] that amyloid deposits develop at the site where infectious material from an animal ill with scrapie was injected into a previously healthy animal.

The nature of the infectious agents that cause scrapie and CJD has been elucidated recently through the research of Stanley B. Prusiner.[72] It now seems that the material that causes infection is not a virus but a previously unrecognized biological form, which Pruisner calls a prion. Prions are distinguished from all other known infectious agents by the fact that they lack both DNA and RNA.[73] According to Prusiner, the molecular structure of scrapie prions contains a specific protein, called PrP, which is required for infectivity.[74] Prions are rod-shaped, 10 to 20 nanometers in diameter, about five times as long, and may each hold as many as one thousand PrP molecules. Prions obtained from animals with scrapie have been highly purified and their ultrastructure examined. Marked similarities to the ultrastructure of amyloid have been noted, including the ability to accept Congo red dye, birefringence, and rodlike shape. Prusiner suggests that "amyloid plaques may represent paracrystalline arrays of prion polymers."[75]

Kuru and CJD prions probably differ from each other in details of protein molecular structure and from those of scrapie. Prions produce more prions through a process not yet understood. The presence of these entities in AD has not been established.[76]

Study of the ultrastructure of prions indicates that they have qualities similar to those of amyloid, although investigators are not prepared to state that they are the same substance. Amyloid may be a residue or sign of the presence of infection without being the agent of disease. As Prusiner points out: "Indeed, amyloid plaques . . . may represent footprints of the infectious pathogen but are not an obligatory part of the disease process."[77]

It is now established that AD, CJD, kuru, and scrapie bear significant clinical similarities, although the courses of the disorders are not identical: The incubation period in each instance is lengthy; pathological brain changes are comparable, although not the same, and include loss of neurons and presence of amyloid; but infectivity has been clearly established for the latter three disorders only.

Despite the suggestive nature of this information, infection as the cause of AD is in dispute. In fact, a body of evidence speaks against this theory. If AD is caused by an infectious process, it is reasonable to expect that it should be transmissible to other human beings or, by experiment, to other species. However, other than for two instances in which brain material from AD patients injected into monkeys produced a disease state similar to CJD, there is no such evidence; and in regard to the study just cited, laboratory error is probably involved since the experiment proved not to be replicable.[78] Further, epidemics of AD have not been reported. Examples of spread to close family members, as in spouse to spouse, are not proven, although genetic factors may be implicated (see the section on genetic origin). Health workers, who often have close and prolonged contact with such patients, do not appear to exhibit increased indices of the disease.

Prusiner's comment is provocative: "Because the existence of prions in Alzheimer's disease is still a hypothesis and the disease is not transmissible to laboratory animals under the conditions studied, it does not seem prudent at this time to regard it as an infectious disorder. . . . Indeed, studies of prions may force us to modify the definition of infection."[79]

Abnormalities of Neurotransmitters

Another possibility under consideration is that AD is caused by a primary abnormality of a factor or factors within the cholinergic neurotransmitter system.[80] Acetylcholine is synthesized by the combination of molecules of choline and acetyl coenzyme A, a process dependent on the catalytic effect of the enzyme CAT.[81] A significant decrease—in the range of 30 to 50 percent or more of control values—in tissue levels of CAT have been found consistently in the brains of AD patients, when these brains are compared to those of control specimens.[82] Furthermore, the brain areas most lacking in CAT, such as the hippocampus and the basal nucleus, are characteristically the same as those in which the well-known neuropathological changes are prominent.[83]

Analysis of brain cell fractions has shown that CAT is manufactured in the body of the neuron and slowly transmitted to the nerve terminals or dendrites, where its functional activity occurs.[84] The question arises: Could the cause of AD be a selective destruction of the enzymatic capacity of the neurons, leading secondarily to loss of both cellular function and structure? The answer is unknown. Note, however, that the dendritic portions of the involved neurons are the most prominent site of destruction in AD. It would therefore appear logical that synaptic function would be lost, regardless of the quantities of choline, acetyl coenzyme A, and CAT present in neurons, or of acetylcholine available to transmit impulses between cells. On the other hand, a genetic abnormality that impacts upon neurotransmitter formation or upon neuronal structural integrity could be responsible.

Genetic Origin

Close blood relatives of individuals with AD have an increased likelihood of developing the disorder. Careful study of family pedigrees provides the evidence, which is obtained only by extending the information base over many decades and several generations. Because AD becomes evident late in life in many instances, frequently used techniques for testing hypotheses of genetic origin are not readily applicable to this problem.[85] When the illness under study is age-dependent, potential patients may die of other causes before the disease picture develops, even though they may be carrying the disorder in latent form. Therefore in some instances AD may appear nonfamilial by artifact because the relatives at risk have died of other causes.

Researcher and neurologist Peter Davies has analyzed family pedigrees and shown that in some instances inheritance of AD follows a clear pattern of autosomal dominance. In these instances, there is a hint of a single abnormal gene.[86] Physicians in Sweden reviewed clinical information about patients who had resided in Stockholm mental institutions and had carried a diagnosis of senile dementia.[87] People admitted to these hospitals over a fifteen-year period were included in the study, and 377 individuals were ultimately accepted as index cases. It should be noted that proof of AD based on pathological examination was not required in this study. First-degree relatives of the selected patients, all living in the community, were sought, and further examples of senile dementia were discovered among this group. The researchers were then able to compare the incidence of this disorder among close relatives to that in the population at large. The increased risk among close relatives was in the ratio of 4.3 to 1.

Long term study of twins has provided useful insights. Clinician and researcher F. J. Kallmann's work,[88] published in the 1950s, was devoted to the study of mono- and dizygotic twins, their siblings, and other relatives over a period spanning decades. In regard to senile dementia, for monozygotic twins, the rate of concordance was 42.8 percent; for dizygotic twins, 8 percent; for siblings, 6.5 percent, and for parents, 3 percent. From today's viewpoint, while this striking study remains broadly valid, it must be questioned somewhat because of the lack of accurate diagnoses of dementia at the time the work was being carried out. In 1973 psychiatrist and researcher Lissy Jarvik and associates sought out the survivors of Kallmann's studies.[89] Seventy-five percent of the survivors without dementia, who were last examined in 1967 and reachable in 1973, remained free of organic brain symptoms. It is worth noting that these survivors had reached a mean age of more than eighty-nine years, strong evidence that advanced age itself does not induce dementia.

Geneticist Leonard L. Heston and associates, working in Minnesota, have undertaken a study of descendants of 125 individuals proven, by study of brain tissue, to have died with AD. The earliest pathological material dates from 1952.[90] Through assiduous effort, as many as four generations of family members have been located and made themselves available for interview and clinical examination. Ninety-eight secondary cases have been found, ninety-two siblings and six children.[91] This unusual opportunity to follow the familial pattern of AD, while not as yet complete, has already shown that inheritability is probably an important factor in an appreciable number of instances: All of the secondary cases studied through 1981 with autopsy-proven AD were relatives of 51 of the original 125 patients. Relatives of the other 74 primary patients appear to be spared. As Wurtman points out, the implication is strong "that about 40 percent of the original patients had a familial disease,"[92] but as we have noted earlier, the likelihood of disease development is related to life-span. According to the genetics studies of Marshall Folstein,[93] if a first-degree relative of a patient lives to age eighty-five, the risk of developing the disease is between 30 and 50 percent. This rate of family-associated disorder is compatible with diseases known to have a genetic basis of an autosomal-dominant nature with age-dependent onset.[94]

Corroboration of the suggestion that genetic/chromosomal abnormalities may be associated with the development of AD lies in its parallels to Down's syndrome (mongolism; trisomy 21).[95] Down's syndrome is the most common human chromosomal disorder, and among its most evident symptoms is significant mental retardation. It is noteworthy that patients with this condition who die after the age of thirty, an advanced age for those with Down's syndrome, upon autoposy reveal neuropathological brain changes of NFTs, plaques, and loss of neurons strikingly akin to those seen in Alzheimer's patients.[96] Heston's work includes a study of a subset of thirty patients with proven AD and their families. Of the relatives, twenty-two themselves developed the same disorder and seven others had Down's syndrome. These frequencies of disease expression far exceed those expected in the population at large.[97]

Donna Cohen and Carl Eisdorfer, researchers and investigators, have extended the analysis of the similarities between these two conditions.[98] It is broadly recognized that advanced maternal age is the major risk factor for development of Down's syndrome. These investigators recognized that it might be fruitful to study maternal age at the birth of people who later developed AD. Information was obtained from the Washington State Alzheimer patient registry, and the histories of eighty people registered consecutively, born between 1891 and 1921, were reviewed. Information obtained included establishment of the presence of AD by definitions of preestablished research diagnostic criteria, although verification by pathologic study of brain tissue was not a prerequisite. Maternal age at the birth of each of the eighty cases was obtained through inquiry of surviving family members, birth certificates, and family records. Median maternal age at birth of the affected individuals was 35.5 years. For comparison, 590 birth records were selected at random for persons born in Washington State in 1907, the first year for which comparable records were available. The median age of mothers giving birth was 27.0 years. As Cohen and Eisdorfer suggest, these data "are provocative." Advanced maternal age may be a risk factor for AD, although the manner in which this manifests itself is not evident. Further study of this association is indicated, as is continued effort at understanding the similarities and differences between the origins and pathological changes of Down's syndrome and AD.

Aluminum Toxicity

Substantial aluminum concentrations have been found in brain tissues of patients with AD, compared with controls. Interest in aluminum toxicity as a possible cause of AD stems from a 1965 report on the formation of NFTs in the brains of rabbits exposed to aluminum phosphate.[99] Subsequent work has defined aluminum-associated brain lesions in a variety of species; identified the nature of the abnormalities produced within brain cells; determined a rough measure of normal concentrations of aluminum in human brains; and recognized the presence of aluminum in brain tissues of patients with a number of rare brain disorders.[100]

A particularly striking finding is that a form of encephalopathy, a degenerative brain disorder, may occur in chronically ill kidney disease patients who require prolonged renal dialysis. This phenomenon, which has been called dialysis dementia, appears related either to ingestion of large amounts of aluminum phosphate as medication or too-heavy concentration of this metallic element in the dialysate solution. These patients have substantial concentrations of aluminum in the cortical areas of the brain.[101]

Despite these intriguing findings, direct evidence that aluminum some-how causes AD is lacking.[102] In fact, significant points challenge any such conclusion: (1) The structure of the NFTs that develop in experimental animals subjected to test doses of aluminum differ from those of AD. The former are single strands; the latter, paired helical filaments.[103] (2) The location of aluminum-induced lesions in the brains of animal subjects differs from those in patients with AD. (3) Human beings who might be expected to show high indices of AD, such as aluminum workers, fail, in fact, to demonstrate increased rates.[104] And (4) the brain disorder known to be associated with aluminum toxicity in chronic renal dialysis patients does not cause the development of NFTs.[105]

The most that can be said in regard to the influence of aluminum on the initiation of AD is that "aluminum cannot by itself give rise to the . . . disease but that its presence contributes" to the development in patients with other risk factors.[106] Even this may be an overstatement. It seems more likely that aluminum tends to collect in cells already damaged, and probably has no causative function.[107]

MULTI-INFARCT DEMENTIA

The concept that narrowing of brain arteries by arteriosclerosis causes senile dementia by decreasing the amount of oxygenated blood that reaches the brain cells is a misperception.[108] While vascular narrowing is a consequence of arteriosclerotic changes, this disorder causes neither damage to cells nor decrease in intellectual function. This point has been established clearly through autopsy studies of demented individuals who were compared with nondemented cases similar in age. The degree of arteriosclerosis was essentially the same in both groups.[109]

Arteriosclerosis of the brain's blood vessels causes the common, major disorder called stroke. Strokes are most frequently manifested by paralysis of one side of the body and are associated with other findings of damage to the brain, but dementia is not part of the clinical picture. Careful examination of stroke patients will reveal that abnormalities of perception, expression, strength, and sensation may exist, and depression as well. Significant cognitive difficulties are usually absent, however. Strokes, also known as cerebrovascular accidents (CVAs), ordinarily result from thrombosis of a brain artery, which leads to the death of brain tissue. Such areas of dead tissue are called infarctions. Less frequently, a vessel may be so damaged that blood leaks through the wall into the brain substance itself. This phenomenon, called cerebral hemorrhage, often causes devastating damage and threatens the patient's immediate survival. CVAs can be caused as well by emboli from the heart that float into the brain circulation and occlude an artery. In each of these instances, a single substantial area of the brain is infarcted.

Dementia as a consequence of vascular disease usually occurs in a different fashion, through the development of multiple areas of infaction,[110] each of which may be small. This condition, called multi-infarct dementia (MID), develops more insidiously than a CVA, and usually is the result of repeated episodes of blood clot embolization from the heart or the large extracranial vessels.[111] Vascular disease intrinsic to the brain rarely is responsible for MID. MID develops, therefore, as a result of multiple infarctions from emboli, each of which alone would not cause a major clinical incident, but which when additive are sufficient to injure intellectual function.[112]

MID is thought to be responsible for about 10 percent of significant dementias in the elderly.[113] There is significant value in establishing the proper diagnosis, because the symptoms of MID will worsen unless the cause is controlled.[114] The common precursors of this condition are high blood pressure and/or abnormal cardiac rhythm. Both are treatable.[115]

Careful observation of patients will allow diagnostic distinction to be made between MID and AD. Neurologist Vladimir Hachinski[116] has analyzed the clinical points that characterize MID. These include abrupt onset, stepwise deterioration, relative preservation of personality, emotional lability, depression, history of hypertension, evidence of associated arteriosclerosis, and focal neurological signs and symptoms.

In contrast, AD ordinarily presents gradually, although "one must not mistake sudden recognition with abrupt onset."[117] Neurological abnormalities such as localized weakness, aphasia, loss of sensation, and reflex changes are usually absent.

A confusing element in the diagnostic evaluation is the possibility that an aged, demented patient is suffering from combined disorders. Of the universe of AD patients, perhaps 10 percent are likely to suffer from MID as well.

The lacunar state is a variant of MID in which numerous small vascular occlusions occur, causing multiple sites of tissue destruction. On pathological examination the damaged areas have the appearance of lakes (lacunae), ranging from 0.5 to 15 mm in size. Dementia in this condition is ordinarily mild, in comparison to AD. Other clinical signs are difficulty in walking and pseudobulbar palsy.[118]

The appearance of patients with the lacunar state is often quite similar to those with Parkinson's disease (PD), although the cause differs. In most instances the two can be distinguished by the stepwise progression of symptoms in the lacunar state as incidents of brain damage occur, compared to the gradual development in Parkinson's; and by the difference in response to levodopa therapy, the definitive treatment for PD.[119]

The lacunar state is relatively common in older patients with hypertension and/or diabetes mellitus. While the dementia consequent to this form of brain damage is not in itself treatable directly, the likelihood of further vascular occlusion may be decreased by proper diagnosis, a search for the underlying precipitating causes, and institution of proper therapy.

SUBCORTICAL DEMENTIAS

The term subcortical dementia refers to a constellation of symptoms, produced by a variety of disorders of the central nervous system, among which dementia is prominent, and in which causative brain lesions are found in subcortical areas. Clinical characteristics are sufficiently clear for careful observers to distinguish these conditions from those dementias caused by damage to cortical areas of the brain. The most prominent of the latter is AD.

Subcortical dementias cause changes in personality and emotional conduct, with apathy a prominent finding, and occasional outbursts of anger; loss of memory; and slowness of thought and action. Vocabulary and ability to use language skills are well preserved.[120]

Among the subcortical dementias that occur with frequency in the elderly, those associated with PD and Huntington's disease (HD) require comment.

PARKINSON'S DISEASE

PD is a disorder of the central nervous system that occurs predominantly among older people. The usual clinical picture includes tremor at rest, often particularly prominent in the hands; rigidity of the muscles, including those of the face, resulting in a masklike facies; shuffling gait, with a tendency to fall forward; and poverty of movement. There is a generalized decrease in muscular action, slow speed of movement, and delay in initiating activity.[121] The primary neuropathological lesion responsible for PD is degeneration of cells in the substantia nigra, an area of the upper midbrain. Neurofibrillary tangles are not found in the brains of patients with the common, or idiopathic, form of PD.

A number of biochemical abnormalities have been discovered in the brain tissues of patients with PD. The most prominent, and evidently the one largely responsible for the symptoms of the disease, is depletion of dopamine consequent to degeneration of the dopaminergic cells of the substantia nigra.[122]

Dr. James Parkinson first described this condition in 1817 and noted specifically "the senses and intellects being uninjured."[123] It is evident, however, from recent studies that an association between PD and dementia exists. Changes in mentation range from minor losses in memory, through episodes of confusion, to frank dementia. Many PD patients superficially observed will be perceived to have intellectual deficits because of slowness of movement and/or depression so often associated with this condition. More careful analysis shows that many patients suffer from difficulties in short term memory and conceptual thinking.[124]

Most analyses report the incidence of significant dementia in PD to range from between 6 and 30 percent.[125] The meaning of these figures is uncertain, however. For example, in some of the studies cited, terms were not defined adequately, the description and classification of dementia was not clear, and the selection of cases was biased toward inclusion of the most demented because institutions provided the analytical universe.[126] It now seems clear that two groups of PD patients can be identified:

> . . . one, a younger group, with an exclusive motor disorder having a longer and more benign course plus a better response to levodopa, and the second, an older group, with a motor- followed by a cognitive disorder, with both a more fulminant course and a poorer response to levodopa. The clinical overlap between these two groups is such that one cannot reliably predict who will become demented.[127]

There is growing evidence of an association between the dementias of PD and AD. The abnormalities of neuropathology and biochemistry are sufficiently similar to suggest a common pathogenesis.[128]

Levodopa, the present most effective treatment for the physical symptoms of PD, may cause mental changes in patients. Further, there is no useful therapy for the dementia of PD. As a consequence, levodopa should be used with great care in a PD patient who already has dementia. The potential value of decreasing the tremor and rigidity must be weighed against the possibility that the drug will itself create a toxic confusional syndrome of "delusions, hallucinations and aggressive behavior."[129]

HUNTINGTON'S DISEASE

HD is an uncommon hereditary disorder characterized by development of slowly progressive dementia, personality changes, choreiform movements of unusual and severe degree, and peculiar posture of the body. In the United States the prevalence of this condition is four to eight per one hundred thousand. HD is a familial condition that makes its clinical appearance in midadult life. The disorder is transmitted from parent to child in an autosomal dominant manner with full penetrance. Thus each offspring of a parent with an HD gene has a 50 percent chance of being affected. In almost all instances the course of HD is one of deepening loss of intellect and bodily disability over a period of several decades. No effective therapy is available.

Brain studies of patients have shown significant loss in the caudate and putamen of gamma-aminobutyric acid (GABA), an inhibitor of neuronal transmission, and of its synthesizing enzyme, glutamic acid decarboxylase. Also, there is evidence of decreased striatal activity of CAT and a reduction in the number of receptor sites for dopamine and acetylcholine. Attempts to treat HD patients with GABA and acetylcholine enhancers have proven futile, however.

While rare in the general population, HD requires mention here because patients tend to be concentrated in institutions. Thus when the causes of dementia are analyzed in institutions, HD makes an impact.[130]

TREATABLE DEMENTIAS

The assumption that confusion or memory loss in an older person invariably implies the presence of AD is erroneous, and may in fact lead to a failure to recognize a treatable disorder. The consequence is all too similar to putting an innocent person in jail.* The search for correctible causes of dementia requires, first, an understanding on the part of the patient and family that a diagnostic effort is essential and worth the effort and cost; and second, an appreciation by physicians and other health workers that methods exist for clarifying the basis of many causes of dementia. About 20 percent of older people with persistent symptoms of significant intellectual deterioration will prove to have a reversible disorder, if carefully studied.[131] Each patient deserves a definitive diagnosis.

· We must clarify further the distinctions between those forms of dementia generally considered to be potentially treatable and those thought to be irreversible. Geriatrician Laurence Z. Rubenstein[132] reviewed several pertinent studies. The disorders with potential for effective treatment included: pseudodementia (depression), found in 7.1 percent of the 406 patients analyzed; normal-pressure hydrocephalus (5.4 percent); mass lesions of the brain removable by surgery, such as tumors and blood clots (3.7 percent); toxic reactions to drugs (2 percent); and a broad variety of other causes (2 percent).

Those causes that Rubenstein considered probably not reversible in-

*A. Lechich, personal communication, 1987.

cluded: presumptive AD (48.5 percent of the patients studied); consequences of acute and chronic alcoholism (10.6 percent)—although, as we shall see, some alcohol-related dementias may, in fact, be treatable in various degrees; and multi-infarct dementia (9.6 percent). The remaining 11.1 percent was made up of numerous disorders, in which HD and the consequences of trauma were particularly noted.[133]

Among the potentially treatable conditions are the broad range of acute medical diseases that affect the general health of the patient and the impact of brain function; more subtle consequences of chronic illness that alter the metabolism of the body; head injury; and side effects of medications, legally prescribed or illegal. It is ironic that many drugs used specifically for therapy of psychiatric or confusional states may in themselves create symptoms of dementia.

ALCOHOLISM

The loss of intellectual function that may occur in people with chronic and severe alcoholism is often not correctible with abstinence. However, dementia consequent to other clinical states in the spectrum of alcohol disease are treatable to varying degrees.[134]

It should be noted, first, that episodes of drunkenness, which would prove simple to recognize in younger people, may escape the attention of observers when the patient is elderly. Alcoholism may simply not be considered as a possibility in the latter age group; the patient and family may use great effort to avoid exposing the diagnosis, from a sense of shame or despair; or, because the presentation may differ in older people, the usual manifestations of drunk behavior may not be seen. Staggering, slurred speech, and somnolence can be passed off by family, friends, or physician simply as evidence of "senility," "arteriosclerosis," or "old age." Even the patient may not recognize that the symptoms come from drinking alcohol, because of the decrease in alcohol tolerance that commonly develops with advanced age. In later life, a little bit of alcohol goes a long way.

Excessive alcohol intake is known to cause a variety of specific disorders, beyond the well-known results of acute alcohol intoxication, that have dementia as a symptom. These include acute auditory hallucinosis, delerium tremens, Wernicke's encephalopathy, Korsakoff's psychosis, and hepatic encephalopathy.

In *acute auditory hallucinosis,* symptoms of hallucination, auditory in nature and deeply frightening in character, may follow withdrawal from heavy, prolonged alcohol consumption. The patient is oriented and therefore not demented. Careful observation will avoid the error of misdiagnosis. Symptoms usually clear spontaneously in several days to a few weeks.[135]

Delerium tremens (DTs) may appear during a decrease in alcohol intake or shortly following abstinence after severe drinking episodes. DTs is manifested by the sudden onset of psychosis, with diverse forms of hallucination, and marked metabolic hyperactivity, with rapid pulse, blood pressure elevation, diaphoresis, fever, and tremor. DTs is known to cause death and may be particularly threatening to older people with preexisting health problems, particularly those of the cardiovascular system.[136]

Wernicke's encephalopathy develops following lengthy periods of alcoholism, particularly when associated with poor nutrition and thiamine deficiency. This disorder, sudden in onset, is characterized by marked confusion, paralysis of the eye muscles, unsteady gait, and peripheral neuropathy. Immediate treatment with thiamine is essential. Although the symptoms will improve under proper therapeutic conditions, they are not likely to clear completely. Without effective treatment, death may occur.

Korsakoff's psychosis is often a consequence of Wernicke's encephalopathy. The distinguishing and major symptom is severe, chronic amnesia. To compensate for profound memory loss, patients with this disorder may engage in confabulation, or the construction of elaborate circumlocutory explanations for their current situation. "Regardless of premorbid personality characteristics, the patient . . . is passive, indifferent, and lacking in affect and initiative."[137]

Hepatic encephalopathy may occur as a result of Laennec's cirrhosis, the major alcohol-induced liver disease. As liver tissue is gradually destroyed, its ability to metabolize and detoxify a wide range of substances is diminished or lost. Brain function is altered, and the patient becomes confused, obtunded, comatose, and at length dies, unless the underlying physiologic abnormalities are treated.

MAJOR INTERCRANIAL DISEASE

Brain tumors, subdural hematomas, and normal-pressure hydrocephalus are three major intercranial diseases that may precipitate treatable dementias.

Through a mass effect on the remaining brain tissue, *brain tumors* may produce significant changes in intellectual function. These include a broad variety of hallucinatory states, confusion, and aberrant conduct. Brain tumors may be benign—the meningioma is a representative example—or malignant, with the primary tumor in the brain or metastatic. Definitive diagnosis is essential, because a cure or amelioration is possible.

Subdural hematoma may follow head injury. This condition is the result of venous bleeding within the cranium, which causes damage to the brain from the mass effect of the ensuing blood clot. Evidence of confusion and obtundation may occur as well as other neurological signs and symptoms. Consideration of this diagnosis is critically important in patients presenting with dementia, because the disease may cause permanent disability or death. Proof of the presence of a subdural hematoma is easily established by means of CT scan of the head;[138] treatment through burr hole drainage is relatively simple and well tolerated. Minor injury to the head, through a matter as ordinary as a fall to the floor at home, may be sufficient to cause a subdural hematoma, so it must be considered a possibility in every case that hints at a loss of brain function.

The following case is illustrative:

RJ was a seventy-five-year-old woman homebound by a previous fractured hip with nonunion [failure of bone ends to unite]. She had a homemaker eight hours per day and used a walker. The patient fell frequently, however, because of generalized weakness and inability to use the walker securely. Over a period of three months, she became increasingly somnolent and uncommunicative, although she would eat and follow directions. She was hospitalized and no evidence of trauma was found. The fundi were not clearly seen because of cataracts. She died within a week. Autopsy showed a large organizing frontal subdural hematoma.[139]

Normal-pressure hydrocephalus (NPH) is a disorder that develops consequent to interference with the flow of cerebrospinal fluid through channels within the brain and over the brain surfaces. NPH is an entity distinct from that form of hydrocephalus which is a disease of infancy. It is caused by a broad variety of conditions that alter the physical structure of the brain or modify the permeability of the brain membranes to cerebrospinal fluid passage.[140]

The origin of most cases of NPH can be identified, particularly through the use of the CT scan. Frequent precursors to NPH include bleeding into the brain (cerebral hemorrhage), tumors, infections such as meningitis and abscess, and direct brain trauma. Distortion within the cranium following brain surgery may lead to this condition as well. In about one-third of cases the cause cannot be determined.

The neurologic symptoms produced by NPH are diverse. Spasticity and unsteady gait (ataxia) are prominent. Urinary incontinence occurs less frequently. Depression and paranoid ideation have been noted, and dementia occurs as well. However, dementia is a late phenomenon in most cases of NPH, and is often mild, although it can develop at a rapid pace.[141] The characteristic nature and development of symptoms permits a clear-cut diagnostic distinction to be made between this condition and AD. Age of patients is another distinguishing factor. Based on extensive autopsy studies, NPH is a disease of individuals largely between fifty and seventy.[142] Differentiating between NPH and PD may be more challenging, because the disturbances of gait in these disorders are the same: shuffling and lack of ability to lift the feet, resulting in short steps; and dementia may occur in both conditions.

Treatment of NPH is based on neurosurgical procedures designed to shunt cerebrospinal fluid past the area(s) of blockage.[143] In 1978 psychiatrist Charles E. Wells cited about a 55 percent improvement rate,[144] but that figure may be changing for the better.[145]

PSYCHIATRIC DISORDERS

The preeminent psychiatric disorder in the aged is depression, a condition now broadly accepted as a cause for symptoms that simulate dementia.[146] Although they are less frequent, late-onset schizophrenia, mania and hypomania, anxiety states, and a broad variety of other psychiatric conditions may occasionally be found in older persons as well,[147] and can produce true dementia.

In surveys of the causes of dementia in the elderly, the frequency of depression as a diagnosis ranges from 6.7 to 24 percent.[148] Depression is an eminently treatable condition. Therefore, our awareness of the possibility that it can be mistaken for AD must be acute, and the diagnosis must be considered in every aged person with symptoms suggesting dementia.

Depression in older people can often be recognized by the presence of somatic symptoms: anorexia, insomnia, and constipation. Beyond these, a constellation of findings may be present that confuse the diagnostic picture and lead the unwary to a misdiagnosis of AD. These include apathy, poor concentrating ability, episodes of confusion, fatigue, withdrawal from ordinary social contact, and hypochondriasis.[149]

The clinical condition in which depression is responsible for symptoms suggesting dementia has been termed pseudodementia.[150] Here, as Wells points out, depression mimics or caricatures dementia.[151] It has been suggested, perhaps a touch ironically, that the diagnosis of depression may be established retrospectively when patients who have "dementia" recover.[152] It is necessary to point out, as well, that when patients who are demented from any cause are able to express their feelings, they have good reason to feel sad and may in fact seem depressed. This sense of loss in the pleasures of life, or anhedonia, must be distinguished from the disease known as depression, the subject under discussion here.

The ability to recognize the distinction between AD and depressive pseudodementia requires that the physician thoughtfully analyze the situation and be aware of the possibility of the diagnosis.[153]

As Professor of Neurology David S. Dahl points out,[154] criteria that tend to distinguish depressive pseudodementia from true dementia can be identified. For instance, in dementia time of onset is often unclear, while in depression a specific event may be recognized as the precipitating factor, or the time of change in the patient's condition can be recognized clearly. Demented patients often may seem unaware of their abnormal state. The opposite is true of depressed people. In dementia patients' recent memory is usually impaired severely, while distant memory may be well preserved. In depression, this finding is far more variable, and the distinctions between recent and distant memory loss are less clear cut. In fact, long term memory in depression is "often inexplicably impaired."[155]

Management of depression with psychopharmaceuticals or electroconvulsive therapy is highly effective and often produces a cure when patients are cared for by physicians experienced in the field. This is a definitive situation in which proper diagnostic effort and use of the available treatment modes can make the difference between years of misery, often in an institution, or a happy and functional life.

REACTION TO THERAPEUTIC AGENTS

Medication reactions are noteworthy causes of reversible dementia in older people. A reasonable estimate indicates that about 2 percent of all cases of dementia in the elderly are caused by drug toxicity; of treatable causes of dementia, this problem is responsible for approximately 10 percent.[156]

Factors that lead to problems regarding medication reactions include excessive dosage; polypharmacy and drug interactions; inaccurate diagnosis and resultant inappropriate prescription of drugs; noncompliance by the patient; and reduced ability of the body to metabolize drugs, leading to unexpectedly high blood levels.[157] A large number of therapeutic agents have been implicated.

Drugs used for treatment of psychiatric conditions, including such agents as haloperidol, tricyclic antidepressants, monoamine oxidase inhibitors, lithium, and phenothiazines, may produce paradoxic effects. Barbiturates, when taken by older people for treatment of insomnia, as calming agents for anxiety, or in therapy of seizure disorders, may produce the reverse of the desired effect: agitation, followed by dementia.

Medications used in therapy of cardiac disorders, including diuretics, propranolol, and methyldopa, may also cause dementia. The existence of the term digitalis delirium is suggestive.

So may *anticancer agents such as 5-fluorouracil,*[158] and *analgesics, oral antidiabetic drugs, anti-inflammatory agents.*[159]

Anticholinergic drugs, such as atropine and related substances, may produce dementia symptoms. In older people, use of these agents may cause worsening dementia for reasons that relate directly to the biochemical and physiologic functions of the brain. Abnormalities of choline-related substances at the synaptic level in the brain appear to be integral in the development of AD and possibly other forms of dementia. Any drug that, when ingested, decreases levels of choline, the pharmacologic substrate of anticholinergics, can be expected to create or exacerbate abnormalities in cognition. Ingestion of such drugs can cause transient symptoms comparable to the memory loss of AD. In these cases, ingestion of choline corrects the problem.

Unfortunately, feeding choline or choline-containing substances to demented patients has not produced any proven benefit, although many investigators have analyzed the possibility.

In order to minimize the likelihood that drugs used in treatment of illness will produce dementia, physicians must be certain, first, that the diagnosis of the disease being treated is correct. A detailed drug history must be obtained from the patient, or through the family, to be certain that all substances being ingested by the person at risk are known. Symptoms may arise due to interactions between drugs that, if taken separately, would not create a problem. For instance, when haloperidol (used in older people for treatment of agitation and anxiety) is taken in combination with the antihypertensive drug methyldopa, it may cause increasing irritability, aggressiveness, and dementia.[160]

Other questions to be considered when prescribing medications for older people are: Is this treatment necessary? Is the dosage correct? It is important to remember that, for older people, effective doses of antidepressant drugs may be one-third those necessary in younger patients.[161] Have plans been made to ensure patient compliance in the therapeutic regime? And perhaps most important, has the patient been observed for the development of new symptoms, and if present, could they be drug-induced? It is clear that drugs can produce dementia and that in most instances the symptoms are reversible upon drug withdrawal. It is an even greater therapeutic triumph to avoid iatrogenic disease in the first place by understanding the risks of all medications, the potential consequences of drug interactions, and the problems of compliance.

DEMENTIA AND ENVIRONMENTAL CHANGE

Striking change for the worse in mental status often follows the placement of an older person in a strange location. People who have held, perhaps tenuously, to a stable life at home may become helpless in a new environment. Habits learned over decades, such as the location of a chair, the bed, the bathrooms, are lost in a hospital or a nursing home. Hospital placement also causes difficulties for the elderly because of the nature of life in an acute care institution. The surrounding people are strangers, the procedures and tests may be painful or frightening, new medications may create difficulties, anesthesia itself may cause problems, and beyond that, the patient is sick or injured. Physicians, nurses, and others whose professional life is spent in inpatient settings obtain from this environment a distorted sense of the frail elderly and of their ability to return to an acceptable level of orientation if they can only get back to their own homes.

It is because people who work in hospitals see many elderly people only in highly aberrant circumstances, situations themselves conducive to confusion and dementia, that arbitrary decisions are made about the fate of elderly patients. They are studied when they are at their most helpless and are sent to chronic care institutions because dementia is diagnosed, when permission to return home might have produced a cure.

GENERAL MEDICAL DISEASES AS CAUSES OF REVERSIBLE DEMENTIA

The aged brain is extremely sensitive to the internal environment. Almost any disorder that alters the environment—cardiac, pulmonary, renal or hepatic failure; endocrine disorders; water and electrolyte disturbances; anoxia, anemia, infections; nutritional deficiencies; and hypothermia or hyperthermia . . . may produce dementia.[162]

Many clinical disorders produce alteration in intellectual function. Those conditions that evidence by abrupt change in mental status have been termed delirium, as opposed to dementia, which is categorized as a more slowly developing form of intellectual impairment.[163] In this discussion we have chosen arbitrarily to define all forms of cognitive dysfunction as dementia, because older people who are symptomatic are likely to be categorized as demented, without further thought. Table 4.1 presents a compilation of medical conditions that have been known to cause dementia.

Because thyroid disease and pernicious anemia are frequent causes of treatable dementia, they require special comment. Both overactive and underactive thyroid states may present cryptically among the elderly. The common clinical signs may be missing, and the patient may appear simply as ill and confused. Hypothyroidism may reveal itself in an older person through apathy, lack of energy, and inertness. Thyrotoxicosis in the elderly can manifest as excitement, manic behavior, delusions, confusion, or the reverse, a condition known as apathetic hyperthyroidism. The proper diagnosis will be suggested to the clinician who has a strong index of suspicion. Treatment is likely to be effective both in restoring an euthyroid state and in eliminating the signs of the aberrant mental status, to the degree that these are caused by the underlying medical condition.

Pernicious anemia is largely a disease of the elderly, caused ultimately, through various means, by vitamin B12 deficiency. Several forms of neurological abnormality may develop, in addition to the megaloblastic anemia that is its hallmark. Damage to the long tracts of the spinal cord, or subacute combined degeneration, is the most frequent consequence to the

TABLE 4.1

Reversible Forms of Dementia in the Elderly

Systemic Disorders
1. Vasculitides—collagen disease (systemic lupus erythematosus, periarteritis nodosa, temporal arteritis, rheumatoid vasculitis)
2. Sarcoidosis
3. Whipple's disease
4. Polycythemia vera
5. Pernicious anemia and other anemias
6. Epilepsy
7. Intravenous drug abuse
8. Hyperlipidemia
9. Hypercalcemia
10. Dehydration
11. Pain
12. Anesthetic reactions
13. Fever

Nutritional/Metabolic Disorders
1. Deficiencies—Vitamin B12, folate, niacin, thiamine
2. Poisoning—heavy metals (mercury, arsenic, lead, thallium); organic compounds (trichlorethylene, toluene, organophosphates, carbon monoxide)
3. Alcoholism—acute; secondary consequences

Diseases of Major Organ Systems
1. Heart—congestive heart failure, consequences of recovery from cardiac arrest, heart block, emboli from heart, arrhythmia; acute myocardial infarction
2. Lungs—chronic respiratory failure, hypoxia, pneumonia, pulmonary embolus
3. Endocrine disorders—thyroid, parathyroid; Cushing's disease/syndrome, Addison's disease; Diabetes mellitus with hyper- or hypoglycemia; inappropriate antidiuretic hormone secretion
4. Kidney—renal failure, uremia
5. Liver—hepatic failure

Malignancies
1. Brain tumors
2. Carcinomatous meningitis

Infections
1. Meningitis, acute and chronic, including viral, bacterial, fungal
2. Encephalitis
3. Bacterial endocarditis
4. Brain abscess
5. Progressive multifocal leukoencephalopathy
6. Lues—general paresis

Therapeutic Drug Intoxication and Drug Interactions
Numerous

Psychiatric Disorders
1. Depression—pseudodementia
2. Manic depressive psychosis

TABLE 4.1 *(Continued)*

Central Nervous System Disorders
1. Stroke; transient ischemic attacks
2. Trauma—subdural hematoma
3. Normal pressure hydrocephalus
4. Multiple sclerosis

Problems of Sensory Deprivation
1. Visual, hearing disorders
2. Isolation; placement in strange surroundings

SOURCE: Blass, J. P. Metabolic dementias. In Amaducci, Davison, and Antuono (Eds.), *Aging,* vol. 13, pp. 261–270; Cummings, J., Benson, D. F., and LoVerne, S. (1980). Reversible dementia. *JAMA, 243:*2434–2439; Damasio, A. R., and Demeter, S. (1981). Dementia due to systemic illness. *Res & Staff Physician, 7:*36–41; Gershon, S., and Herman, S. P. (1982). The differential diagnosis of dementia. *J Am Geriat Soc, 30* (suppl.):58–66; Larson, E. B., Reifler, B. V., and Featherstone, H. J. (1984). Dementia in elderly outpatients. *Ann Intern Med, 100:*417–423; Luxenberg, J., Feigenbaum, L. Z., and Aron, J. M. (1984). Reversible long-standing dementia with normocalcemic hyperparathyroidism. *J Am Geriat Soc, 32:*546–547; Lynch, H. T., Droszcz, C. P., Albano, W. A., et al. (1981). Organic brain syndrome secondary to 5-Fluorouracil toxicity. *Dis Colon Rectum, 24:*130–131; Small, G. N., Jarvik, L. F. (1982). The dementia syndrome. *Lancet, 2:* 1443–1446; Steel, K., and Feldman, R. G. (1979, March). Diagnosing dementia and its treatable causes. *Geriatrics,* pp. 79–88; and Wells, C. E. (1979). Management of dementias. In R. Katzman (Ed.), *Congenital and acquired cognitive disorders.* New York: Raven Press.

nervous system. Symptoms include loss of balance (ataxia), abnormalities of sensation, and occasionally paralysis. In addition, confusion may occur, and true dementia may also be noted.[164] Decreases in cerebral blood flow, oxygen consumption, and glucose utilization[165] accompany cognitive impairment in pernicious anemia and other forms of dementia, including AD. As pernicious anemia presents such a variety of symptoms, medical observers often make an erroneous diagnosis because of failure to consider this disease as a possible cause of dementia.

Accuracy in defining the origin of the problem may be hampered by the fact that anemia may not present until relatively late, following by a considerable period of time the appearance of neurologic symptoms. Treatment with parenteral vitamin B12 is definitive and may result in total cure of the disease if initiated early in the condition. If therapy is delayed, neurological abnormalities may persist.

THERAPEUTIC APPROACHES TO DEMENTIAS

Careful effort should be made to distinguish treatable forms of dementia from others. For people with loss of intellectual function, which at this time appears untreatable in a formal sense, such as for those with AD, we must look to amelioration. AD now causes fully 50 percent of placements in long term care facilities, such as nursing homes. The disease will continue to produce stress upon patients, families,[166] health care services, and financial resources. Establishment of a broad variety of programs and resources to deal with AD is implicit in the concept of a long term care spectrum.

A recognized viewpoint holds that AD "is difficult to diagnose, impossible to cure or arrest in its course, and poorly understood."[167] This being so, it remains a formidable goal to overcome the sense of despair, the general feeling of negativity, that threatens to overwhelm people who work in the field of care for the elderly. And yet there is genuine opportunity to assist patients with dementia and their families.

It is worth recognizing that a set of interactions must exist in order for effective planning and treatment to take place in matters as complex as dealing with dementia. Patients themselves—their rights, wishes, and authority over their own life decisions—must remain the first consideration, insofar as reality and good judgment allow. The needs, concerns, and anxieties of the family are a matter of legitimate interest, and should enter the planning and decision processes as well. Patient and family, then, require the availability of health care workers knowledgeable in the field of dementia, who will share the development of appropriate plans of care.

THE PATIENT

As psychiatrist Loic Hemsi indicates, "only the person with dementia lives with the dementia itself." Further, the demented person is a human being, not a disease, and has remaining significant individual characteristics, "a personality, a biography, a lifetime of relationships and interactions [and] . . . it is only by taking them into account . . . that a proper understanding can be obtained of the situation of a person with dementia."[168]

Any plan of care must recognize that demented patients are particularly susceptible to changes in environment. Since they hold tightly to familiar clues in their living situations in order to function, treatment programs must respect this point. It is wise, however, to avoid requiring that patients be confined to their own rooms for fear that any change will be harmful. Interesting, even moderately challenging experiences can be sought to make life attractive. A familiar accompanying person may serve as the necessary anchor to reality and allow patients to visit relatives or enjoy community activities. A sensible balance between the need for protection and the stimulation of the outside world should be sought.

In general, demented people are known to retain old memories but forget the more recent. This point can also be interpreted to mean that ability to learn is lost, but that which has already been learned is kept.[169] While variations on this insight are without limit in individual cases, it remains a useful rule. Demented patients will do relatively well with daily life and old habits in their own homes, and poorly if asked to take on new tasks. For example, a patient may be able to eat and perform bathroom functions at home, but be unable to travel alone to an unfamiliar destination, even with written directions.

It is reasonable to expect reactions to the evidence of dementia from symptomatic people. A person who recognizes that memory and control of life are being lost will be distressed, anxious, and depressed. A frequent and understandable compensatory psychological recourse will be denial and/or confabulation.

THE FAMILY AND OTHERS

Those people intimately involved with demented patients, and who are concerned to help, need to appreciate the complexity of the issues. A husband or wife, children, siblings, friends, neighbors, may need education and guidance about their own conduct.

> ... there is an equilibrium between the patient and her environment, human and material. At its best, this results in a secure, contented and calm person who happens to have core disabilities of dementia. That adjustment can be broken by the actions of others. Distress and abnormal behavior can be induced, possibly without necessity. This indeed is what would happen with any person subjected to strain beyond her ability to tolerate. . . . What is different [in the patient with dementia] is the drastically reduced threshold to stress and the excessive degree of reaction.[170]

Thus when external forces—people or the environment—exert stress on the patient, a worsening of symptoms may well result. A cycle then evolves in which, because of the patient's more demented conduct, additional stressors are added, including institutional transfer, and all is lost.

On the other hand, people in the network of family and friends are in a position to help, by understanding the patient and the nature of the problem.[171] If contentment of the disabled person and maintenance within the home are the goals, those individuals in regular association with the patient are a critical resource.[172] These members of the informal support network are not bound by professional dicta or work rules, nor by government regulation. Training by health workers can compensate for what they lack in formal training or experience. For example, group sessions for those concerned, conducted by a trained leader, have proven useful.[173] Group work both improves the technical and empathic skills of those who must provide care for patients and satisfies a major need for mutual support and understanding.[174]

Disputes among relatives are a commonplace in these situations, and often produce severe threats to families because of the strain imposed upon financial and personal interrelationships that may be fragile. Displacement of feelings onto others, such as the professional establishment or even the patients themselves, may be the recourse of relatives under strain. The latter situation may result in assault upon the demented person. In England the term granny-bashing has evolved for this phenomenon.[175] Through group discussion sessions, damaging feelings of anger and rejection, followed by guilt, may at times be averted or resolved.

PROFESSIONAL TREATMENT APPROACHES

Health workers responsible for demented people have a twofold task. First, protection of the health and rights of the patient is an absolute standard. Second, for effective therapy, assistance to and involvement of other people close to the patient is of major importance. Those professionally in charge must engage the family in a therapeutic network that is a force for good, and also help to deter the negative feelings that often arise. These feelings can destroy changes for stability and improvement.[176]

The physicians, nurses, and social workers involved must persist in the view that the patient's interests are paramount.[177] "A common error is to identify with normal people around the patient, thus seeing the problem only through their eyes. . . ."[178] The first objective, then, is to assure the patient's comfort, maximize the potential for independence, and develop sufficient protection to minimize the chances for accidents, wandering, or fires.

To help the family and others involved with the patient, group work, psychological counseling, and sensible planning for the sharing of tasks are pertinent functions of health care staff. Honest recognition of the fact that the patient is unlikely to improve, and in all probability will worsen, is fair and necessary.

The major workload in effective systems for care of demented patients often falls upon paraprofessionals such as home health care aides. Success of the plan clearly then requires that the aides be trained and that attention be paid to their well-being.[179] Aides often must spend hours alone with demented patients. Frustration, anxiety, and agitation may result. Group sessions for aides of elderly patients have been found effective in maintaining these employees on their jobs in good rapport with their charges.[180]

The specific therapeutic modes available for demented patients are modest. They include judicious use of psychotherapeutic drugs for control of secondary symptoms, such as anxiety and agitation. It is important to realize, however, that such drugs are often abused, particularly in institutional settings, in order to make patients more manageable.[181]

Reality orientation is a set of techniques designed to place demented people in touch with details of daily life. All those involved with patients suffering from memory loss can and should engage in informal reality orientation. Emphasizing of names, dates, time of day, the calendar, the face of the clock, and the identification of everyday objects has proven useful.[182]

Reality orientation has also been developed into a formal therapy. Gerontologist J. C. Folsom defines it as "a group-oriented, psychotherapeutic technique for assisting confused, disoriented elderly individuals (frequently diagnosed as having Alzheimer's disease) to learn and practice techniques that help them cope with the problems caused by their confusion and disorientation."[183] In principle, the technique consists of having staff or trained family members use contact with the patient to help restore identity. Identity is defined for these purposes as awareness of time, place, and person. Responses to be anticipated from patients vary with degree of dementia, but it is useful to expect an appropriate reaction.

Most reality orientation experiences have taken place in institutional settings. However, recent work suggests that this form of treatment may also be effective in day care programs[184] or in the home.[185]

Day care and respite services created by motivated persons in indigenous community-based settings are being developed across the country. Sponsored by a variety of local agencies and volunteer groups, they are designed to assist patients with dementia and their family members.[186] Programs of this nature are likely to become a significant component of a long term care spectrum.[187]

Chapter 5

Alcoholism and Older People

"Alcohol is a pervasive clinical and social presence in our society."[1] While a virtual library of information exists about alcoholism in general, only modest attention has been devoted to the problem among older people. This is perhaps to be expected, considering that the issue of alcohol abuse in the aged combines two complex subjects about which there is more controversy than fact. It is difficult to define alcoholism or aging clearly and with broad agreement.

As we attempt, then, to develop an effective understanding of these issues, leading to diagnosis and treatment, a critical insight follows. Older people who misuse alcohol have two interrelated concerns: old age and drug abuse. "These problems have the quality of a mathematical progression, with the result far exceeding the sum of its parts."[2]

This discussion considers the phenomenology of alcoholism in the elderly, with particular emphasis on factors that set older persons apart from others. We review first the variables that require elaboration in assessing alcohol use in the aged. This is followed by analysis of diagnosis, demographic and alcohol use patterns, medical and social consequences of alcohol-related problems in the elderly, and treatment issues. In addition, we develop a typology of age-specific factors required to classify alcohol abusers. These factors include: genetic, familial, social and societal history; physical settings in which patients live; health status of the person; diverse therapeutic approaches that have been advocated; concerns of spouse, family, friends; and attitudes of health workers toward older people and toward alcoholism.

Older alcoholics tend to be hidden from view, for reasons that are in part understandable. These include both patient's and family's feelings of shame and embarrassment, the fact that physical disability often requires older people to drink alone, and health workers' failure to recognize the problem. Beyond these reasons, and key to understanding of the alcohol/old age double-bind, is the fact that ingesting small amounts of alcohol can cause large problems in aged persons. Moderate drinking, in amounts that would not fit any common definition of alcoholism, may damage older bodies already in a borderline state of health.[3] As people reach advanced age, they change in their sensitivity to acute alcohol ingestion, development of physical dependency, and tolerance to its effects. Evidently the adaptability of the brain to any form of insult at later ages broadly decreases, and this adaptability may be further damaged by exposure to alcohol.[4] It is a general truth that because of decreases in their ability to metabolize the drug, older people do not exhibit the classical features of addictive alcoholism. They cannot, by and large, tolerate large amounts of alcohol.[5] As a result the manner of presentation differs from that of younger drinkers. Older people are more likely to demonstrate a problem through a combination of physical, mental, and social symptoms: self-neglect,[6] falls causing fractures, confusion, and behavior leading to family quarrels.[7]

Why do people drink? This remains a subject unresolved in alcoholism research. As psychologist Brian Mishara and associates point out,[8] one view holds that alcoholism is a disease that results from the chemical nature of alcohol, combined perhaps with a genetic predisposition and the individual nature of personality. Others stress the social and cultural background of the drinker, emphasizing events in the life of the person involved.

Why do *old* people drink?

As unattractive as the picture of the bottle-addicted old person may be, one might continue to ask what realistic alternatives are available in a society that so often places care and concern for the elderly near the bottom of its social priority list. While this line of reasoning is not intended as a defense for alcohol abuse in old age, it does suggest that some caution be exercised before automatically concluding that the use of alcohol in old age is itself a fundamental problem. It can be seen instead as a simplistic and less than optimal response to other problems that are much more fundamental. From the practical standpoint, the latter view might lead to more attention being paid to the identification and alleviation of the causes of alcoholism rather than the problem drinker per se.[9]

Older persons must bear, to a degree more than others, loneliness, isolation, alienation, and lack of self-esteem. For people faced with life in an institution, gerontologist Robert Butler's phrase "houses of death" for nursing homes[10] perhaps makes the point. In this situation, drinking may be seen as one of life's few remaining joys, behavior that makes life bearable when all personal control is removed.

The following case report from the files of the Chelsea-Village Program[11] is relevant:

LL, a sixty-eight-year-old musician, lived a life confined alone to his room because of shortness of breath due to emphysema. On our visits he was regularly drunk, and liquor bottles, full and empty, were prominent. The presence of malnutrition, extensive soft pitting edema, and multiple contusions were noted. The nurse, social worker, and physician reiterated the harmful consequences, and the patient agreed that he should stop, but he failed. His reasoning: "I'm trying to think of something else I can do which will give me any pleasure in life."

We recognize that the body must inevitably age, but personality, interest, and appetites do not.[12]

Just as each person has his or her own developmental history, so does each generation.[13] Attitudes toward drinking are created in part by the milieu into which each of us is born and reaches maturity.[14] For instance, people who lived their early lives prior to World War I reacted to different social mores than did those who grew up during the prohibition era: "We all live in different worlds according to our age."[15] Recognition of this cohort effect is essential to an understanding of each older patient's background, and it has direct implications for individual and group treatment. Further, it complicates considerably plans for therapeutic approaches toward alcoholism and the elderly, now and in the future. We may find that people who were young during the depression will differ considerably from the post–World War II generation, when money for purchase of alcohol was more available.

Within each racial, social, or ethnic group, and between men and women,[16] further distinctions clearly exist. For instance, psychiatrist Irvin Blose points out that in some native American populations, the Plains Indians in particular, "excessive use of alcohol is not common or seen as a cultural necessity among [those] . . . who survive to become elderly":

There is a common respect for the person, a sense of community and a sharing of all material things, a subsequent respect for the aging, and consideration of various times of life and life processes as a condition of nature. The aging native American is not subjected to the kinds of sterotypes and the need for pathological narcissism, or to various other environmental forces that exist in white society.[17]

Another striking basis for variation is based on genetic differences.[18] For example, about 85 percent of Oriental people often note strong dysphoric reactions to alcohol, in the form of flushing and malaise, with ingestion of even small amounts.[19] High acetaldehyde levels in the blood evidently are responsible for this phenomenon. Acetaldehyde, toxic to the body, is the major degradation product of alcohol metabolism. People with the flushing syndrome lack one of the isoenzymes of aldehyde dehydrogenase, which leads to an inability to reduce acetaldehyde promptly into its less harmful by-products.

We must also relate the attitudes of health workers to this complex of biological, social, and societal issues if we are to plan effective treatment for older alcoholics: "The culturally rooted aversion among mental and public health personnel in general toward devoting themselves to care of the aged does not yield simply and automatically to the call for action, nor should it be expected that geriatricians would readily overcome their resistances to working with alcohol-related problems."[20]

In general, agency personnel in alcoholism programs express a low level of concern about older drinkers.[21] Most such organizations focus on younger alcoholics in trouble with employers, the legal system, or the family. Only 3 percent of enrollees in Alcoholics Anonymous (AA), the preeminent treatment program, are aged sixty-five or older.[22]

The relationship between old age and alcoholism is influenced by the multitudinous variables of life. These include the health status of the individual; the interactions between medications and alcohol, and the associated multiple drug use, or polypharmacy, to which older people are often subjected; loneliness; and the consequences of institutional placement. There is a general understanding among workers in this field that a susceptibility to alcoholism is inherited.[23] To suggest, however, a straightforward process of intergenerational passing of the bottle is simplistic. Taste perception, sensitivity to alcohol, metabolic variation, individual characterological differences, societal distinctions, and cohort effects all have an influence. A review of these points requires us to recognize that the origins of alcohol abuse are multiple, the consequences varied, and treatment challenging.

DIAGNOSIS OF ALCOHOLISM

BARRIERS TO DIAGNOSIS

Problems in diagnosis constitute perhaps the greatest barrier to effective treatment of older alcoholics. Inherent to this discussion is the fact that older drinkers do not fit the alcoholic stereotype and may escape recognition. The diagnostic effort is complicated further because many older people avoid contact with agencies that care for alcoholics, break off relations with caregivers before the diagnosis is established, or receive treatment for other conditions while their problem with alcohol remains undetected.[24]

The issue is sometimes clarified when patients are hospitalized and alcohol use ceases suddenly. Withdrawal symptoms may develop, and provide the diagnosis.[25] Among other clues for the recognition of this problem among the elderly, beyond the obvious discovery of empty bottles under the bed, are: unexplained depression; change in ability for sexual performance, or in interest; impotence; confusional states; appearance of withdrawal symptoms; staggering, falling, or injuries; loss of appetite or decreased interest in food; an attack of gout; and agitation, anxiety, or insomnia.

MIXED ETIOLOGIES

The physician's tendency to neglect alcoholism as part of a differential diagnosis is compounded by a general lack of knowledge about the effects of alcohol on elderly patients. Behavior that would identify alcoholism in younger people may be passed off in the elderly as eccentricity. Problems caused by alcohol abuse blend into pathological states that arise from the sociological or physical consequences of aging. The interconnections between alcohol and depression, use of multiple medications, and the stresses of late life thus serve to cloud diagnostic efforts.

Among these older patients, alcoholism must be distinguished from dementia. Memory loss is often a presenting complaint of the elderly. Problems in diagnosis arise because alcohol abuse is one of many potential causes of memory deficit;[26] alcohol may cause confusion in older patients who do not appear to be drunk, because tolerance to the drug has developed; and in their early stages most dementias fluctuate in degree of expression.

A cycle of difficulty may arise in these situations. Alcohol that is ingested to relieve feelings of anxiety caused by memory loss aggravates the very problem for which it is used. The steps from early dementia of any origin, to anxiety and depression, and then to drinking are understandable.[27] It is therefore mandatory that clinicians think about alcohol abuse as an underlying or contributing factor in any older patient who presents with dementia.[28]

The potential for suicidal behavior in older drinkers requires comment. When combined, the effects of alcohol and depression seem to create a significant suicide potential, no matter which was the initiating cause. Alcohol abuse has a part in about 30 percent of suicides.[29] Further, the suicide rate is increased in older people—23 percent of successful suicides occur in people sixty and over, but this age group makes up only 15 percent of our population.[30] Older drinkers may possess all the stressors that lead to suicide. In addition to advanced age and alcoholism, these include social isolation, loneliness, and the likelihood of recent bereavement.

CHARACTERISTICS OF OLDER DRINKERS

NUMBERS

The precise degree of alcoholism in the elderly is not known. A summary of the best evidence indicates that alcohol problems affect about 1.6 million persons among the 20 million individuals sixty-five years and older living in our country.[31]

There are high rates in certain subgroups of the elderly: widowers, individuals with medical problems, those who are hospitalized, the brain damaged, people in long term care institutions, and individuals in trouble with the police.

About 20 percent of people in nursing homes, in general, fulfill the criteria for alcoholism.[32] It is particularly noteworthy that studies of some nursing homes show that the proportion of residents with alcohol problems is in the range of 40 to 60 percent.[33]

The impact of this problem upon the health system is striking. Fully 10 percent of people who come to emergency rooms for alcohol-related problems are age sixty or more.[34] Studies of older medical patients in general hospitals show that from 15 to 49 percent have disorders influenced by alcohol.[35] While these figures include Veterans Administration patients,[36] most of whom are male, the extent of the problem is broad and highly significant.

In a study of people who telephoned a central alcohol information clearing house in New York City, about one-third were concerned with a person over fifty-five years of age. Most of the calls were from relatives.[37] Other similar surveys confirm that up to 30 percent of calls to such agencies pertain to the elderly.[38]

The extent of alcoholism among older people has been commonly cited to be 2 to 10 percent. This information is based on a community survey, circa 1965, limited to males in New York City.[39] (See table 5.1.)

Although this information is now more than twenty years old, it appears to remain valid and is supported by more recent studies.[40]

Among these is a 1986 analysis carried out by Dr. Pearl Lefkowitz and associates at Saint Vincent's Hospital in New York.[41] One hundred eighty-

TABLE 5.1
Percent of Probable Alcoholics by Age Group

	% of Probable Alcoholics
Age	
45 to 54	2.3
55 to 64	1.7
65 to 74	2.2
Marital Status	
Single	2.9
Married	2.5
Divorced/Separated	6.8
Widowed	10.5

NOTE: Numbers refer to percentages of the total in each age group.
SOURCE: Adapted from M. P. Bailey, P. W. Haberman, and H. Alksne. (1965). The epidemiology of alcoholism in an urban residential area. *Q J Study on Alcohol, 26:* 19–40.

one homebound patients with a median age of eighty-five were studied through chart review for evidence of alcohol abuse.[42] Through this evidence, 19 (10.6 percent) were considered to be alcohol abusers. Of the 181, 104 were interviewed with the CAGE questionnaire, a previously validated screening tool for alcohol abuse. By this technique, 15 of the 104 (14.4 percent) were deemed to be alcohol abusers.

Nineteen (18.3 percent) of the 104 interviewed identified by *either* chart review or CAGE questionnaire had alcoholism-related diagnoses such as liver disease or seizure disorders. Three others had overt evidence of alcohol abuse, such as empty vodka bottles, in their homes.

The high-risk groups for alcoholism in this study included males (22 percent of males abused alcohol), cigarette smokers (24 percent), divorced or separated participants (38 percent), benzodiazepine users (27 percent), people who fell habitually (33 percent), and patients with signs of self-neglect (38 percent). Eighty-six percent of elderly alcohol abusers identified in this study were early-onset drinkers, beginning at age thirty or younger.

AGE OF ONSET

Broad studies indicate that, starting at about age fifty, people begin to drink less.[43] (See table 5.2.) There are a number of possible explanations for this.

First, *sampling may be faulty.* Perhaps older people surveyed understate their drinking more significantly than people in other age groups. This may be a result of deliberate or unconscious denial. Or there may be a bias in the research technique.

Second, *alcoholism may be a self-limiting disease.* Heavy drinkers may die early. Table 5.2 suggests the ironic fact that abstainers are the next to die and that moderate drinkers live longer. As we will see, this may be a factitious indication.

Third, *people may, in fact, genuinely drink less as they get older.* Causes underlying this explanation for data include the body's inability to tolerate previously acceptable levels of alcohol ingestion; a deliberate attempt to decrease alcohol intake because of concern about the consequences; or loss of the social atmosphere that previously encouraged drinking.

Fourth, *older people are disproportionally female,* [44] and women are less likely than men to be heavy drinkers.

Finally, *cause of death may be incorrectly designated on death certificates,* in order to avoid social stigma.[45]

Another explanation is related to the extent that drinking is a consequence of stress. According to geriatrician Kenneth Weiss, stress, in broad biological terms, is based on drives for territory, mates, and competition within the species. In humans, these problems decrease with age. "Thus, there is a natural life-cycle reduction of the kinds of anxieties that lead people to drink."[46]

It is reasonable to believe that people who start drinking heavily early in life tend to die early. Best estimates indicate that this group loses ten to fifteen years of life expectancy or more compared to its nondrinking peers.[47] Few Skid Row men began drinking relatively late in life. Of the ninety-four Bowery men sociologist Howard Bahr[48] interviewed, a mere 7 percent began heavy drinking after age forty-five. Other studies[49] confirm these figures.

Among elderly heavy drinkers, three groups can be identified: the few survivors of many years of heavy drinking, intermittent heavy drinkers, and reactive problem drinkers. The few survivors are people who have alienated their family and friends, have medical problems as a result of drinking, and are likely to be identified through community surveys rather than through their own efforts to seek help. The intermittent drinkers have consistently lapsed throughout adult life in response to pressure. And the reactive problem drinkers managed to cope earlier in life but started drinking under stresses of advancing age. Certain ambiguities arise in accounting for this group. If, for instance, retirement can be considered a cause of drinking, it also appears to be a cause of abstinence. Since, as table 5.2 reveals, there is a marked decrease in heavy drinking at about age sixty-five, as many people probably stop drinking as start following job loss.

Explanations for this statistical dip lie, perhaps, in "wisdom of the body."[50] Studies show that, for the same intake, older persons develop higher blood alcohol levels than younger people.[51] This phenomenon is

TABLE 5.2

Degree of Alcohol Intake by Age of Drinkers

Age	Numbers	Percentages			
		Abstainers	Infrequent	Light or Moderate	Heavy
Men					
21 to 24	(100)	16	8	54	22
25 to 29	(116)	17	8	51	24
30 to 34	(109)	12	7	51	30
35 to 39	(134)	16	12	50	22
40 to 44	(150)	18	8	54	20
45 to 49	(114)	25	7	38	30
50 to 54	(116)	25	13	41	21
55 to 59	(81)	30	14	34	22
60 to 64	(82)	30	5	41	24
65 and up	(175)	38	16	39	7
Women					
21 to 24	(112)	32	20	39	9
25 to 29	(144)	29	21	45	5
30 to 34	(156)	29	23	42	6
35 to 39	(189)	27	22	44	7
40 to 44	(189)	35	16	43	6
45 to 49	(144)	36	14	40	10
50 to 54	(147)	51	16	32	1
55 to 59	(118)	50	14	35	1
60 to 64	(110)	47	20	31	2
65 and up	(257)	60	15	24	1
TOTAL Sample	(2746)	32	15	41	12

SOURCE: D. Cahalan, H. Cisin, and H. M. Crossley. (1969). *American drinking practices.* New Brunswick, NJ: Rutgers Center of Alcohol Studies.

related to age changes in the body composition (to be discussed later). Older people may therefore sense that less is enough. Furthermore, concern about difficulties in speech, locomotion, and equilibrium may be more disturbing to older persons; and the favorable effects of alcohol, such as feeling high, euphoria, and uninhibited behavior, may be less attractive than before.

GENDER

For some older men, the double loss of spouse and job may precipitate heavy drinking. Elderly widowers are a high-risk group.[52]

A sudden decrease in drinking is noted in women when they reach age fifty (see table 5.2). This drop may be accounted for by the assumption that ages forty-five to forty-nine, when drinking in women reaches its peak, is the period when commonly understood midlife crises occur. After this age, women have less need to drink because of changes in the expectation of female sexual roles and conduct.

The prevalence rate of alcoholism in aged women is obscure, but understanding of the cohort effect suggests that it is probably increasing.

While in every age category men are more likely than women to have identifiable alcohol problems, it is important to recognize that a significant number of women are included in all studies.[53] Professor of social work Eloise Rathbone-McCuan,[54] citing research gerontologist Edith Gomberg, reviews myths and stereotypes about alcoholism, age, and women (see table 5.3).

Beyond the intellectual failure that all stereotyping reflects, this way of thinking blocks effective treatment.

ECONOMICS AND CLASS DISTINCTION

Economic class breakdowns are noteworthy. A study in which people categorized themselves by income revealed that 80 percent of the "prosperous" group ingested alcohol, 70 percent of the "average income" people drank, and 48 percent of the "poor" used alcohol.[55] A study in which people categorized themselves by social class revealed that 83 percent of those in high social position used liquor, compared to 51 percent of those in the lowest category.[56] These analyses, it must be understood, refer simply to any use of alcohol, not to abuse or alcoholism. They indicate, however, that availability of money influences drinking.

TABLE 5.3
Myths and Stereotypes About Alcoholism, Age, and Women

Female Alcoholics	Elderly Alcoholics
1. are sexually promiscuous.	1. don't live into advanced age.
2. are young when they seek treatment.	2. can't change their behavior.
3. live in a social world that fails to recognize their problem.	3. characteristically live on Skid Row.
4. find greatest help from their physician.	4. are all long term chronic alcoholics.
5. are poorly educated.	5. have no family ties.
6. represent a single personality type.	6. all have organic brain impairment.

SOURCE: E. Rathbone-McCuan and L. A. Roberds. (1980). Treatment of the older female alcoholic. *J. Addiction and Health, 1:* 104–128.

GENETIC BASIS

"Drunkards begat Drunkards."

—PLUTARCH

People who start early in life are thought to have a genetic basis for their drinking, influenced of course by many other factors. As alcoholism researchers Marc Schuckit and Paul Pastor point out: "A series of investigations employing family studies, twin studies, animal investigations and genetic marker studies are all consistent with the genetic hypothesis but are not able to separate the relative importance of heredity and environment."[57]

For those who start drinking later in life, it is reasonable to believe that there may also exist a predisposition toward drinking that had remained under control earlier. Genetic vulnerability, pressures of later life, and the extent of defenses against alcohol abuse interact.

For some individuals, the stresses of increasing isolation and failing health associated with aging may make them much more vulnerable than did the stresses of developing a life occupation and raising a family. The more rigid patterns demanded by job and family may serve as a protection . . . [against] . . . allowing drinking to get out of hand—a defense that disappears as the family grows or retirement nears or is achieved.[58]

UNDERSTANDING THE EXTENT OF THE PROBLEM

All analyses of alcoholism in older people have built-in errors and limitations. As Gomberg points out:

There is a complicated interweaving of demographic variables: gender, socioeconomic class, religious affiliation, race or ethnicity, size and location of one's community within the United States, which relate to *whether* and *how* older persons will drink. Among older populations, to summarize, women are less likely to drink, poorer people are less likely to drink, people affiliated with ascetic Protestant sects are less likely to drink, et cetera.[59]

Three main problems affect our analyses: lack of data, inadequate terminology, and obscuring of the diagnosis by physical illness.

First, only limited data are available that relate alcohol use/abuse to the wide number of demographic variables. Studies generally fail to discriminate functions of sex, economics, ethnicity, geography, family/isolation, and work/retirement.

Second, inadequate and inconsistent terminology affects comparability across studies. How do we distinguish among social drinkers, heavy drinkers, problem drinkers, and alcoholics? Information is often subjective. For example, note the problem of a retiree whose drinking patterns at work, not observed by his wife, were acceptable; but martinis at lunch under her eye are objectionable. Note the mother, now living with her adult children, whose "nightcap," previously unknown to them, causes concern.

Third, physical illness often obscures the diagnosis of alcoholism. Hospital studies are based on diagnoses recorded at time of admission. Alcoholism may not be listed, because the physician is unaware, because it may be a secondary problem, or for self-evident social reasons. The same data-collection problems arise in nursing home studies. Thus indices of alcoholism tend to be underreported.

Validity of survey instruments are suspect in general, because people tend to give "acceptable" answers.[60] A natural result is that the degree of alcohol abuse is in dispute. Case finding is a necessity if we are to measure the extent of the problem. Older people pose special difficulties in this regard. Those in trouble with alcohol do not enter the health care system in the conventional manner.[61] They tend to avoid seeking care until they are in crisis. They are less likely than younger people, for instance, to be involved in problems with the law for public disturbance or drunken driving; and when such incidents occur, they may often be released out of pity or mistaken kindness.

Furthermore, aged drinkers are rarely found in detoxification centers because the amount of alcohol they are able to ingest rarely causes a need for detoxification. They tend to avoid AA, possibly because of fear of public exposure. When they encounter physicians, in emergency rooms or private offices, the diagnosis is often missed because physicians confuse the signs of alcoholism with those of aging. "Indeed, the medical profession is no different from any other: Its members are, for the most part, ordinary empty-headed dolts, ready to see what is not there and to deny the obvious."[62]

Finally, family fear of stigma produces a conspiracy of silence.

In sum, as psychiatrist Dan Blazer and epidemiologist Margaret Pennybacker[63] point out, older patients seen in treatment may differ substantially from unrecognized cases in the population, and the methods of reporting employed by many studies, combined with strict case definitions, may miss a substantial number of older alcoholics.

DEFINITION OF TERMS

By alcoholism, do we mean heavy drinking and intoxication? Or drinking in isolation? Does our definition refer to problems caused to other people in the drinker's environment? Is it a matter of harmful interactions with medications taken by an older person who drinks moderately? Are we concerned with dangerous effects on health?[64]

Lack of adequate, consistent definitions of terms tends to bring into question the validity of studies done to date.[65] This is a particular concern regarding aging and alcohol because the standard definitions are based on findings in younger alcoholics.

For instance, the major criteria for diagnosis of alcoholism established by the National Council on Alcoholism[66] include:

1. Drinking a fifth of whiskey per day, or its equivalent in wine or beer, for a 180-pound person.
2. Alcoholic "blackouts."
3. Withdrawal syndrome: gross tremors, hallucinosis, convulsions, delirium tremens (DTs).
4. Blood alcohol level greater than 150 mg per 100 ml without the appearance of intoxication.
5. Continued drinking despite medical advice.
6. Family and/or job problems caused by drinking.

Psychiatric terminology, as listed in the DSM-III,[67] is equally inapplicable to older people. For alcohol dependence (alcoholism) to be established as a diagnosis, the presence of both a pattern of pathological alcohol use or alcohol-related impairment in social or occupational functioning and signs of either tolerance or withdrawal are required.

Unfortunately, these definitions are inappropriate for the population under study. Most older alcoholics lack an opportunity for occupational malfunction because they are no longer employed; many are not evident social misfits because they are isolated; and many older people in trouble with alcohol cannot ingest enough to develop tolerance.

Dr. Sheldon Zimberg[68] has developed a scale of alcohol abuse (see table 5.4) that is helpful in definition. According to the scale, alcoholism is ordinarily "less severe in elderly people. There are generally less physical sequelae and less evidence of signs and symptoms of alcohol addiction."[69] Level 3 is the maximum degree of severity reached by most elderly alcoholics.

Perhaps the most useful approach to defining problem drinking among older people requires that we discriminate between the expected conse-

TABLE 5.4

Range of Alcohol Abuse

Degree of Drinking Severity	Qualities
1. None	No drinking, or only occasional drinking.
2. Minimal	Drinking is not prominent. No associated social, family, occupational, health, or legal problems.
3. Moderate	Frequently drunk, up to two times per week; and/or evident harm to social, family, or occupational activity. Evidence of physical impairment related to drinking, such as tremors, frequent accidents, poor appetite. No history of delirium tremens (DTs), cirrhosis, or hospitalizations associated with drinking.
5. Severe	Steady drinking. History of DTs, cirrhosis, chronic brain syndrome, neuritis, or nutritional deficiency. Major loss of social or family relations. Hospitalizations related to drinking.
6. Extreme	All of the above plus loss of home and/or inability to maintain self on public assistance.

SOURCE: S. Zimberg. (1978). Diagnosis and treatment of the elderly alcoholic. *Alcoholism: Clin & Exp Research,* 2(1): 27–29.

quences of normal aging and the problems that arise from excessive drinking in later years.[70] Alcoholism as a clinical condition must mean loss of control over drinking and a state of dependence on alcohol, but because the lifestyles of older people differ distinctly from those of younger people, criteria must be appropriate.

A sensible definition for older drinkers should be pragmatic and combine the criteria of physical and psychological addiction, societal norms, and social problems.[71] The following cautions must be recognized, however. First, physical addiction, by definition, requires the presence of specific signs when the patient withdraws from alcohol use. These range from hangovers, through tremors and alcoholic hallucinosis, to DTs. A weak aspect of definition here is that signs such as tremulousness and anxiety may be ongoing conditions in the elderly, not related to stopping alcohol use. Second, psychological addiction assumes the presence of a compulsion to drink. This part of the definition is subjective and is therefore hard to measure. Third, variation in societal norms exist within subgroups of the population. In each such group, older people whose social behavior resulting from drinking is beyond accepted bounds may be recognized as alcoholic.

CONSEQUENCES OF ALCOHOLISM IN OLDER PEOPLE

I may be forgiven for saying, as a physician, that drinking deep is a bad practice, which I never follow, if I can help, and certainly do not recommend to another, least of all to anyone who still feels the effects of yesterday's carouse.

—ERYXIMACHUS, in Plato, *The Dialogues*

From the earliest days, people have sought substances to increase pleasure and deaden pain. Alcohol is probably the agent used most extensively over the millennia to achieve this goal, and wherever available there have been those who have taken it to excess. Ancient Chinese manuscripts contain records of drunken behavior; in the Vedas there exist prayers to the gods asking them to join their worshippers in drunkenness so they might grant the prayers of the supplicants, which they would refuse if sober. The Old Testament notes the widespread use of alcohol and of the evils derived therefrom.[72] Galen, the eminent Greco-Roman physician of the second century A.D., called alcohol "the nurse of old age."[73]

The establishment of pubs in nursing homes and homes for the aged has been suggested as a cure for loneliness and depression through the socialization encouraged by communal drinking.[74] For many years physicians have prescribed *spiritus frumenti* in hospital orders for unhappy or withdrawn older patients, although in fact the depressant qualities of alcohol may produce the reverse effect.

Further, studies of heart attack frequency suggest that there may be medical benefit to moderate drinking.[75] A 1979 report[76] showed that consumption of two ounces of alcohol daily was inversely related to coronary death, in a study of 568 married men with matched controls. Dr. William L. Haskell and associates of the Stanford University School of Medicine reported in 1984 that moderate alcohol intake seemed to protect against the development of coronary artery disease, but found that the benefit was not the result of a fall in serum high-density lipoproteins.[77] One suggested explanation is that moderate levels of blood ethanol may inhibit platelet aggregation.[78] A substantial body of information counteracts these positive qualities of alcohol use for older people, as we will see. The beneficial effects of alcohol in the elderly are modest at best, and the possibility for harm is significant.

CHANGES IN BODY MASS

As people age, nutritional demands for maintenance of optimal health decrease. Seventy-year-olds need, in general, only 70 percent of the calories that forty-year-olds require. Any excess is stored as fat. As early as age fifty-five, men's lipid content increases to 36 percent of total body weight, compared to 15 percent at age twenty. For women the figures change from 33 percent to 48 percent respectively.[79] As the percent of body fat rises in older people, there is a concomitant decrease in lean body mass and an associated fall in total body water, both intracellular and extracellular. Total body water falls 15 percent between ages twenty and eighty.[80] Bone mass is also reduced. As a result of these changes, old people have decreased reserves of sodium, potassium, magnesium, calcium, and phosphorus.

Despite this, although it has reduced physiologic capacity, the normal aging body is able to function adequately. However, with the superimposition of chronic disease, alcohol abuse, or multiple therapeutic drugs, capacity to adapt is diminished and a cycle of deterioration can ensue.[81]

As mentioned, blood levels of alcohol are increased in the elderly, compared to younger individuals, following ingestion of the same amount. This is a direct consequence of the fact that older people have relatively smaller amounts of body water. Alcohol is diluted in a lesser volume of body liquid and reaches the organs at a higher proof.[82] The inevitable consequence is that the elderly are relatively intolerant of alcohol. Women are at a higher risk than men because of their greater fat content, smaller total body water pool, and lesser body size.

It has often been observed that younger people tend to drink larger quantities of alcohol, although less often, and the elderly to ingest lesser quantities, but drink more frequently.[83] Quantities that appear to cause few problems in younger people clearly can produce untoward effects in the aged, and there are decreases in individual drinking capacity over the years as well. The following news story from the *New York Times,* reporting on a fire at Hampton Court, provides an example. Retired retainers of the royal family are housed in this sixteenth-century palace fifteen miles outside London.

The March 31 [1986] blaze, which heavily damaged the palace, killed Daphne Lady Gale, the 76-year-old widow of Gen. Sir Richard Gale, commander of Britain's Sixth Airborne Division in World War II. Although the cause of the fire has not been confirmed, fire officials have said they believed that it began in or near Lady Gale's apartment. Neighbors said Lady Gale was accustomed to having a drink by candlelight before she went to bed.[84]

HEALTH-RELATED PROBLEMS

The effects of alcohol consumption and aging are similar in that they both may result in impaired cognitive behavior and death of neurons, although the focus and severity of this loss may differ. Both can cause various molecular changes that influence responsiveness to drugs. It is equally true that subtle changes with age in neuronal sensitivity, hepatic enzyme activity, kidney function, and reduced lean body mass may influence responsiveness to alcohol.[85]

Alcohol interacts with a variety of sedative and hypnotic drugs in a manner that decreases the threshold at which effects occur. Consider the likelihood that an older person who drinks alcohol unwisely and develops an unanticipatedly high blood level will be harmed by concomitant use of barbituates, benzodiazepines, or chloral hydrate.

It is noteworthy that, of the one hundred most frequently prescribed drugs, more than half contain an ingredient known to act adversely with alcohol.[86] Here women may be at greater risk than men, for it appears clear that women are heavier users of tranquilizers and other psychoactive drugs[87] and that this pattern continues into advanced age.[88]

Former U.S. Surgeon General Julius Richmond, in a communication to physicians in 1979, offered the following advisory, worth review at this time.

1. Routinely document the history and scrutinize the pattern of alcohol consumption for individual patients to determine the possible relationship between presenting complaints and mixing drugs with alcohol.
2. Be alert to the possible interaction of prescribed, over-the-counter, or illicit drugs—singly or in combination—with alcohol.
3. Pay careful attention to the section in the package insert that deals with drug-alcohol interactions, and consult the current medical literature and references for specific problems.
4. Limit as much as is practical the quantity of drugs dispensed with any one prescription and monitor the patient with regular follow-ups for unexpected reactions to the medication.
5. Consider, both in the choice of therapy and in the evaluation of the patient, the likelihood of the patient's adherence to your admonition (and that of the warning label on the prescription) against using alcohol while taking medication.[89]

TARGET ORGANS

As a simple function of age, because older alcoholics have insulted their organs for a longer period of time, they have more tissue damage than do younger drinkers. Each additional increment of damage is more pernicious, because the organs are already compromised by disease and age.[90]

Acute Effects

Immediate harmful effects of excessive alcohol use in elderly people include:

- *Drug interactions* with psychoactive medications, leading to stupor, coma, and death.
- *Tendency to stagger and fall,* with the possibility of fractures; the associated risks of automobile driving and pedestrian injury.
- *Acute urinary tract obstruction* in men with borderline prostatic hypertrophy (see discussion under "Diuresis").
- *Sleep apnea and respiratory arrest.*
- *Potentiation or inactivation of numerous therapeutic agents,* leading to aggravation of illness. Tricyclic antidepressants, antihypertensives, anticonvulsants, and antibiotics are included. The potentiation of the aspirin anticoagulant effect is especially notable. It may lead to gastrointestinal hemorrhage consequent to gastritis from heavy drinking.
- *Increase in cardiac rate and output, and increase in systolic blood pressure.* Shunting of blood to peripheral vessels through cutaneous vasodilation, leading to loss of body heat and the possibility of accidental hypothermia.
- *Acute gastritis and pancreatitis.*
- *Starvation-associated metabolic ketoacidosis* consequent to preexisting poor diet, vomiting, and concurrent illness.
- *Hypoglycemia.*
- *Attacks of gout.*
- *Masking of the pain of angina pectoris,* a result of the analgesic effect of alcohol, and thus the loss of a warning signal of cardiac distress.

Effects on the Brain

Neuropathological changes in the brain characteristic of chronic alcoholism combine with those of advancing age in an additive fashion. A common result in older drinkers is loss of neurons beyond the threshold of the reserve capacity inherent in all major organs, and the consequent failure of intellectual and other brain functions.

Further insults to the brain may follow as secondary effects of chronic alcoholism. These include reductions in cerebral blood flow, poor nutrition, head injury, traumatic epilepsy, increased incidence of stroke,[91] alcoholic confusional states, and DTs. It is simple to perceive that the decline of cerebral function will thereby be accelerated.[92] The cognitive deficits that result include decreased short term memory, lessened capacity for abstract thinking, hampered ability to carry out complex tasks requiring memory, and disordered visual-spatial relationships.[93]

Anatomic and biological changes in the central nervous system caused by aging or alcohol are similar, insofar as can be determined by the current state of investigational art. Neuroscientist Gerhard Freund points out: "When destruction is so extensive that compensatory processes are insufficient, behavioral deficits will result. A small amount of additional anatomical or biochemical destruction may then cause a great degree of behavioral deficit."[94] We should note, then, that drinking may be devastating to an already intellectually impaired older person.

Both aging and alcohol abuse can also have profound effects on a substantial number of neurotransmitter-neuromodulation systems within the brain,[95] as can withdrawal from alcohol.[96] Normal aging, for instance, produces only moderate decreases in brain serotonin system functions, whereas it causes severe loss in the capacity of the catecholamine systems. Alcoholism, on the other hand, causes marked loss in both of these systems. In brief, both aging and alcohol exert substantial effect on brain catecholamine functions, but differ in their effect on other systems.

In any analysis of these matters we must recognize that alcohol/aging interactions are merely putative, not proved. For example, nutritional controls are largely absent in the various technical studies. Therefore the distinct actions of alcohol or aging are not easily distinguished when measured against partial starvation, debility, or concurrent illness.

In an attempt to explain the neurophysiological and behavioral consequences of alcohol abuse in older people, four theoretical models are proposed: the premature aging model, the right-hemisphere dysfunction model, the generalized dysfunction model, and the frontal-limbic-diencephalic disruptian model.

The premature aging model. Although the point is not absolutely established, there are similarities of behavioral changes in aging and alcohol abuse that suggest that alcohol may advance the clock of aging.[97] This concept is based in part on the observation that older nonalcoholic controls and detoxified alcoholics who are ten to twenty years younger seem to share a number of specific cognitive effects. Evidence for this hypothesis includes (1) a study that showed similar learning curves between thirty-four- to forty-nine-year-old alcoholics and fifty- to fifty-nine-year-old controls[98] and (2) tests of abstraction ability in which older alcoholics performed worse than younger ones. In these tests younger alcoholics were equal in ability to younger controls, but older alcoholics performed worse than older controls. These findings suggest that an interaction between age and drinking could explain older alcoholics' impaired performance, while allowing for the adequate capability of younger drinkers vis-à-vis their control group.[99] Brain tissue obtained from autopsies was tested for reactivity to alcohol. Specimens from older persons were more responsive than those from younger individuals.[100] This information, limited though it may be, tends to suggest that older brains are at greater risk from *contact* with alcohol.

The right-hemisphere dysfunction model.   This model asserts that abnormalities of intellectual function found in alcoholics are lateralized essentially to the right hemisphere of the brain. Numerous studies supporting this point have shown that the verbal skills of alcoholics remain more intact than do those of motor performance.[101] The left brain is known to be responsible for verbal ability, including the capacity to carry out well-rehearsed, practiced, and repetitive tasks using words. The right brain is known to control nonverbal, visual-spatial, and visual-motor functions. This concept has proven to be less sophisticated than the generalized dysfunction model.

The generalized dysfunction model.   This model holds that the toxic effects of alcohol lead to a generalized or diffuse state of cerebral dysfunction. We have noted that in some studies alcoholics seem to preserve verbal as opposed to motor skills, but more advanced research shows that the verbal performance of alcoholics is in fact harmed. Areas of verbal learning, problem solving, and memory are particularly affected. These deficits, when added to those already described in nonverbal abstracting, perceptual-spatial, and motor tasks, appear to support the concept that both right- and left-brain hemispheres become damaged.[102]

Computerized tomography (CT) scans consistently show diffuse enlargement of sulci and ventricles in the brains of alcoholics, indicating the presence of brain atrophy. These findings exist in 50 to 95 percent of alcoholics studied.[103]

In evaluating the validity of the generalized dysfunction model, it is important to note that brain atrophy is a normal finding in CT scans of aged people.[104] No study available distinguishes age versus alcohol as a cause of atrophy. However, since younger chronic alcoholics and normal older people both show atrophy, this information appears to support the premature aging hypothesis.

The frontal-limbic-diencephalic disruption model.   The frontal lobes, limbus, and diencephalon of the brain are known to function in an integrated manner. The disruption model emphasizes the parallels in clinical behavior between chronic alcoholics and patients with frontal lobe and/or limbic abnormalities. There is a relationship between these lesions and the number of years over which patients abuse alcohol.

Neuropsychological studies reveal similarities in organizational ability, capacity to incorporate new information in order to improve performance, spatial scanning in maze tests, and inappropriate social behavior. This includes impairment of restraint in concealing emotion; boasting and self-aggrandizement; expression of hostility and puerility; and limitation of intellectual synthesis ability, including distractability, retention of knowledge, and ability to learn.[105] Further, there is evidence both from CT scans[106] and autopsies[107] that in alcoholic patients with cerebral atrophy the abnormality is predominantly in the frontal lobes.

There is insufficient evidence to support any one of these models as definitive. It is clear, however, that, as it ages, the brain becomes increasingly susceptible to the toxic effects of alcohol. This suggests "a more serious prognosis in elderly alcoholics than in their younger counterparts and that the curtailment of further alcohol abuse in this age group" is important.[108]

Effects on Other Organs

A multitude of harmful consequences to the body from alcohol abuse is recognized. Because old people have old bodies and old organs, it is understandable that their limits of tolerance have become marginal. The following brief review assumes that we are relating the findings to aged individuals.

The liver. Cirrhosis means scarring and shrinking of the liver. In advanced cases, the liver may be reduced to the size of a fist. Resulting signs and symptoms include fatigue, anorexia, weight loss, jaundice, bleeding, gynecomastia, testicular atrophy, and muscle wasting. When hypertension occurs within the portal system, intraperitoneal fluid (ascites) may develop along with peripheral edema, esophageal varices, splenomegaly, and hepatic encephalopathy. Cirrhosis is a common cause of death in this country, often a specific result of massive gastrointestinal bleeding.

Changes in breast tissue and the testicles, evidence of feminization, are evidently a result of the fall in testosterone production and defects in the hypothalamic-pituitary axis. In addition, alcohol has a direct toxic effect on the testicles. Decreased libido follows, with fall in sexual interest and performance.[109]

Liver damage from alcohol starts with simpler and more reversible clinical problems. Cirrhosis is the final stage. A single large binge, or dose of alcohol, can produce a significant fatty change in liver cells. Repeated alcoholic insults make these changes chronic, but fatty liver remains an abnormality that will clear with cessation of drinking.

Acute alcoholic hepatitis is a more threatening development. This is an inflammatory process of the liver cells that develops consequent to severe drinking episodes. It is characterized by malaise, nausea, vomiting, abdominal pain, jaundice, tenderness of the liver, and elevation of the white blood count and hepatic enzymes.

Cardiovascular system.   In addition to acute affects on cardiac performance and blood pressure, alcohol used to excess on a chronic basis has a direct toxic effect on the heart. As a result, disorders such as cardiomyopathy, cardiac fibrosis, and microvascular infarctions may occur. When poor nutrition is added, a common state in chronic alcoholics and in some old people, additional damage to cardiac muscle may take place. This can lead to viral invasion, vitamin deficiency disorders such as beriberi, and alteration of the immune defenses.

Gastrointestinal tract.   The stomach is a particular target organ for alcohol. Ingestion causes a prompt increase in gastric acid flow and a fall in pepsinogen production. The result is a loss of the mucosal barrier to autodigestion, increased permeability of the stomach wall, and erosive gastritis leading to hemorrhage.

Lungs.   Patients with chronic pulmonary diseases such as emphysema or bronchitis are placed at additional risk by alcohol abuse. They are particularly sensitive to the diminished respiratory drive caused by the depressant effect of alcohol on the brain.

Other Consequences

Gout.   Lactic acid levels in the body rise following excess alcohol intake. This is due to the interruption of the enzymatic pathways required for normal metabolism of lactic acid. High levels, in turn, inhibit the secretion of urates by the kidney, leading to hyperuricemia. The acute form of arthritis known as gout develops when urates crystallize in the joints in the form of uric acid.[110]

Diuresis.   Alcohol ingestion causes a decrease in the pituitary gland's release of antidiuretic hormone. The kidney therefore absorbs less water, and an increase in urinary output results. Elderly men whose lower urinary tracts are already partially obstructed by prostatic hypertrophy may exhibit a sudden inability to urinate. This is a medical emergency.[111]

Subdural hematoma.   Obtundation and staggering may lead to falls and head trauma. Subdural hematoma is among the more subtle forms of intracranial injury and may occur without external evidence of damage. It is an insidious process in which venous blood accumulates inside the skull, forming a mass that causes slowly increasing pressure on the brain. If diagnosis is established in a timely fashion, effective treatment is available.

However, in elderly alcoholics who may be perceived as brain-damaged for other reasons, this chance may be lost, and death may occur. The likelihood of subdural hematomas is made evident by Dr. M. M. Glatt's study[112] in an English geriatric hospital. Two-thirds of the patients who were admitted because they were alcoholics showed evidence of injury from falls.

Malnutrition. The acute and chronic effects of alcohol ingestion may severely affect people's ability to maintain normal nutritional standards. This phenomenon results from confusion, depression, decreased appetite, poor absorption, and altered metabolism of nutrients.

Older people who drink are particularly susceptible to the consequences of poor nutrition. The degree of the problem is dependent largely on the extent to which normal nutrients are replaced by those in alcohol.[113]

PHYSICAL DEPENDENCE, TOLERANCE, AND WITHDRAWAL SYMPTOMS

Persistently elevated blood levels of alcohol can produce physical dependence and craving, or addiction.[114] These symptoms result primarily from the results that occur when alcohol use is suddenly stopped. That is, patients feel a compelling urge to drink in order to avoid the anxiety, sleep disturbance, nausea, vomiting, and weakness that accompany falling blood-alcohol levels. It is important to note that a mere *fall* in blood level, rather than complete absence of alcohol in the blood, is often sufficient to create withdrawal symptoms. This clinical picture results from a central nervous system hyperexcitability directly related to decrease in the amount of alcohol bathing the brain cells.

Withdrawal phenomena occur when blood levels of alcohol fall, or when people stop drinking. Severity of the phenomena is closely related to the length of time the patient has been drinking excessively and to the quantity of alcohol ingested.[115] While the symptoms are the same for persons of all ages, the danger of pernicious physical results is greater in older individuals. Symptoms range from commonplace hangover headaches and malaise, through tremors and shakes, to alcoholic hallucinosis, grand mal seizures, and ultimately to DTs. DTs is a serious illness, manifested by confusion, high fever, massive diaphoresis, hallucinations, and major stress upon the cardiovascular system. Significant tachycardia and blood pressure elevations are noted. Death rate is in the range of 20 percent.

Chronic alcohol abuse produces tolerance. People who have become physiologically tolerant must achieve a higher alcohol blood level in order to become intoxicated than at earlier stages of drinking. People who must ingest ever more alcohol in order to achieve their goal place their bodies at increased risk of damage. Internal organs and tissues suffer from the resultant elevated alcohol level; this is especially true for older people, who have lost margins of safety. It must be emphasized that tolerance allows people to function while blood-alcohol levels are high, and that bodily harm proceeds apace.

Great and dangerous cross-tolerance exists between alcohol and other sedative-hypnotic agents. Attempts to calm down an aged person who has a high alcohol blood level through the naive use of such drugs may prove fatal.[116]

APPROACHES TO TREATMENT

GOALS

As Edith Gomberg has put it:

On the basis of the information we have now, alcoholism among older persons exists and needs to be addressed. The data . . . about outreach and response-to-treatment suggest that this is a population . . . [highly] responsive to treatment programs. Above all, we have a moral and ethical obligation to older persons to offer the opportunity to live their sixties, seventies, and eighties with some peace and dignity, which problem drinking undermines.[117]

The harmful effects of therapeutic nihilism pervade the field of alcoholism treatment.[118] When we add negative feelings that health workers may hold about working with older persons,[119] it is possible to understand why this combined set of problems is difficult to resolve. As alcoholism researchers Carlo DiClemente and Jack Gordon point out, "The assumption seems to be that children grow, develop and change but that adults only grow older. How much does this pessimistic view color our stereotype of the elderly as either unable to change or too old to have valuable treatment resources wasted on them?"[120] In fact, older alcoholics are treatable and curable—in general, they are more likely to be successful in this effort than younger people.

Based on the available information, sobriety appears to be a wise and prudent goal for older alcohol abusers. In planning for treatment, we must first understand why the patient is in trouble.[121] What is the driving force behind the call for help? The motivation will ordinarily be either physical distress or the concern of family members. Whatever the reason, action must be taken and a coherent approach developed.

A major test of success for any treatment program lies in finding the people at risk. The challenge here is that alcoholism, in general, is an underreported problem. Gomberg states: "It is estimated that *all* facilities dealing with alcoholism: clinics, hospitals, Alcoholics Anonymous, et cetera, see only about 10% of alcoholics in the United States."[122] Older drinkers are more elusive and less apparent than others. Reasons for this phenomenon, which directly concern case finding and treatment efforts, include: denial; the need to lie, in writing, in order to have patients accepted by long term care facilities, such as nursing homes; attitudes of agency personnel, because older people rarely fit into treatment categories where successful outcome such as return to work can be demonstrated; problems with transportation and finances,[123] which limit the ability of older people to seek treatment; the need to include therapy of medical illness as part of the plan, a resource often missing in alcoholism programs; and the paucity of programs directed specifically to the needs of older drinkers.

This litany of negatives is particularly unfortunate, because workers have had considerable success in helping elderly alcoholics.[124] Certain programs have shown that almost twice as many patients over age sixty complete the course of treatment than do those of younger ages.[125] One explanation offered for this finding is that people who develop alcoholism when older have fewer major psychiatric disorders than long term drinkers.

Even for the latter group, alcoholism is not immutable. The cases of 197 former alcoholics were reviewed[126] when the average age of the group had reached seventy-four, twenty-five years after their first psychiatric hospitalization for alcoholism. Almost two-thirds of these people showed a significant decrease in alcohol consumption. There was also a marked decrease in previously noted psychiatric diagnoses such as depression, mania, and aggressiveness. The social situation had stabilized for many of the former alcoholics. Although they continued to lead relatively dependent lives, they now experienced much less interpersonal conflict. Approximately two-fifths were judged to be in "satisfactory" or "good" condition from the psychiatric standpoint, and only one-fifth showed clear psychiatric pathology.[127]

Therapeutic planning for older alcoholics must incorporate areas of special vulnerability: state of physical and mental health, coordination of tasks, particular attention to social services, and vocational and avocational opportunities. Treatment principles must include, as well, the following components:

1. *Confrontation.*
2. *Clear and transmittable views about abstinence as a measure of success.* There are inevitable disputes about this point. Alcoholics Anonymous perceives abstinence as the only goal, without particular concern for other aspects of life. Other programs seek abstinence but require additional improvements as well; and a third view looks basically for life enhancement without requiring abstinence.
3. *Detoxification,* often in the hospital. Close observation is needed to control withdrawal symptoms, which may be particularly hazardous in the elderly.
4. *Recognition of the risks associated with the use of central nervous system depressant drugs in the detoxification process.*
5. *Rehabilitation and education,* including patient and family.
6. *Long term therapeutic contact,* individually or in groups.
7. Also, consideration of the involvement of patients with AA.

TREATMENT METHODS

A number of treatment methods are now in use for dealing with problem drinking. Current approaches include some that are strictly medical, others that emphasize social and/or group work, and some that are mixed.

Persistent interest pays off, as the following case summary from the files of the Chelsea-Village Program[128] shows.

The patient was an elderly white woman who had had a successful career as a show business agent. She began drinking in her fifties in order to meet the evident social requirements of her male peers. When our staff first met her she was homebound by chronic obstructive pulmonary disease, diarrhea, and weakness. She could not walk and used a wheelchair. Her physical appearance was frail. She ate poorly and evidence of alcohol use was obvious. There was usually a smell of alcohol on her breath. She denied the correlation of her obvious physical deterioration with drinking. "Don't talk to me about that. I'm seventy-six years old and I've been drinking for a long time. I'm not interested in hearing your lecture on drinking. It relieves my boredom and I will give it up as soon as I feel better. . . . I've been drinking a bottle of port a day and it isn't a problem. . . . [My] family never believed in letting our emotions come to the surface."

Our concern was expressed regularly on repeat visits to the patient. She became increasingly paranoid in her thinking, fell several times trying to transfer from bed to wheelchair, and grew demanding and alienating in her behavior. As the situation worsened, the following was recorded:

NURSE: "Do you know you're killing yourself?"

PATIENT: "Yes (crying). You're making me cry. . . . I've got to hold together.

. . . I don't want to talk any more or I'll come apart. I'm very dependent on alcohol to dull the pain of life."

Shortly thereafter she accepted hospitalization for treatment of depression and alcoholism. On our first visit after her return home she looked well, discussed her plans for visits to AA by ambulette, was alert and sparkling in her conversation. "You know, I stopped drinking because . . . well, just look at me. . . . It's not worth it."

A note six months later states that the patient had taken no alcohol in the interval. She had continued her weekly participation in an AA group. "The first time I had an urge to drink was yesterday when I heard that a friend who's an actor was going to my favorite restaurant for lunch. If I was there I would definitely want a drink. I find it quite a relief not having to decide whether I want a drink or I don't want a drink. I just don't drink."

Drug Therapy

The logic behind the medication approach to treatment is the assumption that alcoholics suffer from a general state of dysphoria, with anxiety and depression. People use alcohol to relieve or suppress their feelings. Psychotherapeutic drugs can be used to replace alcohol for this purpose.[129] Evidence for the efficacy of this approach is lacking. Furthermore, as we have noted earlier, drug therapy causes special risks in older people.

Disulfiram (antabuse) treatment programs have achieved success as a preventive for some patients. This drug is completely distinct in its effects from tranquilizers and hypnotics. When taken regularly, it results in severe and threatening physical consequences for people who then drink alcohol. It has no effect otherwise. The disulfiram reaction starts with feelings of heat and flushing of the face and body. Tachycardia follows, with the sensation of palpitation. Then patients note shortness of breath and the need to hyperventilate, followed by nausea and vomiting. These symptoms commonly produce marked feelings of anxiety.[130] Because of the severe physical effects, disulfiram programs seem unwise to recommend for older people, whose health may already be marginal.

Psychosocial Therapies

The principle approaches to psychosocial treatments are based on guidance and counseling. It seems clear that many older alcoholics benefit from a supportive social network in which other people are engaged to help at each stage of treatment and recovery.[131]

Family therapy may be an especially useful concept for older drinkers. It answers the need for social support and works toward resolving isolation and loneliness. Leaving the family out of the treatment program, in contrast, serves to reinforce disengagement and alienation between patient and family.

By its nature, individual psychotherapy must address the patient's main

defense mechanism, denial.[132] Such a treatment lacks pertinence with people of advanced age. Psychotherapists in general seem to recognize this
point and are often reluctant to accept older alcoholics as patients.

Group therapy, on the other hand has proven its value.[133] In groups of
alcoholics, "the sharing of experiences by similarly afflicted persons promotes the development of meaningful insight."[134] Group work has a secondary value as well. It creates a new social network for its members and
relieves the boredom and sense of abandonment that may have led to
alcohol abuse.

AA uses group therapy as its basic concept and is the most effective
available resource for large numbers of alcoholics. AA brings together
people in trouble; it fosters a spirit of mutual understanding and empathy
by peers. AA encourages development of responsibility for others through
one-to-one sponsorships and thereby enhances feelings of self-worth. The
only goal for AA members is abstinence. Excuses, explanations, or ration-
alizations are not accepted.[135] AA welcomes all alcoholics, including the
elderly, and many members are in midlife.[136] Unfortunately, people of
more advanced age are not well represented.

Institutional Programs

Detoxification in acute care hospitals and psychiatric facilities will work.
Then what? Older patients who wish to stay sober may engage in the
variety of therapeutic approaches just discussed. However, for those people too frail for independent life, options are slim. Nursing homes tend to
reject problem drinkers. They are perceived as unwelcome guests who
cause management, health, and social problems. Administrators try to keep
their institutions alcohol-free, but alcohol abuse remains a serious, often
unrecognized and untreated disorder in nursing homes.[137] Incarcerated
patients may use great imagination to sustain their addiction. We know of
an aged amputee in a New York City home who kept his bottle hidden in
his prosthetic leg.

Institutions can be developed into therapeutic sites. The well-known
efforts taking place at the Queen Nursing Home in Minneapolis are a good
example. Until 1973 Queen was a typical nursing home, but over the years
the staff began to recognize that many residents were alcohol abusers
despite efforts to screen them out. "We were caring for people with a
drinking problem anyway, but all we were doing was emptying bottles."[138] Now this nursing home seeks out elderly alcoholics for admission.

Patients are referred to Queen from detoxification centers, hospitals, and
occasionally the courts. The personnel include trained alcoholism counse-
lors. When patients are ready for discharge into the community, careful
plans are made for continuing treatment and support in outpatient programs. Unlike the situation for most nursing home residents, reentry into
society is a genuine goal for these older alcoholics.

CONCLUSION

Examination of demographics, drinking use patterns, and medical consequences of alcohol abuse in the elderly reveals age-specific phenomena that require consideration in diagnosis and treatment. These very factors, along with personality inventories,[139] are already recognized as the basis for classifications of alcoholism in the general populace. However, alcoholics and alcohol abusers have not been categorized according to age-specific factors.[140] This is despite assiduous attempts, some dating to the late nineteenth century, to construct all-inclusive definitions of alcoholism.[141] Dr. E. M. Jellinek's approach to a typological synthesis of alcoholism, published in 1960,[142] appears to have received broad recognition as valid.[143]

There remains a gap in the typology of alcoholism for old persons. It must be recognized that factors specific to advanced age influence the presentation of alcohol-related problems, their manifestations, and the severity of health-related consequences from the ingestion of alcohol. The diagnosis and treatment of alcoholism among the aged requires special training.

PART THREE

HOME CARE

Chapter 6

Long Term
Home Health Care

Most frail older people, when allowed a choice, prefer to remain in their own homes.[1] This judgment is more than a truism about the meaning of home. It is based on fear and hope: fear of the danger of moving to an unfamiliar environment, of placing one's intimate needs in the power of others, and hope of maintaining the independence and the dignity that are essential to controlling one's own life. Charles Dickens makes the point: "Mrs. Gamp's apartment was not a spacious one, but, to a contented mind, a closet is a palace."[2]

Even in the best of nursing homes, residents must generally live by the same clock, eat the same food, and share the same activities. Infantilization is almost an inevitable result and is often associated with confusion, depression, and physical failure.[3] For those people who have a degree of dementia and are able to survive at home because of deep familiarity with the environment, transfer to another location is often devastating.[4] How does one find the bathroom at night? How to get a drink of water? Whom to ask for help among strangers?

When an older person is removed from home for a long time, it is hard to return. The forces that pressed for transfer still exist: family desire, professional opinion, and financial factors. The older person's former home may no longer be available. Even more potent may be the sense of defeat that people feel under these conditions, the idea that all is lost. It takes unusual spunk to keep fighting for independence. The following letter was received by a long term home health care program:

> Dear Sir: I have been trying to get out of this Nursing Home for eight months. They won't let me out. I am 93 ½ years old. I have to find someone I can trust to mail these letters. They took my SSI check away from me. I borrowed the money for these stamps. I wish I had never come here. This is an awful life in here. I don't want to stay here the rest of my life. I want to be at home. I can live cheaper and happier.[5]

Programs that offer long term health care at home for older people allow the spectrum of services to flower at a crucial point in the patients' lives. Assistance is given just when the idea of transfer to an institution is most likely to emerge. Family members and neighbors who may have attempted, on their own, to maintain a safe life at home for the person at risk can become exhausted, afraid of danger to the person's health or survival, and concerned about their degree of responsibility.[6]

Frail older people themselves may be tempted to give up an independent life solely for the security and access to care that an institution offers. The full range of professional services made available by an effective home health care program can make the critical difference. Further, such programs encourage the patient's informal supporters, who may have been frightened away or have urged institutional placement, to return. These people also need assistance and guidance in order to sustain the confidence necessary for sharing in the plan of care.[7]

Recently long term home health care for the aged has been thought of and described as an alternative to institutional placement. This viewpoint is now outdated. It is more appropriate to consider a life at home the desired, natural, and expected mode of care for frail older people. A move to a nursing home is the alternative mode of care.[8]

For effective care of frail older people in their own homes, a competent and motivated team of professional personnel must be engaged, a group with comprehensive skills and experience. The homebound aged are likely to suffer from a complex and multifaceted set of problems, beyond the ability of any one health worker to resolve. The combined efforts of the team members, however, can often make the difference between successful maintenance of the older person at home and transfer or death.

Further, the goals of the staff members must include an overt desire to understand and fulfill the wishes of older people under their care. Health workers, especially physicians, are tempted to impose forcefully their own standards on the weak, ill, and elderly, people who are too passive or afraid to resist. Many an inappropriate or unwanted nursing home admission has been a consequence of the sense that the doctor knows better than the patient what that person's fate should be.[9] This is a potential pernicious factor in such programs, as it is in all of medicine. The paternalistic (perhaps we should also say maternalistic) temptation must be recognized and rooted out. The patient ordinarily knows best, as the following illustrates:

Early in the twentieth century a nursing home was maintained by New York City on Welfare Island, a spot of land in the East River. A physician at Bellevue Hospital, then as now an acute care hospital, had arranged transfer of a gentle, timid, confused, aged woman to Welfare Island. She no longer needed hospital care. The physician approached his elderly patient and told her that she was going to Welfare Island. She looked up at him, anxious and frightened, and said, "But doctor, I don't want to go to *Farewell* Island.[10]

DEFINITION OF TERMS

The field of home care is plagued by problems of definition. Terms like certified home care, home care agency, homemaker, home health aid, housekeeper, long term home health care, and hospital-based and community-based programs are in regular use, although their meaning is imprecise.[11]

Long term home health care programs bring health care workers into the homes of the homebound elderly. A frequent program design incorporates nurses, physicians, and social workers into teams that, through their combined efforts, establish and maintain the health, safety, and stability of the patient.[12] The social worker team member arranges for the assistance of paraprofessionals such as homemakers. The clear goal of such programs is to work with patients over long periods of time, perhaps years, in order to assist aged people to remain at home.

Such programs have been established by the individual initiative of pioneering groups in various localities and thus exist randomly across the country. They may not be supported by the patients' Medicare entitlements. There is thus great variability in their structure, function, funding, and success.

Certified home care programs, on the other hand, exist broadly across the United States, are largely based in acute care hospitals, and are supported by Medicare, Medicaid, and various private insurance carriers, including Blue Cross. State certification of such programs permits these forms of reimbursement. The programs' basic intent is to shorten hospital stays. Typical certified home care patients are discharged with the expectation that nursing and rehabilitative services provided at home will speed their return to normal functioning. They are expected to get well. To exaggerate slightly for effect, the classic home care patient might be a young man who fractures his femur skiing. He may be able to leave the hospital several days early if a home care program provides physical therapists and visiting nurses. In general, these programs are limited to short term care for people who have been hospital inpatients and who, by various government definitions, are deemed to require skilled nursing care.[13] These restrictions make certified home care programs of limited value for aged homebound people, who are likely to require help over prolonged periods of time and, in fact, may never return to functional good health; are usually found in the community rather than in hospitals; and need a range of professional services beyond the scope of such programs. A potent irony of this situation is that Medicare's skilled nursing requirement itself is a bar to care for the chronically ill because the current definition equates "skilled" with "acute." Thus long term nursing care cannot also be "skilled."[14] (See chapter 2 for further discussion of the skilled nursing requirement.)

Paraprofessional services are those given by home attendants, homemakers, home health aides, housekeepers, and other similar employees. Long term home health care requires the availability of such staff members. Certainly the frailest patients need the presence of another human being, merely for the sake of safety, and if no family member or volunteer is at hand a paid employee must be found. For those older people who can help themselves to a degree, assistance may be in order for shopping, cleaning, cooking, bathing, and all those functions generally considered as activities of daily living.

The distinctions between the various forms of paraprofessional care are discussed in chapter 7. However, despite whatever skills such persons can lend, paraprofessionals alone cannot create the essential qualities that allow the frail elderly to remain at home. They require observation, on-site training, and even personal counseling and guidance in order to function effectively.[15]

Emergency response systems have been developed that permit older people living alone to call for help easily. These systems include portable call buttons, which, when pressed, alert a selected person or a twenty-four-hour switchboard, and devices attached to the body that are activated by a change in pulse or respiratory rate. Long term care programs can contract with such systems for their patients.

Various *therapies*—such as physical and occupational therapy and nutritional counseling—may occasionally be useful. Sometimes it is mandated that personnel with these skills be included on the team (see "The Nursing Home Without Walls" section for a discussion of how this works). It should be recognized, though, that forcing the services of such therapists on very old, chronically disabled persons may lead to frustration and pointless expense. The judgment of the basic professional team members who know the patient best, along with that of the patient and family members, should guide the decision about seeking this form of service.

The same questions arise in regard to the use of *high-technology services.* It is now possible to provide advanced life support at home through renal dialysis, mechanical ventilation, and parenteral nutrition. Complex forms of cancer chemotherapy and other drugs can be provided through permanently sited cannulas inserted into the great vessels.[16]

In fact, with these high-tech developments it is possible to create a minihospital for each homebound patient, complete with equipment and the necessary technical staff.[17] Furthermore, because these forms of treatment are considered acute care, Medicare will pay their costs. The availability of these technologies suggests a developing paradox. It is encouraging that an ever sicker and more disabled group of patients can receive essential care at home. In this sense perhaps we can say that home care has come of age. On the other hand, the use of advanced technology in the home, especially as it may be applied to the frailest of old people, is disturbing. It seems to threaten some of the tenets that have made the original long term home health care programs distinctive: concern for human needs, the quality of life, and prudent use of resources and funds.[18]

Once again we face an irony in which substantial sums are spent on advanced treatment of end-stage disease, while at the same time modest expenditure is denied for simpler long term care services needed to keep the frail elderly from institutional placement. Moreover, high-tech service opportunities have attracted entrepreneurs who have devised methods for tapping Medicare and promoting their wares so that profit, rather than humane care, is the goal. The proper way to incorporate technological advances into home care thus remains an unresolved issue. Most important, we must be certain that older people control the course of events and not allow them to become objects plugged into machines for the benefit of others.

VALUES AND SIGNIFICANCE OF LONG TERM HOME HEALTH CARE

Despite these various efforts, the nature and structure of long term care services for the aged in this country are generally perceived as unsatisfactory. Gerontologists Rosalie and Robert Kane point out[19] that the control of spending for the current set of programs, almost entirely attributed to expenditures for nursing home care, has become an intractable problem. Long term institutional costs in 1984 were estimated to be in the range of $26 billion, paid for about equally by public and private sources, and are expected to reach $76 billion by 1990. Because of the demographic imperative, pressure for expansion of nursing home services continues and, at the same time, is strongly resisted by those who will be required to pay the costs. State governments in particular, which usually must bear at least half of Medicaid expenditures, struggle against the creation of more nursing home beds, often through the tactic of denying certificates of need. Note that Medicaid is the most prominent source of public expenditure for nursing homes because people who must pay the cost themselves, estimated to be about $30,000 per year, usually become impoverished rather quickly. At this point Medicaid eligibility is reached, and the state must pick up the tab.[20]

With few exceptions,[21] the federal government has remained aloof from developing policies and programs to support long term care at home. Medicare, which would seem to be the logical vehicle for this development, has remained almost entirely an insurance program for acute care.[22] Over the last decade legislation has repeatedly been discussed and introduced before Congress to amend Medicare and to alter its focus. These attempts have been thwarted by anxieties about costs.[23] In fact, the degree to which home care programs save money, if they do, remains in dispute. Depending on the needs of the respondent, these programs may or may not be cost effective.[24]

The major concern is that, with a revamped Medicare, people who have somehow been surviving at home without looking to the government for support would be entitled to financial help. There is fear that families that have been coping and caring for their aged relative would now perceive the task as the government's. There exists the risk that proprietary businesses would enter the professional home care field in order to capitalize on the new monies and devise means for milking the system.

In fact, it is evident that there are large numbers of older people who could benefit from professional home health care, homemakers, and/or home health aides. The Department of Health and Human Services estimates that for every resident of a nursing home, there are two or three persons living in their own homes who are fully as disabled.[25] These people have resisted nursing home placement, even though in due time their care would be paid for by Medicaid, because they do not wish to pauperize themselves and because they value deeply the ability to control their own lives.

EXEMPLARY LONG TERM
HOME HEALTH CARE PROGRAMS

Over the last fifteen years long term home health care services for the frail aged have been developed across this country. A wide variety of organizations have sponsored these programs, including indigenous community groups, medical schools, hospitals, and government at various levels, usually with the goal of bringing help to those who need it.²⁶ Financially motivated enterprises have appeared as well.²⁷

The means to support these programs have been equally various. In some instances the combination of sweat equity, volunteer assistance, payment in kind, and private philanthropy has served. Other programs, developed by innovative legislators, have used state-controlled funds, such as Medicaid, to create and sustain these efforts. The federal government, while maintaining a strict view of Medicare as an acute care insurance program, has supported examples as research demonstrations. In these instances multiple purposes are served: Lessons are learned about policy, techniques, and costs of long term care at home; because demonstrations are limited in time (usually to three or four years), no permanent federal commitment is implied; some older people actually receive significant services; and those people in the health care field pressing for change are placated, albeit temporarily. In only one instance—the Social/Health Maintenance Organization (S/HMO)—has consistent federal support been placed behind a long term home health care program.²⁸ Thus we face a quandary: Most frail older people prefer to live at home; our various layers of government now pay substantial sums for nursing home care; the need for long term care services is increasing and will continue to grow; and yet any significant move to change policy is thwarted by fear of yet further costs.

To resolve these concerns, a number of projects have been developed and conducted in recent years. Through these efforts, we now have substantial information about the nature, structure, costs, need, and value of long term home health care, but the courage for legislative and executive action generally remains lacking.²⁹

THE NURSING HOME WITHOUT WALLS: NEW YORK STATE'S LONG TERM HOME HEALTH CARE PROGRAM

New York State Senator Tarky Lombardi, Jr., who developed the Nursing Home Without Walls legislation, has said:

Now think about it. What type of program would you want to be in? Would you want to be in an acute care bed? Would you want to spend the rest of your life in a nursing home bed? Or would you prefer to spend the rest of your life at home, with your own family, with your own friends, with your own neighbors, with your own community? . . . I, for one, don't want to be in a nursing home if I can avoid it. I hope to live out my old age and die with dignity in my home if I can . . . with my family with me.³⁰

During the mid-1970s, Lombardi developed the concept of Medicaid-supported long term care legislation.[31] The driving force behind the creation of this effort was Lombardi's strong personal feeling about the manner in which older people were treated, combined with a logical theory and rationale designed to correct a number of the obvious aberrations in the existing long term care system. These included excessive expenditure of public funds, frequent instances of inappropriate institutionalization, fragmenting of care in those situations where attempts were made to keep the elderly at home, a reimbursement system that clearly favored institutions over home care, and lack of focus on discharge planning and case management.[32]

Lombardi's innovative proposal thrived partly because of New York's history of approving and assisting pioneer developments in health care. Examples of this, which have led to changes on the national scene, include support of the Montefiore Hospital Home Care concept in the late 1940s;[33] revision in nursing home policies, following the reports of the Moreland Commission on the scandals in the industry, during the 1970s;[34] and leadership in development of prospective reimbursement rate setting in the 1970s and 1980s.[35]

The intent of Lombardi's legislation was to create the opportunity for people who were candidates for nursing homes instead to remain in their own homes. This goal was to be achieved through the establishment of Long Term Home Health Care Programs (LTHHCPs) throughout New York State. His bill delineated the specific services that homebound persons could receive and included a cap on costs. It was approved by the New York legislature and signed in 1977 by then-Governor Hugh Carey.[36] Support for this initiative was provided, in part, by the federal Health Care Financing Administration (HCFA), through a waiver of the Social Security Act, which permitted reimbursement under Medicaid for certain services to patients that were not previously allowed.[37]

At the heart of Lombardi's concept was the view that it made sense for the state to help older people remain in their own homes, if they so desired and were otherwise eligible for nursing home placement, and if the costs to government were not higher than those that would be incurred through nursing home care. Thus the program allows a broad range of professional services for people in their homes; establishes eligibility criteria that permit participation only for those people who also meet state standards for nursing home placement; requires that case management be the responsibility of a single provider; and provides that expense to the state be controlled by the establishment of a 75 percent cap on the costs for each person kept at home under the program, compared to the cost of institutional placement for the same individual. The Lombardi programs are particularly distinguished from all other long term home health care programs because services are provided permanently and as an entitlement to eligible patients and are paid for by government. Table 6.1 lists the services available.

CASE MANAGEMENT

The Lombardi legislation required that case management services be available to each enrolled patient twenty-four hours a day. Thus someone who knew the patient was always on call to deal with any issue. When the regulations for implementing the Lombardi programs were subsequently developed by the New York State Department of Health, case management functions were somewhat obscured. On the one hand, oversight responsibility, which was regularly interpreted as control over some elements of case management, was mandated to employees of the local health departments; on the other, program staff members, particularly the social workers, whose skills and experience were critical to proper care, clearly knew each patient best. This bureaucratic engima has gradually worked out so that the professional staff members are truly responsible for decisions about health care services and government employees are usually limited to oversight of budgets and the requisite monitoring of program organizations to affirm their probity.

ENROLLMENT AND ELIGIBILITY

The original financial requirements allowing individuals to enroll in Lombardi programs were identical to those for Medicaid entitlement, and only people who would *require* institutional placement were acceptable.

TABLE 6.1
Services Provided by the Nursing
Home Without Walls Program[38]

Required Services	Optional Services
Skilled nursing	Physician care at home
Social service case work	Respite care
Respiratory therapy	Day care
Nutrition counseling	Home repairs and improvements
	Social transportation
	Meals-on-Wheels
	Assistance in moving
	Laboratory services
	Medical supplies/equipment

Over the years these guidelines have become somewhat more liberal: People are permitted to enroll if they are deemed medically *eligible* for institutional placement; and private payment is allowed, so that people who have income or assets marginally above the Medicaid limits can pay a share of the costs and be given care.

CONTROL OF COSTS

The legislation and regulations require (with rare and brief exceptions) that the annualized cost for services of an enrolled patient not exceed 75 percent of the cost of institutional care for someone with a similar degree of disability. The theoretical basis of this decision lies in the assumption that about 25 percent of institutional costs are attributable to provision of shelter and food, expenses that the enrollee at home would bear regardless of program participation. Hence the name Nursing Home Without Walls is appropriate. The dollar value of the cap varies with the locality of the individual program within New York State and is designed to reflect local cost differentials.

By mid-1986, financial analysis of the patients enrolled in the Lombardi programs across the state revealed that total costs averaged slightly less than 50 percent of institutional costs in the local area.* In 1981, the first nine pilot programs were established. By mid-1986, sixty-eight had been created spottily across the state, and more are in the planning stage. A total of 7,317 individuals were under active care at home as of June 1986.[39] Although hampered by rigidity within the bureaucracy, the Lombardi programs represent legislative initiative at its strongest. The programs are the best available example of how a national long term home health care program could be planned and implemented.

LONG TERM HOME CARE DEMONSTRATIONS: MEDICARE AND MEDICAID WAIVERS

In the 1970s and through the 1980s the federal government, sometimes in association with the states, supported a variety of experimental long term home care programs.[40] These projects were funded largely through waivers that allowed payment for services usually prohibited under Medicare and Medicaid regulation.[41] The programs varied widely in geographical base,

*Office of New York State Senator Tarky Lombardi, Jr., personal communication, October 13, 1986.

number of patients served, length of time in operation, number and nature of waivered services, and overall degree of success. They were similar only in their focus on ways to integrate services to older people as a means of helping them remain in their own homes.[42]

The demonstrations can be divided into two general types: the brokerage model and the consolidated direct services model.[43] Connecticut's Triage program was the most prominent of the brokerage type and the On Lok Community Care Organization for Dependent Adults in San Francisco continues as a highly successful example of a consolidated service program.

THE TRIAGE PROGRAM IN CONNECTICUT

Triage was a model program that served to coordinate the provision of health and social services for the frail, homebound elderly in a seven-town region of central Connecticut from 1974 to 1981. The program focused on overcoming the problems inherent in obtaining a variety of assistance piecemeal for each client. This patchwork approach demands that older people summon strong organizational skills, energy, and knowledge simply to pull together and execute a coherent plan of care for themselves. For instance, home-delivered meals, Medicare entitlements, Medicaid eligibility, local transportation resources, all must be sought and obtained separately. Triage, through its control over the allocation of all pertinent resources, was able to function as a broker.

> The patchwork of funding sources for health care services only mirrors the fragmentation of services within the broader health care system. At Triage we refer to this health care system as the "non-system system." People who can afford to pay for available services often do not know how to get to them. . . . [To] manipulate the various systems through which services are provided is frequently frustrating for the individual . . . [who] often gives up and goes without a needed service rather than cope with the red tape required.[44]

Joan Quinn, the conceptual force behind and leader of Triage, has summarized the project's objectives:[45] (1) provide a single-entry mechanism to coordinate delivery of institutional, ambulatory, and in-home services for older people; (2) develop appropriate preventive medicine and supportive services; (3) establish an integrated local service delivery system; (4) obtain public and private financial support for the full service spectrum; and (5) demonstrate the cost effectiveness of coordinated care, including prevention of illness and disability, support for independent life at home, and use of resources appropriate to demonstrated need rather than according to reimbursement restrictions of third-party payers.[46]

During the seven and one-half years Triage was in operation, it served 2,628 people with an average age of seventy-eight; they were largely frail and predominantly widows who lived alone and had minimal financial resources. A substantial additional number regularly remained on a waiting list. The usual reason that help was originally sought was that problems in providing care at home and/or in obtaining needed services were swamping family, friends, other local agencies, and the clients themselves. During the program's first several years, entry into Triage simply required that the applicant be sixty years of age or older, Medicare eligible, and a local resident. Later, because of growing demand, those accepted had to demonstrate that they were at high risk for institutional placement.

The extensive range of services available through Triage included: paraprofessional assistance; nurse and physician visits; psychological and financial counseling; transportation; home-delivered meals; arrangements for nursing home placement when indicated; assistance with chores; obtaining medications, supplies, and equipment; and physical and other therapies. The Triage staff functioned as a coordinator in obtaining these services for patients, rather than as provider of direct, hands-on care itself, and had relationships with about three hundred different agencies.[47]

Finance and Waivers

Triage, and the supportive services that it arranged, was largely supported by Medicare waivers. These were granted in 1975 by the Department of Health, Education, and Welfare, under the authority provided by the Social Security Amendments of 1972. Among the allowed waivers were those for duration, amount, and scope of services; the omission of deductible and coinsurance payments by patients; and the skilled nursing requirement. From 1979 to 1981, patients were asked to share in the costs, when feasible, to compensate in part for the expense of the waivered services. During these latter years, Triage enrollees contributed almost $400,000, or about 10 percent, of the cost of care, all of which was returned to the Medicare Trust Funds.

The Medicare waivers were of critical value to the theoretical principle and daily function of Triage.

[They] made it possible to authorize payment for many ancillary and supportive services not traditionally covered by Medicare, such as pharmaceuticals, dental care, mental health services, homemaker services, glasses and hearing aids. Moreover, many specific Medicare requirements such as deductible and coinsurance, as well as several restrictions on home health care, were waived.[48]

Transportation

During the first years that Triage was in operation, patients often had to wait long periods of time for transport. Subsequently, through the development of a mix of arrangements, the difficulty was moderated. Voluntary agencies, such as the Red Cross, gave some help. Other resources, including commercial taxis and liveries and ambulette/ambulance services, were obtained through contract.

Financial Relations with the Government

Triage struggled from start to finish to maintain its financial viability. The various federal agencies involved over the years included the Administration on Aging (AOA); the HCFA, which funded the Medicare waivers; the Public Health Service; and the National Center for Health Services Research. Each had its own goals, and Triage was required to alter its own intent and change course frequently in order to meet federal agency requirements.

Ultimately, the ending of Triage must be explained by the government's perception that all demonstrations must have a relatively brief life.

Results

The functional status of Triage patients and the total of costs incurred in their care were compared with those of a control group. Triage patients had notably smaller nursing home costs but greater expenses for home care services and acute inpatient hospital care than the controls. On balance, the total cost for both groups was about the same. It must be recognized that the registered patients received substantial services and that regular review of their health status was a consistent element in the program. The controls, on the other hand, made virtually no use of paraprofessional help, such as homemaker, chore, and companion services.[49] Presumably lack of access to these and other services inevitably led the controls to evidence both smaller costs for home care services and higher rate of nursing home placement.

In her summary of the Triage experience, Quinn makes the following points: (1) The brokerage model of long term care service development can be an effective means of controlling costs; (2) the costs of providing access to a comprehensive array of medical and social services for the frail elderly are not significantly higher than the provision of fewer services given "in a haphazard manner in the traditional system"; and (3) the idea that a community agency can function effectively as a broker for services has been established, is viable, and is replicable.[50]

Despite the fact that major effort was placed upon individual counseling, when the Triage program was terminated, many people lost access to care and guidance. Quinn noted that the traumatic effect of the termination process on Triage clients and their families or supporters should not be underestimated.

The Department of Health and Human Services conducted the National Long Term Channeling Demonstration[51] between September 1980 and

June 1986. This was a large-scale research project designed to test whether a carefully managed approach to providing community-based long term care could help control overall long term care costs. Initial data provide equivocal results.[52] Unfortunately, lessons learned from earlier efforts such as Triage were not fully incorporated into the Channeling demonstration, so a continuum of knowledge is lacking. Instead in Quinn's phrase, another "island of research inquiry"[53] may have been created.

ON LOK SENIOR HEALTH SERVICES

On Lok is a free-standing agency in San Francisco that offers a full range of services to older people. It is the product of efforts by a group of concerned individuals in the Chinatown-North Beach-Polk Gulch area of the city who, in 1966, began to be concerned that local aged people, many of whom did not speak English, lacked effective access to health care, housing, and social services.[54] The need for services is explained: ". . . tucked away behind the stores, in the hotel rooms above the nightclubs [of this world famous area of San Francisco] are 18,000 older adults, many with limited incomes . . . and more than a few physically impaired and confused—sometimes too frail even to seek help."[55]

The founders of On Lok, in their original planning, took particular note of the varied needs and diverse ethnic mix of the population they wished to serve. Goals from the start included both meeting the desires of each older person and, at the same time, holding down costs. All services were to be controlled centrally, through a consolidated model of care.[56]

On Lok emphasizes the need for the caregivers to have full control over assessment and provision of services and also the incorporation of teams of professionals into the program so that multiple disciplines are involved. All personnel, including paraprofessionals, share as equally as possible in decisions about clients.[57]

History

On Lok's staff recognizes the growth of the agency as taking place in three phases.

During phase 1, from 1972 to 1975, the initial component, a day health center, was planned, established, and staffed by permanent professional employees, supported by a grant from the federal AOA. Its first home was a nightclub renovated to serve as a storefront day center. The success of this venture subsequently encouraged the state to make adult day health center care reimbursable by Medicaid across California. Those individuals without Medicaid coverage might have been forced out by the new regulations.

In order to help its local residents placed at risk by the advent of Medicaid support, the organization sought new funding from AOA. During the years of phase 2, from 1975 to 1979, these new monies, supplied under a Model Project on Aging grant, allowed the organization to recognize that an entire continuum of care might grow at On Lok. Perhaps the most striking development of these three years was the completion of plans to establish a congregate housing facility for the frail elderly. The building, called On Lok House, was constructed *de novo* with funds supplied by the federal Department of Housing and Urban Development. Section 8 waivers were obtained, and first occupancy took place in the fall of 1980. It is perhaps this event that best fulfills the definition of the Chinese words *On Lok* as "happy, peaceful abode."[58]

In phase 3, from 1979 to date, the design of a full-service program nearly reached fruition at On Lok. However, the ability to control all services that clients might need was still lacking. The goal for phase 3 thus focused on finding the means to integrate physicians, hospitals, and nursing homes with day health and social services into a single system of care for each enrolled person and developing a payment system that would make the entire program viable.

The organization received support from the federal Office of Human Development Services for a four-year plan to develop and study a full spectrum of long term care services for the elderly. The project, entitled Community Care Organization for Dependent Adults (CCODA), was provided with Medicare Section 222 waivers for the hands-on service component by the HCFA. Through CCODA, On Lok moved toward a balanced, flexible distribution of services that attempted to give equal weight to social and support need of clients.[59] Enrollment was limited to 180 persons, and during the four years of the project, almost five hundred individuals were served.[60]

Home Care in the CCODA

On Lok strives to bring all patients to its day health centers for medical care. Even when patients are acutely ill, the preference is to use its transportation resources to move the patient rather than to send the staff into the home.[61] Professional staff members rarely make home visits.

Other forms of home care, those given by paraprofessional employees in particular, are a more substantial part of On Lok. From the start, some services were supplied to patients at home as a supplement to the day health centers. Examples include delivery of meals, help with chores, and assistance from attendants. When, under CCODA, the home care component became reimbursable, the set of services expanded remarkably and increased by a cost factor of ten between the first and fourth years. On Lok now employs twenty-six health workers/attendants for in-home support, along with supervisors. This groups makes up about one-quarter of the organization's total staff.[62]

Although On Lok continues to perceive its day care centers as the focus for health services, the variety of resources offered to homebound clients has grown. Despite the program's original design, growth in the direction of home care has developed at On Lok. Reasons for this may include: increased age and fraility of the clients, the wishes of the clients themselves, the fact that under On Lok's latest formulation these services are reimbursable, and the common sense of the staff, which recognized a need that had not been anticipated in the program design.

On Lok has worked toward financial self-sufficiency while at the same time trying to remain a resource for all people who need help. Clients not eligible for the new waivers could have caused a dangerous financial drag on the agency. Thus in 1983, during the final phase of government-guaranteed reimbursement under CCODA, plans were made to offer non-Medicaid clients the option of cost sharing, through copayments and service charges. When the services allowed under new federal laws started, a cadre of clients, about two-thirds of whom were determined to have personal financial responsibility, were ready to receive services and to pay for them. Some clients left the program rather than pay. The On Lok staff had learned that:

> . . . in our current political and economic system, services that are "free" to the health consumer. . . . are unrealistic except in a time-limited demonstration situation. Participants, as well as other funding sources in the traditional system such as Medicaid and private insurers, need to be involved in paying for community-based long-term care if [it] is to be available on a broad basis.[63]

The Post–CCODA Period

In 1983, when the four-year demonstration ended, a financial crisis reemerged. On Lok told the federal government that it was willing to risk assuming fiscal responsibility for its own operation, subject to the receipt of Medicare and Medicaid waivers, which, with a certain quantity of self-pay income, would be sufficient for viability. This time, however, HCFA failed to come through. As a result, On Lok took the unusual step of seeking a special congressional bill that would allow the needed waivers; even more unusual, it succeeded. The key legislative provision reads as follows:

> Section 603[c] of the Conference Report on the Social Security Amendments of 1983 provides the Secretary shall approve "the risk-sharing application of On Lok Senior Health Services for [Medicare and Medicaid] waivers . . . in order to carry out a [thirty-six-month] demonstration project for capitated reimbursement for comprehensive long-term care services."[64]

In 1986 Congress approved legislation making Medicare and Medicaid support to On Lok available indefinitely. The organization has started to help other agencies across the country carry out similar risk-sharing ventures.[65]

THE CHELSEA–VILLAGE PROGRAM,
ST. VINCENT'S HOSPITAL AND MEDICAL CENTER OF NEW YORK

The Chelsea-Village Program (CVP) started its work in 1973 and is distinguished from other long term home health care developments that have been discussed by its theoretical and philosophical basis and its means of financial support. The CVP is a component of the Department of Community Medicine at St. Vincent's Hospital and Medical Center of New York. As such, it exists in order to carry out the hospital's mission to care for the sick poor.[66] St. Vincent's, which was founded in 1849 by the Sisters of Charity of St. Vincent de Paul, continues to serve this mission even though it has become a modern, eight hundred-bed tertiary care institution.

The CVP has among its goals overcoming barriers to care for its frail, homebound aged patients. Thus requiring payment for its professional services would be antithetical. All CVP patients, most of whom lack adequate funds of their own, receive services without reimbursement to the program from any formal source.

Finances

Financial viability of the CVP stems from three roots. St. Vincent's Hospital itself has been, from the start, the stalwart support of the program. Despite the potent forces at work in New York State that have threatened the very existence of not-for-profit hospitals since the early 1970s, St. Vincent's has paid relevant administrative and professional salaries and provided the staff with offices, equipment, and supplies. A portion of a New York State Health Department grant to the hospital's Department of Community Medicine, allocated to the CVP, provided valuable assistance for several years. Finally, financial contributions from foundations and private individuals have been offered consistently. Money has been available for the program to sustain itself and in fact to thrive. No patient has ever been turned away because resources were lacking, and each year the number of aged people under active care at home has grown. Further, since the CVP is not regulated by government, there are no arbitrary restrictions on eligibility, duration of care, or nature of services.

Observations made in the hospital's emergency room in the early 1970s led to recognition that aged people, particularly those living alone and too disabled to reach out for help, were a medically unreached group.[67] They were regularly brought in by ambulance, either moribund or dead on arrival. Two physicians, a nurse who was a Sister of Charity, and a social worker/community organizer developed what seems now to be a simplistic, hearts-and-flowers view that teams of professional staff members should seek out the frail aged in the local community—the Chelsea and Greenwich Village areas of Manhattan—and help them before help was too late.

As the number of persons referred increased over the first six months, the CVP was required to seek more staff members. The demands for help soon outstripped the capacity of the original team. At first, volunteers within the hospital's social service department provided casework assistance, but a full-time staff member with social work skills soon became essential. By 1986 the paid CVP staff had increased to six: two social workers; a nurse, who has been with the program from the start; a van driver, who doubles as an electrocardiogram technician; a homemaker; and a coordinator.

Physician Involvement

It is noteworthy that all physician services to CVP patients over the fourteen years of its existence have been volunteered, and no program doctor has ever accepted any form of financial reimbursement.[68] The first medical services were provided by young attending physicians and medical residents; thus, since most were on salary, they were in a sense supported by St. Vincent's Hospital. However, these doctors assumed CVP workloads in addition to their ordinary duties. The physician volunteer effort continued to grow, so that by 1987 about fifteen different physicians, some in private practice, participated during a typical week. In addition, in the same spirit of service, subspecialists from all major disciplines have made themselves available for the home care of patients.

Why have doctors been willing to sustain their interest and concern in this work? The following comments from a CVP staff conference are pertinent:

ATTENDING PHYSICIAN: What good does it do you, in your development as a physician, to work in this kind of program?

MEDICAL RESIDENT: I think it does three things. It gets me out of the hospital and out of the structured part of the training program, both of which give me a very parochial view of medicine. Also, it introduces me to homebound old people, an opportunity I wouldn't get any other way. This is important because I intend to practice Internal Medicine, and I need this experience. And, number three, it gives me humility—it teaches me about old people and their problems and what I can and can't do as a doctor.

FELLOW IN COMMUNITY MEDICINE: The perspective in the hospital is limited. When we take care of a patient inside the institution, it's hard to look beyond the hospital environment. In this program we see the patients in the outside world, and we interact with the reality of their eating habits, their living space, their neighbors, their connections with people around them—or their lack of connection. This is valuable to me, because people live in the real world. They don't live in the hospital all the time.

MEDICAL RESIDENT: In the hospital I have a tendency to look at patients on paper. I see a lab result, and add medicines here, and add a test there. I've learned in this work that it isn't always necessary to do just that in order to care for patients adequately. Some of my patients who are living in their own environment are getting along very well. I find there's not such a great need to correct everything on paper if they're functioning well as people. There's a great old man I've seen up on Greenwich Avenue who has slight swelling of his legs. In the hospital situation I would give him a diuretic, but this would make him miserable at home because he can't get to the bathroom easily. At home, I just have him elevate his legs, and he's doing fine.

FELLOW IN COMMUNITY MEDICINE: I had a chance to work in the outside world, and now I'm back in the inside world again. As house officers, we're unrealistic about illness. We tend to think that if the patient isn't having a myocardial infarction and in cardiogenic shock, he doesn't belong in the hospital, and that ends our concern. But most illness is not that way. This is not necessarily what you see when you become a doctor in the real world. In this program we're very much in that world.

ATTENDING PHYSICIAN: The value of this work to me is the opportunity it gives for fulfillment of deep personal and professional goals. I'm able to pay back to the society I live in some of the debt I feel for being given the chance to be a doctor. And also I find a lot of gratification in knowing that my skill and experience are useful to helpless old people who might otherwise be dead or in a nursing home—and who don't want to be. I'm really happier when I'm working in this program than in any other part of my professional life.[69]

The secondary gains are perhaps more significant than money. The following letter received by the CVP from the son of a patient, himself a physician, who had died at home while under the program's care suggests the feelings that are at work.

It has been a month and a half since dad died, but I still think back on his 90 good years and his two years of hell. To him hell was reflected in his saying, "I used to be a doctor but now I'm just a schmatte." To him being a doctor meant loving and caring for and about people.

TABLE 6.2

*Age and Sex
Distribution upon
Entrance to the
Chelsea-Village
Program*

Decade	No. of Patients
20 to 29	4
30 to 39	11
40 to 49	17
50 to 59	49
60 to 69	193
70 to 79	508
80 to 89	606
90 to 99	123
100+	6
Unknown	0
TOTAL	1,517

NOTE: men = 535; women = 878.
SOURCE: Department of Community Medicine. (1987). *Chelsea-Village Program 14-Year Report.* New York: St. Vincent's Hospital.

TABLE 6.3

*Marital Status on Admission
to Chelsea-Village Program*

Marital Status	Number	% Male	% Female
Unknown	48	47	53
Single	394	39	61
Married	297	62	38
Widowed	670	20	80
Divorced	70	42	58
Separated	34	50	50
Other	4	0	100

SOURCE: *Chelsea-Village Program 14-Year Report.*

For me the warmest memory I will carry in my heart is that of a sick, tired, and not always coherent old man reaching up and kissing his doctor. This was his benediction on a doctor who loved and cared as he did. That which will live with me forever is the gentle kiss which was returned to him.[70]

Results 1973–1986

In its first fourteen years of service, the CVP and its staff have made more than eighteen thousand home visits and cared for about fifteen hundred patients. Their average age is eighty-three; two-thirds are women; two-thirds live alone; all have been homebound on admission to the program. Tables 6.2 through 6.6 delineate their characteristics, based on statistics from January 1973 to December 1986.[71] The program continues to use teams of professional staff members in making home visits and has grown so that it operates forty hours per week, with about 160 individuals under care at any one time. Patients can always reach a CVP physician via an on-call system.

Lessons have been learned. Among them, according to CVP staff, is the necessity for entry requirements that make common sense. From the start, in order to receive help, patients simply needed to be homebound by reasonable definition, geographically reachable, out of contact with the health care system, and willing to accept the CVP team. The latter point deserves emphasis. CVP staff members learned quickly that some older patients avoided contact and rejected much-needed care because of concern that they might be manipulated. Their fears were focused, it seemed, on being placed in an institution and losing their independence, their own homes. The comment of a ninety-two-year-old woman, on the team's first visit to her, is considered representative: "The only thing I'm worrying about is keeping out of a nursing home."[72]

TABLE 6.4

Degree of Isolation of the 1517 patients
on Admission to Chelsea-Village Program

	Number/Percentage
Living Alone	*905/59.66*
Living with others	*612/40.34*
Spouse	260/17
Child(ren)	167/11
Parent(s)	13/1
Other relatives	99/7
Same-sex roommate	45/3
Opposite-sex roommate	28/2

SOURCE: *Chelsea-Village Program 14-Year Report.*

TABLE 6.5

Primary Causes of Homeboundedness

Disability		Number of Patients
Orthopedic:		*374*
Arthritis	153	
Previous fractures	105	
Intervertebral disc	4	
Paget's disease of bone	11	
Amputation(s)	31	
Other orthopedic	70	
Neurological Disease		*176*
Cerebrovascular accident (stroke)	96	
Parkinson's disease	20	
Poliomyelitis—old	4	
Spinal cord tumor	2	
Multiple sclerosis	14	
Peripheral neuropathy	2	
Other neurological	38	
Medical Disorders		*693*
Chronic pulmonary disease	98	
Cardiac disease	139	
Chronic alcoholism	20	
Cirrhosis of liver	3	
Obesity	14	
Anemia	3	
Peripheral vascular disease	31	
Generalized debility and weakness	184	
Blindness	22	
Malignancies	70	
Lung	21	
Breast	11	
Gastrointestinal tract	18	
Prostate	20	
Other medical	109	
Psychiatric—Psychosocial Disorders		*183*
Dementia	113	
Mental retardation	8	
Psychosis	17	
Anxiety	14	
Other psychiatric	31	
Other		*28*
Not homebound		*63*
TOTAL		1,517

SOURCE: *Chelsea-Village Program 14-Year Report.*

Based on these early experiences, the CVP's goal evolved: to help aged people remain independent, in their own homes, out of institutions, and in the best possible state of health.

CONCLUSION

Human beings are most fulfilled when they are able to use all their personal resources—strength, intelligence, drive, and life experience—independently. It is especially characteristic of our pluralistic country to strive for this kind of freedom. People of greatly advanced age are likely to have decreasing authority over their own lives, a situation most dramatically exemplified by loss of their own homes. This may occur in the most arbitrary of ways—for example, through institutional placement without permission. It is far more common, however, for older people to be trapped subtly by the paternalistic and maternalistic feelings of those around them. The consequences range from an overly cushioned life at home, with power to make decisions removed, to nursing home placement, which assuages family guilt and fear about the costs of freedom for the older person.

Elderly people must be asked for their own definitions of life's goals, and

TABLE 6.6
Sources of Referral to Chelsea-Village Program

Source	Number of Referrals
Settlement house	90
Community service agencies(includes 115 from Visiting Nurse Service of New York)	272
Government agencies	73
Church-related	34
Community individuals	304
Hotel managers	8
St. Vincent's hospital referrals (Includes 73 from Certified Home Care Department and 265 from hospital physicians)	705
Other hospitals	31
TOTAL	1,517

SOURCE: *Chelsea-Village Program 14-Year Report.*

we must serve them as they seek those goals. The alternative, to inflict on them our own ideas of what is right, is pernicious.

Long term home health care programs help the most frail of older people maintain a significant choice: where to live. Most such persons will be strong candidates for nursing home placement; at the same time, most will have a desperate wish to remain independent, in their own homes and communities, and out of institutions. The goals of these programs are, simply, to allow older people the choice. This is accomplished by creating a comprehensive network of professional, paraprofessional, and community services that make viable a life at home.

Chapter 7

Paraprofessional Workers

Home care programs, both the traditional sort, which serve over several weeks, and those designed for long term care, depend substantially on paraprofessional workers. These employees usually are assigned under care plans approved by physicians and are supervised by nurses. Therefore they function through a relationship with formal health workers, are responsible to them as well as to their patients, and have genuine paraprofessional duties.

Homemakers, home health aides, home attendants, housekeepers, chore service workers—terms and definitions abound—are often the people most critical to the fulfillment of the plan of care for the patient. Beyond this, for many people of greatly advanced age, the aide is the only human contact available.

Homemaker programs, to be safe and effective, must be integrated with other forms of service. However, it must be recognized that these workers often constitute the glue that binds together a fractured life and that many older disabled people would be institutionalized or dead without their aides: "We have seen homemakers provide eyes and ears for the social worker, the psychiatrists, the physician and nurse with a kind of carefulness and continuity that can never be achieved through single home visits, office consultations, or even in the institutional setting."[1]

HISTORICAL BACKGROUND

The modern history of programs to help ill people at home in this country dates back to the late nineteenth century, when Lillian Wald and her associates volunteered to give care to impoverished immigrants, largely women and newborn children, on the Lower East Side of Manhattan. Their efforts grew into the Visiting Nurse system as we now know it in the United States.

Employment of lay staff to work with professional personnel in the care of patients at home began through a small program in New York City's Family Services Bureau of the Association for the Improvement of the Poor. This agency focused on nursing the ill, but in 1903 added "four women for the purpose of lifting temporarily the simple everyday burdens from sick mothers." Reports from this agency in later years noted that these employees, called "visiting cleaners" or "visiting housewives," assisted in home repair and taught housekeeping skills.[2]

A further advance in the field took place with the establishment of a formal homemaker service by the Philadelphia Jewish Welfare Society in 1923. These homemakers served primarily as "substitute mothers" when a mother was disabled or hospitalized.[3]

Major evolution in employment of paraprofessionals took place during the Depression years of the 1930s. The Works Progress Administration (WPA) hired *housekeeping aides* "to attend families with overwhelming problems and hopefully prevent family breakups."[4] While by 1940 there were about 38,000 homemakers in the country, there was little growth in the field during World War II.

Growth began again with the development of the Montefiore Hospital (New York) home care program in 1947. (See chapter 6 for further discussion of this program.) Its premise assumed that family members would be available to give basic care between professional visits; but from the start housekeeping employees were included.[5]

A CHANGING, GROWING FIELD

From its beginnings until after World War II, the preponderance, almost 80 percent, of paraprofessional service was for the care of children. Today, however, far more than 80 percent of paraprofessionals' time is given to care of the elderly. In parallel with this shift, a vast increase in the need for these workers has taken place. The demand, while perhaps not always fulfilled, is manifested by a growth in the number of agencies employing such personnel.

As recently as 1958, only seven hundred elderly people were under the care of publicly financed paraprofessionals in the United States.[6] By 1962, according to the National HomeCaring Council,[7] there existed approximately three hundred homemaker-home health aide service programs in forty-four states, employing about 3,900 people.[8] By 1972 there were 3,700 such programs in all states, and by 1982 the National HomeCaring Council estimated that about 240,000 people were so employed.[9] Today there are more than 350,000 individuals working as employees of some eight thousand agencies.[10]

The paraprofessional field has become organized, through the creation of national lobbying and support organizations. In 1939 the National Committee on Homemaker Service was established. At its annual meetings, appropriate terminology was developed, surveys of need and number promoted, and methods to develop support for this work sought. In 1960 the group produced the first national guidelines for homemaker job descriptions. These were followed by establishment of standards for paraprofessional training and supervision. Two years later a National Council for Homemaker Services was created. The council's goals were built upon earlier work, and pressed forward standards for accreditation, training, monitoring, and supervision. The name of the national group has been changed several times. In recent years it was known as the National Home-Caring Council,[11] and in the fall of 1986 it merged into the National Foundation for Hospice and Home Care.

Entrepreneurs began to recognize the profit potential of deploying paraprofessional workers through proprietary agencies several years ago. The states have gradually amended the necessary laws and regulations to permit competition between voluntary agencies and profit-oriented businesses. New York State, among the last to capitulate, removed the barriers in 1986. As of March 1986 there were 1,947 proprietary agencies certified to bill for care of Medicare patients across the country. An unknown number of others function without certified status.*

Thus the field of paraprofessional care has proceeded to change and develop as opportunity became evident. This form of service began with the casual employment of a few women to assist in housework and child care, through establishment and growth of substantial not-for-profit organizations, to the present day. Now voluntary, not-for-profit agencies exist in parallel with proprietary companies in most localities. Because they receive some charitable income specified for this purpose, voluntary agen-

---

*V. J. Halamandaris, National Association for Home Care, Washington, D.C. Personal communication, April 1986.

cies are more likely to be able to help poor people who lack access to entitlements, such as Medicaid. Proprietary companies seek clients with sufficient funds to pay for paraprofessional workers out-of-pocket. Both types of organizations compete for patients who are covered by any form of insurance.

DEFINITION OF TERMS

The federal government and the states have promulgated regulations defining the various forms of paraprofessional service. Two general categories of employees exist. Homemakers, home health aides, home attendants, and personal care workers are permitted to give direct health-related services through physical contact with patients, under professional supervision. Housekeepers and chore service workers, however, are limited to household tasks, shopping, cooking, errands, and other functions in which they have no physical contact with the patient.[12]

A *home health aide* is a person who has completed an approved basic training program in personal care, to provide selected aspects of patient care under nursing supervision for patients receiving services from a certified agency.

A *personal care worker* is someone who has completed an approved training program and assists a patient at home, under a nurse's supervision, with personal hygiene, dressing, feeding, and household tasks essential to the patient's health.

A *homemaker* is an employee who meets established standards and assists persons homebound because of illness, incapacity, or absence of a caretaker/relative in managing and maintaining a household, dressing, feeding, and incidental household tasks.

A *housekeeper/chore service worker* is an employee who meets established standards and does light work or household tasks such as cleaning, laundry, and meal preparation for homebound persons, in the absence of a caretaker/relative, in situations that do not require the services of a trained homemaker.

In this text we have usually chosen the word homemaker to stand for all paraprofessional employees.

Workers defined by these standards are ordinarily recruited for patient care through contact by family or case manager with an agency or program certified by government. This agency is responsible for assuring that the employee is appropriately trained, determining the nature and hours of service, monitoring the quality of work, and paying the salary. In general, if payment for service is to be derived from a government-supported source, the worker must be obtained through a certified agency. If the patient and/or family recruit a paraprofessional worker privately, payment will in all likelihood come from personal funds.

So much is clear in theory. In practice, definitions in the paraprofessional world are enshrouded in fog. The functions of the variously titled classifications of workers inevitably overlap. It is no more feasible that a housekeeper will never assist a patient in a health-related matter than that an aide will never cook a meal or clean up a mess. If lines so arbitrarily drawn were in fact enforced, the current cumbersome system would become unfeasible.

The distinctions between categories of worker are derived from a convoluted history and often maintained for the benefit of the agency rather than the worker. They are in effect enforced by government regulations that control payment. For instance, home health aides are reimbursable under four of the major government programs, Medicare, Medicaid, the Social Services Block Grant, and Title III of the Older Americans Act. Personal care can be paid for only under Medicaid, and chore services only through SSBG and Title III.[13] A more detailed discussion of financing is provided later.

Thus if a patient needs paraprofessional help at home, the first unofficial task of the case manager, home care department, or agency will be to determine the nature of the individual's entitlements. If Medicare is available and the patient can be deemed to require so-called skilled nursing services, hiring of a home health aide can be supported. If, on the other hand, the basic need is for long term assistance at home, beyond the highly limited Medicare allowance, a homemaker must be sought. This employee can be paid for only through SSBG or Title III. It is often irresistibly tempting to design the evidence for need to meet the case of the patient's legitimacy for support under a particular funding source.

This is made practical by the overlapping of job descriptions and functions among all types of paraprofessional workers. H. D. Hall, executive director of the San Francisco Home Health Service, points out[14] that all require professional supervision and are expected to provide reports to the supervisor about the patient; with few exceptions, they receive payment from a source other than the patient; they may serve temporarily for brief emergency periods while the patient's natural supports are absent or unavailable; or they may be the only human resource for an individual for a relatively long period of time; they all give personal care to some degree; and they all carry out tasks that can be defined as chores.

What is clear from the above similarities is the basic assumption that the social, environmental, and health needs are inseparable, that each need must have attention, and that each need is related to the others. Job descriptions and tasks of the chore person, homemaker, home health aide, and home attendant are not basically different. . . . Attempts to differentiate the functions for each type of in-home personnel are . . . tied to funding sources rather than to needs for service.[15]

Paraprofessional job descriptions tend to be overly specific, causing vagueness about responsibility for particular tasks in particular circumstances. A literal fulfillment of regulation would produce inane results. Hall illustrates:

> If the home health aide is out of the house and the homemaker or chore person is there, what happens if the patient needs help to get to the bathroom? Must the homemaker watch as the patient evacuates his bladder in bed?
> Does the home health aide not close the living room window in a rainstorm because it isn't the bedroom?[16]

Here we see a situation characteristic of many ossified bureaucracies. Rigid standards are established and unofficial mechanisms promptly arise through which commonsense goals of humane patient care can be achieved by evasion. Of course, vast inefficiencies result, and costs are inevitably increased for no practical gain in patient care.

SPECIFIC PARAPROFESSIONAL FUNCTIONS

The duties of these workers fall naturally into the categories of domestic chores, personal care, and paraprofessional health services. The overall goal, however, should be integration of skills in the interests of each patient. The specific duties of these workers are noted in the following sections. It is important to recognize that, fully as significant as any list of tasks, the very presence of the homemaker is valuable. She is a fellow human being who reduces the older person's isolation, maintains morale, and averts depression.

DOMESTIC CHORES

Aged people are often unable to maintain a reasonable standard of upkeep in their homes. Occasionally the cause is loss of intellectual function.[17] More often, people who are very old may simply lack the strength, energy, and agility to clean the house, do the laundry, prepare meals, shop for food, take out the garbage, pay bills. No family member or friend may be available. Therefore the homemaker becomes a critical resource for independence simply by taking over some of the household tasks. When relatives or neighbors are able to share in these tasks, the homemaker serves a valid respite function.

This point requires emphasis, as Hall indicates.[18] People in government responsible for paying the costs of home health care fear the spread of paraprofessional services. The concern is that family members will cease their unpaid efforts, back away, and abuse the opportunity to obtain a worker supported by others. However, there is evidence to the contrary. Without a degree of help families may have to give up the attempt to care for an elderly person at home and opt for institutional placement, because they are overwhelmed. Home care does not void family involvement; it makes it feasible.[19] With some help from a paraprofessional, through a well-organized home health care program, a sharing of work load and responsibility often occurs. The family members are then able to sustain their portion of the tasks.

PERSONAL CARE

We have noted the arbitrary distinction drawn in law and regulation between responsibility for the patient's environment and the patient's body. Any simple analysis of personal care reduces this matter to an absurdity. For instance, is meal preparation and assistance with eating a housekeeping or a paranursing function? Personal care services can be carried out well by workers who are properly trained, provided they are closely supervised.

Personal care tasks generally include assistance with care of teeth and mouth, grooming, bathing, transfer from bed to chair to commode to walker, walking, dressing and exercise, and preparation of special dietary meals. Each of these matters may appear simple, but mistakes can be painful and costly to the patient's health.

HEALTH CARE

Paraprofessional health care is the conduct of routine health care tasks or of specialized aspects of personal service. It is particularly important that the paraprofessional be thoroughly trained and supervised by the program nurse responsible for the patient. Workers in this paraprofessional area are usually called home health aides. They may be considered nurse's aides transferred to the home setting. Once the professional personnel establish the patient's plan of care, those tasks that can be carried out appropriately by the aide are clarified. These may include assistance with prescribed skin care and prevention of body deterioration due to prolonged periods in bed (back rubs, exercises, and simple massage are included); help in the use of support devices; dressing changes; observation and recording of vital signs, such as temperature and pulse rate; general monitoring of the patient's condition; irrigation of an in-dwelling (Foley) bladder catheter; change of colostomy bag; administration of medications; and application of heat or cold.[20]

As high technology in home care becomes more commonplace, aides will be needed to carry out increasingly complex health-related tasks. These functions may include participation in home renal dialysis, total parenteral nutrition, administration of oxygen, and use of potent medications.

The criticism may arise that paraprofessional services are obtained for patients and paid for by the taxes of the general public, when the need is not genuine. In effect, is there appreciable expense simply to supply maid service for the elderly? Surely, some examples of abuse can be found. However, most of the aged who are disabled and not in institutions receive basic and essential help from spouses, children, other relatives, and friends, rather than from paid employees. According to the 1982 Long Term Care Survey[21] about 4.6 million disabled elderly people live in the community. Almost 70 percent rely exclusively on unpaid helpers. Other studies support this finding.[22]

However, it is unclear whether the current natural support system can remain intact. The capacity of children to help parents of extreme old age may decrease because of the advanced age of the children themselves. This phenomenon will grow as the demographic imperative advances. Further, the current and growing trend for women to be employed leaves fewer people available at home to take care of the elderly. Thus gaps in the network of care will become more likely as more very old people exist and as they require more help. An answer may be for paraprofessionals and informal supports to share responsibility more frequently than is now true. (See chapter 8 for further discussion of informal supports.)

The physical, social, and household needs of frail elderly people are interrelated, and therefore the job descriptions, training programs, and placement of paraprofessional helpers should be made appropriately flexible. Regulations of the various government programs that pay for these services should therefore be amended to allow development of what could be called the generic paraprofessional. Perhaps the term homemaker is apposite. This development is in the interests of effective patient care within the home, prudent use of available funds, and workers' careers. Such a move would eliminate the existing arbitrary distinctions between allowable tasks of home care workers and "deliver us from the current dilemma about who shall wash the face and who shall wash the floor."[23]

STANDARDS FOR PARAPROFESSIONALS

The summary statement of a national conference of homemakers in 1937 included the charge of "thinking through satisfactory standards of service."[24] This goal was pursued by the National Council for Homemaker Services. Shortly after its establishment in 1962, the council produced a code of standards, and by 1965 over fifteen thousand copies had been distributed throughout the United States and Canada. The standards contain concepts that are equally valid today: Patients require proper assessment and case management; and paraprofessional employees deserve adequate training, wages, and benefits.

As the National HomeCaring Council noted in 1981, "All the standards are interrelated, and each must be understood in the context created by the others. Together they protect the interests of consumers and give consumers a basis for judging the competence of an agency that provides in-home service."[25]

The virtue of holding to honorable and sensible standards such as these is unarguable. However, the goal remains unreached. Poignant testimony by Janet Starr, until 1987 Executive Director of the Home Care Association of New York State, is pertinent. She noted in a 1982 report of her association: "The person who purchases services directly from an agency and pays the full cost of these services is not protected by any standards. The care he receives may be very good, or it may be substandard care provided by untrained workers."[26]

Sexual bias is a persistent problem in engaging serious government consideration of enforcing standards in this field. Ann Mootz, director of United Home Care, Cincinnati, Ohio, notes:

> In past years, when advocates of standards . . . approached legislative committees to seek support for training and supervision, they were often met with the "good old boy" response, "Any woman knows how to do all of that." However . . . many legislators now recognize the need for special preparation for homemaker(s) . . . and for regular backup by professionals . . . they have read of scandals, neglect, and abuse in home care programs around the country and realize that this is a field ripe for trouble.[27]

New York State, through new legislation (Chapter 959 of the Laws of 1984 of the State of New York), has attempted a remedy through the means classically employed by government: licensing. The new legislation requires that virtually all agencies providing nursing, home health aide, and personal care services be licensed and monitored to guarantee compliance with standards designed to ensure that care is given safely, by competent trained personnel. Since New York is a leader in the home care field, other states are quite interested in the results of this attempt to control quality of care. What are the prospects for success? As Starr indicates:

> It will take legislation and years of effort to amend aging, social services, mental health and mental retardation laws to ensure that common, basic standards for paraprofessional services are met. . . . [Also] we have not given adequate attention or recognition to the persons who provide this vital service. In many respects we have exploited them. We have sown seeds for a potential scandal. We have ignored the escalating human resource needs in the paraprofessional services while we have continued to delegate more care to them, and put more demands on them.[28]

TRAINING

One risk of increased government oversight is excessive emphasis on written documentation and parallel loss of time and energy for concern about the genuine interests of patient and employee. It is worth a moment to stress this point. The ultimate purpose of the homemaker is to help patients meet home health and social needs. The employees must be trained and supervised, and their standing as a prime outside force in the lives of their patients must always be recognized. The homemaker is the eyes and ears of the health care team, able to report on patient status when others are not present, while at the same time carrying out domestic chores and personal and paraprofessional duties. The homemaker serves a valuable function simply by monitoring, because she is in intimate service with the patient and is in good position to note change. Her ability to report alterations in the patient's condition to her professional supervisor is important.

However, many paraprofessionals enter the field lacking the necessary skills and sensitivity, despite evidence that "solid job skills, which form the basis for safe, reliable care, depend on adequate training."[29] The critical task of training programs is to develop the capacities of new workers in these areas. In the training process the goals of cleanliness, punctuality, responsibility, and team cooperation are pressed. A proper attitude toward the patient is vital, one in which the dignity and privacy of the older person are respected.[30] The homemaker must understand that she is not the ultimate authority or decision maker. This responsibility belongs, first, to the patient and/or appropriate family members; and then to the doctor, nurse, or social worker.

The homemaker must avoid becoming emotionally entrapped in the patient's problems while at the same time being sensitive and responsive. She should try to incorporate the patient in decisions about personal care and for maintenance of the environment, and maintain a sense of flexibility. She must remember that she is in the home of another person.

Largely through the persistent effort of such organizations as the National HomeCaring Council and its predecessors,[31] formal training of paraprofessionals has become a federal requirement in some situations. All home care agencies and projects that operate under the Medicare Conditions of Participation for home health aides must use trained paraprofessionals. It is not a requirement for Medicaid-supported personal care workers or those employed under Title XX or the Older Americans Act. Therefore the states maintain an option as to whether training must be mandated.

A good case can be made for extending the training mandate. Florence Moore and Emily Layzer have carefully reviewed the subject and point out:

Without appropriate basic training, workers can cause themselves and the consumer serious bodily harm by using incorrect procedures to perform such hands-on activities as lifting the ill or handicapped person. Safe care for the consumer is jeopardized further when the worker has no basic training in preparation of special diets, transferring patients from bed to chair, and other activities required of these workers.[32]

In most instances, patients are friendly, cooperative, and courteous, and their difficulties center on physical disorders, limitations in activities of daily living, finances, and isolation. However, emotional illness, dementia, and exaggeration of preexisting pernicious character traits may also exist. These qualities offer an especially challenging task to the homemaker who is required to spend many hours, often alone, with the patient. Training that provides paraprofessionals a degree of insight and understanding in how to work with angry, hostile, and combative patients is important. Supervision of the worker in the home by professional agency staff is imperative, for the personal support it offers and also to ensure that the relationships in the home are sound.

The National HomeCaring Council developed a model training curriculum.[33] Newly hired paraprofessionals receive about sixty hours of classroom and laboratory instruction and fifteen hours of field practice. The cost of employee turnover is high in many ways. Agencies that carefully screen and train their workers will serve their patients and themselves more effectively, because good levels of staff retention will be more likely.

The council attempted to develop an accreditation program for home care agencies. The first initiative, in 1971, was an approval system following a self-evaluation by agencies. In 1976 a full accreditation process began, based on a site visit to the agency under consideration. In attempting to promote its accrediting system, the council argued that an agency can use the designation as a marketing device. Despite this, relatively few took the trouble.[34] Nevertheless, the effort has been favorable for the development of the field. At least a dozen states have used portions of the council's standards in their own accreditation process for home care agencies; and in several instances the federal government has accepted accredited status by an agency as sufficient evidence that it meets federal conditions for receiving funds.[35]

ETHICAL MATTERS

RESPONSIBILITY

Ethical issues arise when a decision is made to keep a frail aged person at home. Patients themselves, when they insist upon making this choice, accept a share of the consequences. So do family members, case managers, physicians, and discharge planners. If paraprofessional workers are to be included in the plan of care, the sponsoring agency assumes a considerable degree of responsibility for assuring the probity, skill, and supervision of the worker. The homemaker herself, of course, carries an important part of the load as well: to recognize that the needs of the patient come first, understand job requirements and limits, and know when to call for help. Plans must exist for quality assurance and for moral support of both the patient and the homemaker.

George Kanoti, of the Department of Bioethics of the Cleveland Clinic, states that the following general principles of ethical medical practice should apply regarding clinical decisions in favor of home care:

"1. Beneficence—do good to your patients,

2. Non-maleficence—do not harm your patients,

3. Freedom—invite your patients to participate in therapy, and

4. Justice—distribute limited resources fairly. When these ethical principles are served, balanced, and monitored, home care will truly be a responsible means of meeting one's obligations to those in need of medical care."[36]

BARRIERS BETWEEN PATIENT AND WORKER

Paraprofessional workers often differ in background and language from their patients. This is a consequence of the cohort effect, immigration patterns, the state of the job market, and limitations on the nature of work available to people of modest education. Ethical issues promptly become integral to the interrelationship. This causes no surprise to any thoughtful observer. It is a commonplace of daily life in the United States, with its vast and polyglot population, that persons of different culture and race approach each other with caution, if not with fear or antagonism. The result may be that the good name and reputation of the homemaker is questioned unfairly. Bigotry toward minority group members exists. Why should the situation in a home care setting differ? After all, the homemaker is a stranger in the home of another person.

The following examples from the files of a long term home health care program are illustrative.

The patient, L, was a sixty-seven-year-old woman, living alone, significantly impaired in intellectual function by dementia possibly induced by chronic alcoholism. Her only relative was a niece who rarely contacted the patient. Care was given by a personal care worker (PCW) referred by an agency after appropriate training, who worked from 8:00 A.M. to 8:00 P.M.

Social worker notes from the patient's record: Patient had burned her legs when she dropped a cigarette on her lap and it burned through her nightgown. Was taken to ER (when discovered) by . . . PCW and was treated there. (She said) "I guess I shouldn't smoke." The PCW is very frustrated . . . because of L's uncooperative nature and verbal abuse. Neighbors are circulating a petition to have her evicted. Very concerned about fire. I discussed with her the importance of not smoking any more. In past she would hide cigarettes from PCW to smoke when she was alone. L agreed, but when I was leaving asked for a cigarette.

Social worker note six months later: Received call from Homemaker Agency. Niece called agency to accuse PCW of causing burns to L's legs.

M has just celebrated his ninety-sixth birthday. He lives alone in a small walk-up apartment. His homemaker has been with him for thirteen years. Social worker note: Spoke to the homemaker. She had alerted M that she will be leaving in two months to [move]. Since that time M has been most abusive to her. It would seem inadvisable for her to continue with him since he knows she will be leaving.

Social worker note (one week later): Conflicts in relationship with homemaker now resolved as patient understands why she must leave. He has already apologized to her for his verbal abuse. He thought that once she left he was going to be forced into an "Old Man's Home."

Social worker note (another week later): Homemaker called me very upset. Apparently M called police accusing her of taking his Social Security check. . . .

she considered leaving patient, and explained that she had taken the check to cash it for him, as usual. She calmed down when I told her I would visit tomorrow.

Social worker note (next day): Discussed above incident with patient, who denied that he called police.[37]

It is perhaps more surprising that the relationship between home care worker and aged patient usually works out well. Two people isolated with each other for hours regularly establish an effective accommodation through necessity if not desire. Often a deep sense of caring and concern grows. The two may anneal in a bond of deep affection.

The quality of caring has been illustrated by L. Eliezer Lerea of Southern Connecticut State College and Barbara F. LiMauro of Waterbury [CN] Hospital in a study of grief among health care workers.[38] They investigated the prevalence and nature of grief in response to patient suffering, loss, or death. Workers were nurses and aides employed in acute care hospitals and skilled nursing facilities. It is reasonable to extrapolate their results to the home care situation. Psychological reactions to grief most often cited by the workers were thinking and talking about the patient, feelings of helplessness, and crying or despondency. The brief comments quoted by these authors are telling:

I remember. . . . I was a mess! I still can't forget that old man. When I came to work and saw that empty bed, I thought I would fall apart. I still think about him sometimes. . . . Sometimes I dream about him.

Mr. L lived at—— Convalescent Center for more than seven years. He was such a kind, dignified man. I watched him go downhill all that time . . . unable to feed himself, incontinent, confused. When he died, it was like I lost my own father. I grieved but I was also relieved.[39]

THE POTENTIAL FOR ABUSE

Despite the fact that most patient-homemaker relationships are harmonious, the opposite may occasionally occur. There may exist an atmosphere of sublimated hostility. Worse, either party may be overtly abused. The frail older patient, especially if without family, friends, or other natural supporters, is an easy victim. An unscrupulous person can steal or carry out other malfeasant acts without the patient's knowledge, particularly if some dementia is present. Even if the patient is aware, threats or emotional blackmail may be used to prevent him or her from asking for help. The patient may be willing to settle for a thief in the home rather than abandonment. Instances of physical abuse are known and tolerated by the patient because needs more imperative than safety and comfort are met.

Addiction to alcohol may, for instance, be a driving force, as the following case summary from the files of a long term home health care program reveals:

AL was a seventy-four-year-old woman referred to the program by a Meals-on-Wheels driver. He had noted accumulated piles of unopened dinner packages in the one-room apartment. On the team's first visit, the door was opened by a homemaker. The patient was a feeble, emaciated and bed-bound woman, who greeted us with: "Why are you here? Leave me alone. I don't want to have anything to do with you." The aide stood to the side and observed. After the passage of a few soothing words, AL permitted a brief physical examination by the doctor. A smell of alcohol on the breath of the patient was evident. Multiple fresh and old bruises on arms, legs, and abdomen were observed. The tone of her conversation shifted between unctuous gratitude and vituperation. A partially full Scotch bottle was seen on the bed table.

The aide was asked about the bruises and replied that she thought they were caused because the patient regularly fell out of bed. The patient herself said she was unaware of the injuries. In regard to alcohol use, the patient denied drinking, and would not explain the bottle. The aide said she couldn't understand where it came from because she had told the local liquor stores to stop delivering.

We asked how long the aide had worked with AL and were told they had been together nine years. The aide was paid with the patient's private funds. We were not able to learn how much money was being paid, or the extent of the patient's assets.

We were immediately concerned that physical abuse was occurring, and found a moment to ask the patient if, in fact, the aide injured her. She denied it, and repeated her lack of awareness of trauma. One week later, on a second visit to AL by the home health care team, the patient seemed weaker, more demented, and possibly jaundiced. We urged hospitalization but the patient begged us not to take her away. Plans for legal action or psychiatric placement were under active consideration when we were informed that AL had been taken to the local hospital in coma and had died in the intensive care unit twelve hours later.[40]

Paraprofessional workers may also be abused. While they are relatively unlikely to suffer significant physical harm, it has been known to happen, particularly if the patient is psychiatrically ill. The following note in a case record from the files of the St. Vincent's Hospital (NY) Chelsea-Village Program is illustrative:

CD is an eighty-nine-year-old woman living alone, known to the program for three years. She has become increasingly resistant to working with the health team to keep herself clean and nourished. . . . When she assaulted her homemaker with a knife (to no avail), psychiatric advice was obtained. The patient has refused to allow homemakers to continue helping her because "they are stealing from me and abusing me." She was described as alert; her mood anxious, angry and depressed; her affect, labile and inappropriate. She has ideas of reference as well as paranoid persecutory delusions about who we are and why we are there. She was not oriented to time or place. She voiced assaultive intent and implied indirectly that she would like to die. . . . Legal steps were taken to bring the patient to the hospital.[41]

Patients who are inappropriately afraid, have aggrandized expectations of the aide, or are unfairly accusatory present grave difficulties for people and agencies who try to help. The older person may be suspicious enough to refuse to be alone in the home with the worker or to insist that the employee remain always within sight.[42] This form of conduct may destroy the possibility of effective home care.

BUILDING MORALE

THE PROBLEM OF ISOLATION

The nature of their jobs often requires that paraprofessional employees spend many hours alone with a disabled aged person. In some instances the work day may be twenty-four hours long; and even in the more usual situation of an eight or twelve-hour shift, loneliness and other challenges to the worker's spirit may arise. Unlike employment in other settings, such as nursing homes or hospitals, homemakers have no peers. The job site lacks the glamor and excitement of an emergency room. Homemaker functions tend to be undervalued, and these workers are often not recognized as full sharers in the plan of care for their patients. Their status is low and they are easy to exploit.[43]

Their circumstances require our special understanding and support. Stamina and morale are critical elements in the success of their relationships with their patients. A variety of approaches is needed to help paraprofessionals deal with the unusual frustrations and tensions of being isolated for hours with patients, some of whom may be uncommunicative, anxious, and/or hostile.

A spirit of collegiality with other agency staff is essential. Professional supervisors must phone and visit regularly. Employees should be permitted, even encouraged to talk about their work situations, to complain and vent their feelings. These workers should be recognized and treated as valued members of the home health care team. This consideration has practical value for morale, employee retention, and quality of care. Even more important, this viewpoint should be sustained because it is honest and just.

The attitude with which the patient and family members respond to the worker is perhaps even more critical. In most instances, a natural sharing of human feeling develops among all parties. Unfortunate occasions exist, however, in which the employee is treated unfairly or discourteously. Worse, the worker may step into a family controversy and become a pawn in the dispute.

SUPPORT GROUPS FOR HOME HEALTH CARE WORKERS

Innovative approaches are needed to help homemakers resolve these concerns. One example, group work for homemakers, is a support concept that has been tried with success. Barbara DiCicco-Bloom and Carol Coven, a nurse and a social worker associated with the St. Vincent's Hospital Nursing Home Without Walls Program (see chapter 6 for further discussion of this program) developed such a group. The purpose was to provide "a supportive learning environment for women who handle emotional and physical needs of elderly patients, and who serve as crucial links between each patient and the health care team."[44]

Stimuli for the formation of the group was evidence that patients and homemakers sometimes adjusted to each other only with difficulty, that tension levels occasionally became so high that workers quit or were rejected, and that squabbles arose between family members and patients in which employees were importuned to take sides. Workers were at times asked to do work far beyond their job descriptions or were verbally abused. Nurses in the program had also noted a tendency of some homemakers to misperceive their own roles, to assume professional responsibilities, for instance, or to dominate and infantilize their patients. The reverse was also seen—workers' unwillingness to take necessary and appropriate action or make any decision.

Three group cycles took place, varying from six to ten sessions in length, and attended by up to ten personal care workers. The nurse-social worker team led the sessions. Permission to take the time to attend group sessions was arranged for the workers with each patient and agency. As DiCicco-Bloom and Coven planned,

The PCW group focused on interpersonal support, attitudinal change (hypothetically assumed linked to personal attitude as well as physical job isolation and pressure) and continuing education. The content outline resulted from an understanding of the importance of exploring personal attitudes in a supportive group setting, as well as identifying myths and facts about the elderly and teaching specific skills. . . .[45]

As is true of all effective group work,[46] an evolution occurred among the regular members as the cycle proceeded. A sense of sharing and mutual support developed and opportunity for learning as well. The following excerpts from DiCicco-Bloom and Coven's work, recorded from the fifth session of eight in a cycle, are characteristic:

> Discussion opened with seven members actively talking about how they handle anger at patients. . . . (A worker) commented, "I walk away when I get angry—I just go into another room." . . .
> The nurse asked what kind of things get workers angry. W answered, "Well, she sometimes doesn't want to get out of bed. I tell her that I'm upset, and then she'll get out of bed for me." D said, "Oh, those things don't get me angry. . . . I get mad when my patient asks for a specific food and then won't eat it when I prepare it." The nurse asked what the worker thought this meant. "I think she's trying to get to me. There's no one else around." . . . The interpretation of anger as a reflection of loneliness and depression was suggested. . . . A possible option for dealing with the anger—talking about it with the patient—was discussed among all group members.[47]

Structured improvisation has also been used as a group work technique at St. Vincent's, in cooperation with Performing Arts for Crisis Training, Inc., to help paraprofessionals handle difficult situations that occur in the work setting. Structured improvisation is a process through which

> dramatizations of crisis and conflict capture the emotional dynamics of issues such as death and dying, substance abuse, family crisis and conflict management, and racial prejudice. Elderly "actor-trainers" are used to portray patients, and trainees (homemakers) participate in the dramatizations.[48]

Through this process, workers can practice responses to challenge in a simulation of real life.

SOURCES OF FUNDING

PRIVATE PAYMENTS

The total sum paid by older people and their families to purchase the services of paraprofessionals in the home cannot be determined with accuracy. The difficulties in establishing a believable figure relate to problems in the definitions of terms for these workers and the likelihood that individuals are often paid for their work off the books. How can we estimate the money spent by people who ask a neighborhood youth to do some shopping or house cleaning? A gross guess regarding the value of private funds used for these purposes could be based on the assumption that a similarity exists with private payment for nursing home care, which reaches about 50 percent of the total national cost. If this is so, individuals and families pay more than $2 billion from their personal funds for paraprofessional help each year.

PUBLIC PAYMENTS

Public expenditures on the services of paraprofessional workers in the home derive largely from six programs: Medicaid, Medicare, the Social Services Block Grant, the Older Americans Act, Supplemental Security Income, and the Veterans Administration Home Care Services. Total municipal, county, state, and federal costs in this area are approximately $2.2 billion per year.[49]

Medicaid

Medicaid is a national means-tested health care program for the poor administered through the states (see chapters 1 and 2). It uses slightly less than 2 percent of its total budget for home care. In 1984 the dollar cost of all forms of home care service to Medicaid was about $865 million.[50,*] A rough estimate indicates that about half this sum was spent on the services of paraprofessional workers. In thirty-nine states home health benefits made up 1 percent or less of their Medicaid expenditures, making the status of New York State in this regard extraordinary. It accounted for about 78 percent of all Medicaid home care costs in 1985.[51] New York City alone uses about 57 percent of the nation's Medicaid home care funds.[52]

The New York City home attendant program. The New York City Human Resources Administration (HRA) conducts a home attendant and housekeeper program for the elderly. In 1986 about 40,000 clients were served, 32,000 by home attendants, the remainder by housekeepers. Virtually all expenses of the program, estimated at $284 million in 1982,[53] $378 million in 1984,[54] and $481 million in 1986,† are borne by Medicaid. Costs are attributed 50 percent to the federal government, 25 percent to New York State, and 25 percent to the city. Eligibility for both Medicaid and home care services are prerequisites for client acceptance.

Because this is a Medicaid program, patient entry must be defended on a health-related basis. The first step, therefore, is the physician's comple-

---

*George Greenberg, Ph.D., personal communication, October 10, 1986. Compiled from unpublished program data from the U.S. Department of Health and Human Services.

†Information in this paragraph was provided by J. Black, Medical Assistance Program, New York City Resources Administration. Personal communication, April 1986.

tion of an assessment form that includes diagnoses and functional limitations. In real life the form is often completed by a nurse or social worker who knows the patient well, to be signed by the doctor. The document is then reviewed for approval by another physician employed by HRA for this purpose. If all is satisfactory, the routine bureaucratic entry process follows.

Home attendants are permitted to give personal care and carry out tasks such as cooking and cleaning and may be employed for an individual client up to twenty-four hours per day, if it is determined that safety requires constant monitoring. Housekeepers work only at household chores, and to a maximum of twelve hours per week for an individual client.[55]

Virtually everyone employed under the HRA program is obtained through vendor agencies. The remainder, about 4 percent of the total, are paid directly by New York City as independent contractors. These individuals are required when the patient's home is in an outlying area not served by a recognized agency.* Salaries are close to the minimum wage.

Home attendant and housekeeper positions are considered to be unskilled and have modest qualifications: Employees must be at least eighteen years of age, in acceptable physical condition, and show that they are permitted to work. Possession of a Social Security card is considered sufficient evidence. At least a moderate amount of prior training by the agency is expected.

Monitoring of the patient's health status is carried out through contract with the Visiting Nurse Service of New York. A home visit is made every six months, to fulfill federal Medicaid regulations, which require supervision by a registered nurse in order for paraprofessional care to be reimbursed. Nurses from the vendor agency visit as well, to guide, monitor, and support the workers.

Various problems have developed, worth noting because they are representative of issues that will regularly arise in similar programs:

1. *Incompatibility between client and worker.* Differences in culture, language, and age may be unbridgeable. The employee is entirely at the mercy of the patient and family, and may be dismissed without cause at any time.

2. *Poor living arrangements.* Attendants who must sleep in the patient's home may be given inadequate quarters. Food may be withheld or insufficient.

3. *Part-time employment.* Workers tend to resist short periods of service, such as four hours in a day, because they want to earn a full day's pay.

4. *Inadequate analysis of eligibility.* Physician involvement is largely or entirely limited to review of forms. Unfair rejections or inappropriate approvals occur. A potential for inequity exists.[56]

---

*J. Black, personal communication.

5. *Patient and employee abuse.* Instances have been cited in which family members brought their laundry from elsewhere for the homemaker to wash.[57]

6. *Difficulties in quality control,* because "service delivery is far flung and behind closed doors."[58]

The Medicaid waivers of 1981. Medicaid's ability to respond to the needs of the homebound elderly as well as it does today is largely a result of waivers allowed by the Omnibus Budget Reconciliation Act of 1981. As O'Shaugnessey and her colleagues indicate,[59] this legislation permitted the states to increase and diversify the federally reimbursed services offered under Medicaid in local communities. The waivers in Section 2176 of the bill permitted for the first time the use of homemaker and chore services.

Health services may be given to Medicaid recipients at home based on the orders of a physician. These orders must be part of a written plan of care reviewed by the doctor at sixty-day intervals. Four types of services are available: part-time nursing, home health aides, medical supplies, and various therapies.

Part-time nursing can take place in the home. However, it can occur only on a part-time or intermittent basis. Ordinarily, nurse services must be provided through a certified home health agency. In parts of the country where no such agency exists, individual arrangements are permitted through which independent licensed nurses may give care.

Home health aides must be obtained through a home health agency. The titles of these workers vary among the states, as does the precise nature of the tasks they are permitted to perform. Thirteen states require that permission be obtained from the government before an aide may be assigned. Other states exert cost control by their unwillingness to authorize the use of homemakers or by restricting the number of visits and/or hours of care.

Medical supplies and equipment certified by a physician as necessary can be obtained and paid for by Medicaid. Authorization by a state office is required in most instances before purchase.

Physical, occupational, speech and hearing therapies are provided to Medicaid clients as options in the states, and have been made available in all but four.[60] Prior authorization is usually required.

Medicare

Medicare is a national program of health insurance largely for people aged sixty-five and over, and in 1984, according to the latest available figures, 27.1 million people were covered.* There exists at this time no

*George Greenberg, personal communication.

means test for eligibility, and levels of payment are comparable across the country. As distinguished from Medicaid, in which there are fifty different state programs, Medicare offers the same forms of coverage for all enrollees.

This program, by law and regulation since its creation in 1964, focuses on insurance for acute illness. Coverage of chronic care services is excluded (see chapters 1 and 2). This limitation is made clear by the fact that in 1984 only 3.1 percent of Medicare dollars, or $1.9 billion, were spent on home care services;* and this sum was used virtually entirely for the care of people in the several weeks after discharge from an acute care hospital. In 1983 per-person payments for all Medicare beneficiaries averaged $1,724. Of this sum, only $47, on average, was used for the services provided by a home health agency.[61]

Home health aides can be paid by Medicare only as regulations permit, and in reality this means only as long as the patient needs "skilled" nursing services. In most instances regulators have restricted this term of care to a period of about six weeks. Thus home care under Medicare is perceived as an extension of other acute services, not long term home health care, as we define it.

The Social Services Block Grant

Title XX of the Social Security Act is a federal program through which block grants are authorized to the states for a broad range of social services to various population groups. Among these are the aged. The proportion of Title XX money to be spent on home health care services is an option of each state. In recent years the span has been great, ranging from California's use of more than 40 percent of available funds to Oklahoma's use of less than 0.4 percent.[62]

Title XX spent about $555 million for homemaker, home health aide, personal care, chore, and home management personnel in 1985.[63] Almost every state included this form of assistance in its Title XX program, and on a national basis about 14 percent of all program funds were so used. Note that the figures cited are for all recipients of assistance under Title XX, not the aged only. Further breakdown of data is elusive. Federal reporting requirements for services supported by the program have been eliminated. Therefore more recent national data on total expenditures and the number of people served are unavailable.

The Older Americans Act

Title III of the Older Americans Act provides grants for state and community programs on aging. By design, the intent of this title is to develop

---

*George Greenberg, personal communication.

and promote programs for the elderly that foster independence. The goal is to be reached through efforts that secure and maintain maximum independence and dignity in a home environment for older persons capable of caring for themselves, remove individual and social barriers to economic and personal independence for older persons, and provide a continuum of care for the vulnerable elderly.

Services given within the homes of older people thus fall logically within its objectives and, in fact, many Title III projects pay for homemakers, home health aides, and chore services.[64] The amount of money provided to each state depends on its relative number of elderly residents. Under this source of funds, grants flow from the federal government to the state agencies on aging and then to 664 area agencies. Each of these local government units is mandated to spend a portion of the grant monies on in-home care.

In 1985 (latest available figures) the total federal appropriation for Title III was $666 million. Of this sum, $265 million (40 percent) was to be used for supportive services. The portion of these dollars spent on paraprofessional services is not known but is estimated to be substantial.[65]

No means test is required in order for an older person to receive help under Title III; however, the focus of assistance is to be on those with the most evident need. In Title III programs, recipients are permitted to contribute their own funds toward the cost of services, but such cost-sharing is not mandatory.

Title III is a relatively small program in terms of funding and thus cannot make a major impact on the growing need for paraprofessional help at home for the elderly. On the other hand, it has important positive qualities.

[It] has the flexibility to fill gaps in services for persons otherwise unserved. Since Older Americans Act services may be provided without the restrictions required under Medicare and without certain income tests specified for by Medicaid, in some cases Title III funds may be used to serve persons whose Medicare and Medicaid benefits have been exhausted or who are ineligible. . . .[66]

Supplemental Security Income

Supplemental Security Income (SSI) is a means-tested cash payment program, authorized under Title XVI of the Social Security Act and administered by the federal government. Money is paid at a standard rate across the country to aged, blind, and/or disabled people so that a minimum income is assured. (See Chapter 2 for a more detailed discussion of SSI.) The states are permitted to supplement the federal SSI benefit in order to support services in their communities for those eligible. It is through such optional supplements, made available in thirty-five states during 1985, that SSI can pay for personal care workers and homemakers.[67]

In 1985 about 4 million people received SSI payments. Of these, 1.5 million were aged sixty-five and over.[68] Somewhat more than half of elderly Medicaid recipients are eligible for SSI.[69]

SSI was recognized as a surprising source of federal flexibility in the famous Katie Beckett case of 1981. At that time Katie Beckett was three years old and had lived in an Iowa hospital for more than thirty months subsequent to viral encephalitis. Her care cost the federal government, under Medicaid, more than $12,000 per month. Home care assistance would total about one-quarter this sum. President Reagan cited the example of this child's fate as characteristic of "mindless" government regulation. At that point the Secretary of Health and Human Services found that it lay within his authority to waive regulations under a Social Security Action section that allows discretion in SSI regulations. Katie went home two days later.[70] The consequence of this specific case has been approval of a regulation in 1982 that decreased the barriers of federal regulation forcing people to remain in institutions in order to receive means-tested benefits, if care at home was feasible.[71]

Almost all SSI funds are used for cash income supplements. The amount available for paraprofessional services to help elderly people under various state option programs is relatively small and cannot be determined with accuracy.

Veterans Administration Home Care Services

The Veterans Administration conducts a broad network of service programs for older veterans. (See chapter 2.) Of these, home care programs are a small component. The VA is authorized under Title 38 of the United States Code to offer home health services for treatment of disabled veterans. The regulatory language is sufficiently vague that the matter of whether or not such disability must be service-connected remains unclear. Because the statutes are not specific in this and other ways, the VA has substantial discretion to restrict eligibility, and has chosen to limit home care services to a twelve-month period after hospitalization.[72]

Despite the inhibiting effect of this regulatory interpretation, a modest but noteworthy home health care program has been established. This effort, known as hospital-based home care, has grown from departments of medicine and surgery in about seventy of the major VA medical centers across the country. Through HBHC programs, multidisciplinary teams of hospital staff members make home visits up to thirty miles from the hospital base. In 1982, when only thirty HBHCs were in action, about 6,500 individuals were cared for in their homes. The program is now more than twice as large.

Medical, nursing, social work, dietetic, and rehabilitation services are available in HBHCs, and case management is included as a specific goal.[73] The degree to which the VA supports paraprofessional services in the homes of disabled aged veterans is unclear, but the dollars so allocated must be small. The VA spends a total of about $830 million on nursing homes, domiciliary care, and home attendant services combined,[74] with the last cited function using the smallest amount of dollars. In 1985 only $14 million was spent on the HBHC projects.

Chapter 8

Informal Supports

Most frail elderly persons who need help are the responsibility of family members and friends[1] or unpaid volunteers—"natural," "social," or "informal supports," in the current jargon (and in contrast to formal programs and paid workers).

That children should help their aged and frail parents seems only right. That spouses should provide each other emotional and physical support also seems right. And, in fact, 60 to 80 percent of care for impaired elderly people is given by unpaid relatives and friends.[2] Further, there is little evidence beyond the occasional anecdote that families abandon their aged relatives in emergency rooms or nursing homes.[3]

The feasibility of a life at home for a frail older person is highly dependent upon the availability of these informal support persons.[4] That close family members are likely to be of critical importance is perhaps self-evident. As the following case from the files of a long term home health care program illustrates, however, others also may choose to serve:

A 104-year-old woman . . . was sent from a hospital to a nursing home and spent three years there. This step had been arranged by the hospital's social service department, on the advice of physicians who felt she would be unsafe on her own. The patient disliked the institution and knew that she wished to return home. She so informed old friends from the neighborhood, one of whom became fully engaged in efforts, ultimately successful, to find an apartment and obtain necessary assistance. Homemaking help was arranged through a local governmental agency, nursing visits from a hospital-based home care program, and overall supervision by concerned friends and neighbors. For an additional two-and-a-half years this woman was able to live independently in her own apartment, where she died in her one hundred tenth year.[5]

Sometimes patients prefer help other than family. One seventy-two-year-old man in the same program had to enter a nursing home when his wife, who had been caring for him, became hospitalized. When she returned home, the husband refused to leave the nursing home. Instead, the wife visited him daily, and their previously strained relationship improved.[6]

INFORMAL SUPPORTERS

The time of crisis often occurs when the older members of the family reach biological senescence. It should be recognized that the children who now must help their aged parents have other stresses too:[7]

The unrelenting needs of an older person may result in feelings of helplessness, resentment, guilt, affection, rage, concern, or depression on the part of family members. . . . Whether the generations are housed together or apart does not seem to affect the basic response to a problem that has disrupted the family pattern of functioning, except that feelings are more intense and that there is more opportunity for open clashes if the generations live together.[8]

Often the situation is far more benign. Most of the elderly have sufficient physical and intellectual ability to be independent.[9]

It is unclear how much family involvement is going to be needed in the future. We know the numbers of people in each age group for decades to come but not what changes in financing of long term care may occur, what breakthroughs in diagnosis and treatment of intractable conditions such as Alzheimer's disease may take place, and what influence the tone of the general economy may have. Karen Davis and Diane Rowland of Johns Hopkins University point out that simple projection of past demographic trends may minimize the extent of future dependency.[10] Factors such as further rises in divorce rates will increase the proportion of aged isolated women; reduction in birth rates will decrease the number of adult children available to help; more women in the work force means fewer available readily to take over care.[11] All this has been described as a "thinning out of the kinship network."[12]

There is, however, a different view. Technical advances may decrease the need for informal supports. Medical alert systems, for example, allow isolated, disabled people to call for assistance by electronic means. Some systems offer equipment that will respond even if the patient has lost consciousness or is helpless, by recognizing changes in the pulse, respiratory rate, or blood pressure.

As for living arrangements, according to a 1983 report from the New York State Office for the Aging,[13] among older people of unspecified ages outside of institutions, 53 percent live with their spouses, 30 percent live alone, 15 percent with other relatives, and 2 percent with a nonrelative.

Certain subgroups have living situations markedly different from those just noted. Information from the Chelsea-Village Program in New York City, through which more than fifteen hundred very old homebound people with an average age of eighty-three years have received care over fourteen years, reveals that two-thirds live alone and that only one-third of the total have regular contact with a relative. Professor of Gerontology Marjorie Cantor and research associate Jeffrey Johnson,[14] on the other hand, studied 1,552 persons aged sixty and more in New York City and found only 15 percent without a "functional kin," and of these, 74 percent had functional neighbors or friends.

Among the elderly in this country, women predominate over men, a phenomenon increasingly evident as older age groups are studied. According to a 1982 report prepared for the United States Special Committee on Aging,[15] women make up 57 percent of those in the age group sixty-five to seventy-four; 63 percent between seventy-four and eighty-four; and 70 percent of those older.

A growing need for assistance to this group is evident. The oldest people, eighty-five and older, will make up 18 percent of the elderly by the year 2000, up from 9 percent in 1980. People of advanced ages are most limited physically, most likely to have chronic illness, and most dependent on others for help in carrying out routine activities of daily living, such as washing, feeding, grooming, escorting, shopping, and cooking. Further, elderly people with extensive requirements for assistance generally remain in the community rather than in institutions. About 5 percent of people aged sixty-five and over in this country live in nursing homes. Eight to 10 percent, similarly bedridden or homebound and equally impaired, continue to survive outside institutional settings, possibly in part because they lack access to benefits.[16]

Most people who give informal support to the frail elderly are women. In the past, daughters had characteristically been expected to care for family members who were ill at home. Today, when many women work until the expected age of retirement, the strain of meeting the obligations of employment and parental care may be considerable.[17] As Cantor has pointed out, this "dilemma of conflicting demands" is usually handled "not by denial of responsibility but through considerable personal sacrifice."[18]

The degree of sacrifice may be growing in its impact on individual family caregivers because the size of successive generations of women is changing. In 1940, 37 percent of fifty-year-old women in this country had at least one parent living. By 1980, this figure had grown to 65 percent, a situation never before noted. One result, as demographer J. Menken indicates,[19] is that, for the first time, women in the United States can expect to spend more years as the child of an aging parent than as the mother of a dependent child.

The myth of family abandonment is derived in part from the recognition that the traditional nuclear family is uncommon. The assumption has followed that supportive family relationships are irretrievably lost. In fact, while close relatives may be scattered and thus not available for immediate hands-on assistance, a new kind of natural support system has evolved. In urban areas particularly, this system consists of a mix of assistance from relatives, friends, and neighbors, joined with formal services from both voluntary agencies and various governmental programs.

[There now exists] a modified extended family characterized by a coalition of separately housed, semiautonomous, semidependent families. Often possessing a quality called intimacy at a distance, these family units—some nuclear, some female-headed single-parent, others composed of nonrelated adults—share with formal organizations the function of family.[20]

The people who share in the network of care for a frail aged person may coalesce out of a new and immediate need or may be old friends and relatives of the same generation, or elderly neighbors.[21] This peer group has been termed a "convoy of social support,"[22] suggesting the image of people who move through life as part of a mutual support network. A convoy member is more likely to receive help if he or she had previously offered support to other convoy members. The personal characteristics and life situations of the members influence strongly the nature and success of the convoy. Ironically, as people age and become more likely to require assistance, their peer group, cohort, or convoy shrinks, through the death of members.

The structure, size, and viability of the convoy, or social set, is multifactorial. For instance, people who have been lifelong isolates are likely to suffer continued isolation in advanced age. Women tend to have larger social networks than men. People who have worked generate a richer network of convoy members than do others. City dwellers have access to different forms of social contact than do residents of rural areas.[23] Family attitudes of responsibility toward the aged vary among ethnic groups. The elderly with large families, especially if there are many children, share in more substantial convoys that span generations.

The practical significance of this human web is noteworthy for health workers. It may take attention and sensitivity to ferret out the most useful members. Further, as the person under care becomes older and more frail, the time frame in which help is required becomes continual and long term, rather than intermittent and crisis-oriented; the patterns of assistance between generations is no longer reciprocal, but instead flows more clearly from children to parents; and the nature of needed tasks changes from ancillary to central, including direct intervention in housekeeping and personal care.

Homebound aged people present a complex set of problems. Relatives and other members of an informal support network will often attempt to work with the mixture of medical, psychological, social, housing, and financial issues that usually appears. However, responsibility is heavy, a life is at stake, and finding solutions is frustrating. Some natural supporters tend to burn out and fade away or to seek the easy solution of a nursing home placement. Others juggle indefinitely. The frail elderly are best served when the strengths, the time, the interest and energy of family members and friends can be used as a supplement or complement to services from formal agencies.[24]

A sense of partnership between employees of a home care agency, for instance, and the patient's spouse or children is desirable, although family members' watchdog function over paid personnel is important and must be maintained. When the situation at home is working well, natural supports can ease the task of the homemaker, visiting nurse, or home health care professional team, but there are ample psychological reasons why such relationships founder. These include guilt, anger, resentment on the part of the family, and sloth, tardiness, or harshness of the paid worker. Both parties, in the interest of the aged patient, should extend themselves to avoid adversarial positions. Cantor has suggested that a new working relationship structured on positive appreciation of both formal and informal sectors is worth seeking.[25]

Using the home care situation as an example, benefits from melding of natural supports with formal programs derive from several facts. First, family and friends have a historical relationship with the persons at risk and know their wishes and idiosyncrasies better than the paid staff new to the scene. Second, they can provide information and immediate support to prevent or decrease the frequency of emergency calls. And third, when the help given by natural supporters can substitute in part for paid assistance, it may have a potent and immediate effect on the success of the arrangement and the avoidance of institutionalization for financial reasons. Government programs that include a cap on costs, such as the New York State Nursing Home Without Walls, illustrate the point.[26] In that program the bulk of costs go for payment of paraprofessional workers. If family members, for example: can be trained to change dressings or regulate oxygen flow; are willing to share in household tasks such as cooking, shopping, and cleaning; or are prepared to handle personal care functions like bathing the older person, feeding, turning in bed, and helping to the bathroom, money spent for care can be lessened. This holds true unless the natural supporters must give up another paid job to perform these duties.

FAMILIES AND FRIENDS GIVE HELP

Family supports are an essential base for any system of long term care.[27] On the level of public policy, without the involvement of natural supporters in the care of the frail aged, costly paid programs would have to be enlarged. On the individual level, participation in the daily care plan by those who cherish the patient is positive.

Over the last two decades, through the studies of Ethel Shanas, Elaine Brody, and Marjorie Cantor, it has become clearly established that the idealized extended family never existed in substantial numbers in this country, and to bewail its loss is fatuous; most older persons retain vigorous control over their own fate, unless they become demented, and cannot be treated arbitrarily; and younger family members in general care deeply about their older relatives, and remain available to help when frailty develops.

People related by blood or marriage remain the prime human resource for each other, at all ages, for emotional and social support, and direct assistance both in crises and over the long term.[28] Sharing the same living quarters does not seem to be the critical factor in the relationship between generations. Rather, it is the bond of feeling between parents and children that is important. When necessary, the elderly seem in fact to draw special attention from the broader family network. Shanas indicates that, when no children are available to help, others in the family function as substitutes. These may include siblings or nieces and nephews. The genuinely isolated older person is uncommon in the United States.[29]

For best effect, and to avoid frustration and failure, family members must understand the need for sharing in the care of the aged with professional organizations; and the staff members of formal programs must appreciate the great value of incorporating natural supporters in the plan of care. It is unwise to assume that simply because family members and friends are supportive, willing, and loving, they will automatically be able to provide continuing assistance to older people with chronic disabilities who are no longer capable of caring for themselves.

Families care for their older members, but the task can be daunting and should not be minimized. The routine nature and the ordinariness of the work tend to result in lack of appreciation for its worth. The average family's means may be greatly straitened to find the necessary resources for effective home care. Recognize that the common family support network for a disabled aged person consists of a spouse, equally old and almost as frail, or a middle-aged child, usually a daughter, who is employed and is needed as well by her own husband and children. Further, as health care consultant Doris Fine indicates, this form of care amounts almost to the equivalent of an unpaid full-time job "accompanied by stress, fatigue, guilt, fear of nursing home placement, and family strife."[30]

IMPACT ON CAREGIVERS

Family members who care for a disabled older relative pay a price.[31] This price may be openly understood and acceptable to all concerned, and involve, for example, having a woman, now in middle age, give up a paid job and take over the care of her mother. However, there are covert costs as well, often poorly appreciated by the people involved and the cause of later stress. Pressures that derive from longstanding family interrelationships may reach a peak when the parent's fate is involved. Which of the children is expected to sacrifice her own life choices? What are the prices paid among caregivers, beyond loss of income and time, in divorce, stress-related disease, and abuse of the older person being helped? What will be done if the principal caregiver collapses? How does the family deal with the emotional impact of seeing a loved and respected person become frail and dependent; and the sense that the burden of care will go on forever, that there is no relief in sight?[32]

One device for estimating the consequences in such a situation is called the Family Coping Index.[33] Originally designed for assessing the skills of public health nurses, it is well adapted for families to use themselves. The parameters cited for evaluation of the principal caregiver's ability include physical independence, therapeutic competence, knowledge of the health status of the person under care, ability to apply the principles of general hygiene, attitude toward health care, and emotional strength. A Caregivers Strain Index[34] has also been developed. The factors included are inconvenience, confinement, family and work adjustments, competing demands on time, change in personal plans, emotional adjustment, ability to handle upsetting behavior, feelings of being overwhelmed, sleep disturbances, and physical and financial strain. Family groups who are sufficiently calm and organized can use both indexes to evaluate the most prudent means for meeting their needs. It is also reasonable to seek outside advice from a case manager/social worker, the family physician, or staff members of a formal home health care program in order to develop a coherent, effective plan of care that does not harm any family member unduly.

These methods of evaluation suggest strongly that family members and others who give informal help to the frail elderly will benefit from technical training, particularly those whose scores show that they are under substantial strain. Training enhances self-confidence, improves quality of care, and decreases the likelihood of burnout. Legislation to fund a demonstration program for family training has been proposed by Senator Bill Bradley (D-NJ).[35]

One clear task that can be delegated to a willing family member not directly involved in care is to find appropriate outside help. This person can establish community contacts through the local Office on Aging, Visiting Nurse agency, or hospital, and bring together the appropriate people for creation of a logical care plan.[36] Once a program is in place that seems tolerable to the family members concerned, likely to remain stable, and palatable to the older person under care, the major caregivers can take the time to consider how best to capitalize further on the strengths of the people involved. A. Bregman, a social worker, studied the home care status of chronically ill children[37] and developed suggestions for management that seem entirely appropriate to the frail aged. We have adapted and summarized these suggestions, which are applicable largely in situations where substantial informal support is available.

- *Focus on today rather than the future.*
  - Schedule the responsibilities of family members on a day-to-day basis.
  - Plan daily activities to fit the patient's condition, interests, and functional ability.
  - Help the patient to set realistic goals.
- *Maximize normalization of family lives.*
  - Maintain regular daily schedules for natural supporters.
  - Give the patient as much independence as possible.
  - Educate others about the patient's abilities.
- *Minimize the vulnerability of the family.*
  - Find and use credible sources of information and support.
  - Seek choices in intractable situations.
  - Solve problems with the patient's interests first in mind.
  - Oversee the work of outside personnel.
- *Capitalize on personal strengths.*
  - Allow time for respite.
  - Acknowledge the facts of the situation.
  - Plan realistic alternatives for various physical and emotional needs of patient and caregivers.
- *Establish a support network.*
  - Discuss concerns with family members and friends, and try to make major decisions by consensus.
  - Encourage expression of feelings in a productive manner.

- Establish and/or participate in support groups.
- Seek help from organizations with special interests in the patient's condition or the family's situation.

GIVING HELP
TO NATURAL SUPPORTERS

Families often slip gradually into care situations without adequately understanding the issues and difficulties involved, which leads to a multifaceted failure, loss of the older person to an institution or death, and long term guilt and recrimination. Various forms of assistance are available to natural supporters. Unfortunately, family members may settle for help that comes easily to hand and thus miss key ingredients for success.[38] A haphazard approach is likely to result in services that are too sparse or excessive, waste money and energy, and cause frustration and tension within the network of caregivers.

Before the days of massive federal deficits and limitations in spending for domestic programs, a spate of suggestions were put forth for controlled means of helping families with homebound relatives.[39] These are worth noting, so that they may be resurrected when the pendulum swings back: direct financial payments for care of their relatives at home, tax breaks, special access to government entitlements and benefits for older people cared for by family members, development of respite and social services for the natural supporters, requirements that families share with government the costs of home care, and means for freeing assets of the elderly for use in long term care, through home equity conversion or new forms of insurance (see chapter 2).

REIMBURSEMENT TO FAMILIES

The matters of financial payments, tax breaks, and social services for families require additional comment. Respite care, issues of entitlements, and freeing assets are discussed in chapters 2 and 9.

Any discussion of paying financial benefits to families for care of aged relatives at home raises two questions: Is it morally right for the government to pay families for what they should in justice and propriety do for their own relatives anyway? How can the government avoid the enormous costs consequent to assuming payment for the care that natural supporters now give for free?

It is easy to dodge the moral issue by noting that the current fiscal climate at all levels of government makes the matter moot. And yet the question persists. There exist methods through which families who are determined, knowledgeable, and well placed can tap public dollars. In the 1970s a New York City congresswoman managed to obtain Medicaid eligibility for her mother so that the state would pay for nursing home placement. If public-paid home care benefits were made available to the general populace, similar events would undoubtedly take place. What share of costs for long term care should in fairness be borne by patient or family? What should be the government's portion? Should eligibility be based on income or assets? Should there be an entitlement based solely on age and/or need?

Two forms of financial benefits to older people and their families have been proposed: tax incentives and cash grants. In each, the purpose of the funding has been to allow choice in the purchase of health and paraprofessional services at home. Tax credits have been proposed in national legislation but never passed. One type would have given older people eligible for nursing home reimbursements under Medicaid and Medicare a tax credit equal to 50 percent of the daily cost of the institution if they chose instead to remain at home.[40] In the 1970s the Maryland Office on Aging proposed a $250 deduction from taxes for any person caring for an aged individual at home.[41] In 1979 Oregon initiated a tax credit for caregivers.[42] A general problem with tax strategies is the presumption that the recipients have a reasonable level of solvency. Without this, the tax credit has little value. Thus such programs are primarily of benefit to middle-income families who lack sufficient funds to purchase services but are not eligible for Medicaid.[43]

Tax proposals of this nature are largely untried. Direct cash grants to families or to older people for the purpose of obtaining assistance at home have a more substantial history. California, Colorado, Florida, Minnesota, Nebraska, Utah, and Washington have used this approach, some with benefits directed toward any family member, some toward the spouse. Coresidence is a requirement in some instances. Perhaps the most prominent effort of this nature is that of the Veterans Administration. The VA gives supplemental funds to disabled veterans who qualify for its Aid and Attendance Program. More than 170,000 individuals receive a cash benefit through this program, enabling them to pay for additional help at home.[44]

SOCIAL SERVICES FOR FAMILIES

Key forms of assistance characteristically offered by social workers are case management, counseling, and group support.

Counseling

Family members faced with the complexities of care for a frail home-bound aged relative often need more than a simple referral to an agency. Guidance is needed over the immediate and long term regarding such matters as the logical division of tasks and authority within the family network, assuring that the older person maintains appropriate control, understanding and handling guilt, and observing the work of paraprofessionals. Counsel from a sage and experienced physician, a social worker trained in the field, or a religious figure is likely to be helpful, and may become an imperative in order to avoid collapse of the home situation.

In a formal sense, counseling usually includes helping people to accept casework for such purposes as obtaining entitlements and/or services. Guidance must accompany all such efforts, as often feelings of pride within the family prevent members from acknowledging the need for such means-tested benefits as Medicaid. Obtaining information for the family or patient and offering practical advice are part of the counseling function as well.[45] The therapeutic value of counseling must also be emphasized. Primary caretakers under stress, and the homebound patients themselves, often value greatly the opportunity simply to talk privately with an objective, caring outsider, to express feelings that custom or propriety demands be hidden from others, or to reminisce.

Groups for Natural Supporters

Bringing together informal caretakers of homebound aged people in groups serves several purposes. The elemental themes are cognitive learning and sharing of feelings for mutual support. Groups are customarily led by a trained person, usually a social worker or nurse, and people who share common difficulties or challenges are encouraged to participate. Groups on the frail elderly have dealt with specific disorders, such as dementia,[46] or have concentrated on general concerns.[47]

Evaluation has shown that participants develop a sense of mutual support from others in the group; learn insight regarding their own responses and those of the older relative enmeshed in a life situation of major stress; gain practical knowledge about the clinical conditions of elderly persons and about the aging process; and sense the group to be "a safe place to share concerns."[48]

Groups have been formed through requests by family caretakers to staff members of formal programs[49] and from concerns identified by staff members themselves. One such group, developed at St. Vincent's Hospital in New York City, grew from the observation by social workers in the hospital's long term home health care program that patients made grueling demands on their relatives.[50] The amount of time the staff spent providing practical and emotional support suggested the value of a group for spouses, adult children, and close friends. The following material transcribed from group sessions illustrates the point:

SOCIAL WORKER: The reason for bringing you together, the whole goal, was to try to keep people out of institutions and in their own homes, and I think the three of you are a very vital part of the program because you are doing that. You are keeping people that you love very much out of institutions, and you have a lot of experience in doing it. We can talk about how you've been helped to do it and how you can help each other to continue to do it.

NP [sixty-four-year-old man, friend of an eighty-two-year-old male patient]: I just want to say that my particular charge was in a very good institution, with wonderful people. That I could see, a very costly place, and after being there for a few weeks, I came to find that he was tied down to the bed. They were worried that he would fall out of the bed, but it seemed to me that they could have put a railing up, or some kind of a safeguard. Instead he was tied down with a sheet. I guess in order that he not be too much trouble in bodily functions. Various pipes were all connected to him. And he kept complaining of the pain that that gave him. He didn't know who I was or where he was. And I started to beg, "Please, release him." "Oh, no, you don't know what you're up against." "Well, let me try. Please release him from those pipes." So he came home; and I can bear witness that in a matter of weeks, being in his own surroundings, with a sympathetic person at his side, the telephone ringing, things of that sort . . .

OR: [forty-year-old woman caring for her seventy-eight-year-old mother]: In other words, he was back in life again.

NP: Yeah, he got all his memory back. He knew what was happening. You have a bunch of people in an institution that are just degenerating into vegetables when they could be leading some kind of normal life in a family group.

SOCIAL WORKER: Okay, do you want to tell us a little bit about your situation?

ST: [forty-five-year-old woman caring for her eighty-three-year-old father] I have always catered to my parents. "Honor thy father and thy mother." All the way. I mean, there was no such thing as entertaining the idea of putting them in a nursing home. Family members assisted as they were able. This was simply expected of the child. And so it's part tradition, part the fear that we have of institutions, of stories that we've heard about them on TV and such. And yet, you know, my father will sit back many a time and say, "Why doesn't Christ take me so that I do not burden you?" and I realize that he *truly* doesn't want to burden anyone. But he's helpless. . . .[51]

The group process seemed to allow individuals the opportunity for personal relationships. The members helped each other by working out feelings and emotions regarding their aged parents.

ST: I think O was just a little bit too emotionally caught up last week.

OR: I was going to be very quiet this week. I felt I dumped my load last week.

SOCIAL WORKER: I'm interested in what you're saying. You think she was too emotionally caught up?

ST: More so than previous times. Normally she isn't like that.

OR: I know I had a trying week. I thought, "Oh, marvelous. I'll go cry on somebody's shoulder." Three shoulders, yet. And be comforted. And everybody can say, "There, there," and go away feeling better. There's a lot to be said for that. . . . What I was trying to say last week is that I wasn't feeling guilty because I was upset. I felt I had a right to be upset. The thing that was so frustrating was there was no way out of it. There's no changing Mother.[52]

FRIENDS

Sometimes a friend wishes to accept great responsibility for a homebound person. ST, a member of the group just discussed, is an example. Instead of providing physical care, however, it is more common that friends accept a share of social functions, give moral support, indulge confidences, and enjoy mutual interests and hobbies. When friends assist during illness, the help is usually short term or sporadic.[53] As the jargon in the field puts it, "Friends are more likely to perform expressive functions rather than instrumental ones."[54]

In situations where the next generation of relatives—daughters and daughters-in-law—have become the major sources of help, friends are the only peers likely to be on the scene. Older persons who have become relatively helpless may feel useless and unwanted. They may recognize that the family members who have gathered around to help do so from a sense of duty. A friend, on the other hand, is present out of desire. Mutual needs are fulfilled in friendship, mutual choice observed.[55] Friends can exchange intimacy of expression and feeling that may be impossible in a family relationship. In fact, if the older person wants to discuss how she is being treated by her family, who better to complain to than a friend? This relationship enhances self-esteem and sense of personal value, and as such offers positive reasons for living, struggling to improve physical disabilities, and maintaining independence. Friendship is the definitive social relationship. It is voluntary, mutual, and a pleasure for its own sake.[56]

Discussions of natural support usually emphasize family relationships, but the involvement of friends, particularly those who are neighbors,[57] often becomes of critical value when the older person has no family, or if they have left the scene. As Cantor points out, a significant proportion of older people, perhaps one-third or more, are in this situation.[58] For these older people, friends may become surrogate relatives, accept long-range responsibilities, share in the making of critical decisions, and accept legal duties.[59]

AN OVERVIEW
OF INFORMAL SUPPORTS

Some families will never give up, others quail at the first adversity, but there is a breaking point in most such situations. Brody's study of two decades ago remains relevant.[60] She sought the major precipitating reasons why applications were made to nursing homes by or for people who had at least one adult child. Of eighty-five persons, thirty-eight were referred because of the applicant's physical or mental impairment; seven because of similar impairment of the applicant's spouse; ten because of the illness or death of the adult child (three because of the death of that person's spouse and two because of multiple deaths in the family); and six for other reasons, such as bad neighborhood, loneliness, and difficulty in relationships.

These results support the view that only a major negative event will compel most families to seek nursing home placement. The health of the primary caregivers among the natural supporters must be preserved in order for the older person to stay at home.

Brody's data also relate to the question of whether families give up their responsibilities if paid sources of care are readily available. Numerous analyses establish that substitution, when it is possible, is used sparingly. Norms of familial responsibility remain strong in our society. Family members tend to respond to the needs of their older relatives, and when they ask for help from service agencies, they tend to be modest in their requests. They want to be supported, not supplanted.[61]

Confirmatory data come from a three-year study of ninety-six elderly people and their families, conducted from 1976 through 1979. The project, entitled the Family Support Program, was funded and administered by the Community Service Society of New York. Caseworkers and homemakers were provided for the enrolled homebound aged persons and were conceived as incentives, as complements, to encourage families to sustain their efforts.

Among the most significant results of the project was the finding that the majority of families maintained the same level of support for their frail and aged relative as had existed prior to the program. This was true despite the introduction of services or their expansion subsequent to the program. Dwight Frankfather, Michael J. Smith, and Frances G. Caro, the investigators, concluded that "it appears reasonable to think that short-range substitution does favor long-range persistence."[62]

In the twenty-three family situations where less involvement was noted during the study period, most had received additional services from the Family Services Program. In fact, the staff encouraged heavily involved families to do less by offering homemaker services, so that periods of respite could be assured. The logic of this approach is supported by a 1983 policy report of the New York State Office for the Aging. Among the major findings are, first, that family care appears to have an important influence in decreasing the placement rate of older people in institutions and, second, that some short term substitution of formal care for that given by families may save public funds because it may permit the family to retain its older members in the community for a longer period than might otherwise have occurred if formal care was absent.[63]

VOLUNTEERS

Voluntary community service is a cherished tradition in the United States. A 1983 Gallup poll[64] showed that 84 million persons in this country volunteer yearly about 8.4 billion hours of service. In long term care, the roster of figures whose contributions have set modern-day precedents include Jane Addams in social reform, Dorothea Dix in care for the mentally ill, and Lillian Wald in public health nursing.[65]

DEFINITIONS

By tradition, a volunteer performs a service without pay. However, the issue of compensation is complex, and opinions vary concerning appropriate and feasible rationales for reimbursement.[66] Payment for service in the form of a stipend for out-of-pocket costs is common. The federal government provides two examples of this approach in the field of long term care: The Senior Companion Program gives stipends, and the Retired Senior Volunteer Program offers reimbursement for incidental expenses. Both are administered through ACTION, a federal agency supporting voluntary services, established under the Domestic Volunteer Service Act.

Volunteers have worked in the homes of those who need help, at institutions such as nursing homes, or as aides to discharge planners within acute care hospitals. Their most frequent service is in providing home help and companionship. Compatibility is vital. Often, as Dr. Allen Spiegel of

Downstate (NY) Medical Center points out, program directors for volunteer services should consider matching for age, occupation, cultural background, and hobbies.[67]

Volunteers have also become advocates on behalf of the elderly. In the East Tennessee Advocacy Assistance Program, for example,[68] trained volunteers assisted the state ombudsman in monitoring and investigating long term care facilities. Results of their efforts have included changing the 4:00 A.M. wake-up call at a nursing home and the release of a patient held against her wishes.

Volunteers usually function within structured organizations, which are often directed by a paid coordinator and governed by a board. In turn, these organizations have formed associations that focus and direct volunteers for effective lobbying and to press for policy changes. An example is the National Citizens Coalition of Nursing Home Reform, founded in 1975 and now composed of 215 organizations in forty states.

FRIENDLY VISITOR PROGRAMS

Friendly visitor programs fulfill needs of homebound elderly people for human contact, chore services, and observation of their physical and mental status. Further, in times of crisis, the friendly visitor is available as an advisor or go-between; and in less stressful moments is a companion and shopper, reader and writer, a sharer of hobbies and gossip.

The Village Visiting Neighbors (VVN) in the Greenwich Village area of New York is a prototype and worth examining in detail because it has worked out many of the parameters of how volunteers function within an organized program. VVN was established in 1972 by a consortium of interested individuals and local agencies, including churches, synagogues, block associations and their members, settlement houses, the Visiting Nurse Service of New York, and St. Vincent's, the local hospital. The founding purpose was to organize a group of volunteers who would visit their homebound neighbors in the community, develop personal relationships with them, and carry out simple tasks. VVN has gradually grown, so that by the end of 1985 it had served 289 clients in a twelve-month period, with a volunteer pool of 210 persons.* [,69]

The VVN board of directors holds legal responsibility for the conduct of the program, its paid coordinator, and the volunteer visitors. Board members are representatives of the original sponsoring organizations, experienced volunteers and aged people from the area. The board has accepted the burden of fund raising, worked out appropriate bylaws, created

*Robin McCarty, CSW, Project Director, Village Visiting Neighbors, New York. Personal communication, July 1986.

a training program for volunteers, and devised proper record-keeping systems and techniques of documentation.

From the start, VVN grasped its responsibility to control the quality of care. Standards of service have been developed, and volunteers are screened and supervised, to ensure that clients are not abused. The VVN guidelines for volunteer activity urge the visitor to reveal the qualities of a friend:

- Be dependable. Do not promise more than you can fulfill.
- Be cheerful, without inappropriate exuberance.
- Make appointments for visits beforehand, and keep them.
- Accept conditions in the home as you find them, barring matters of immediate safety.
- Encourage the client to maintain confidence in the professional health workers involved in the plan of care.
- Engage the cooperation of other household members, if any.
- Respect the confidences of the client.
- Keep relations on a friendly, cheerful, dignified plane.
- Sustain interest and enthusiasm. Realize that you bring fresh perspectives from the outside world.

Certain prohibitions are emphasized as well:

- Do not give medication or offer medical advice.
- Do not suggest treatments.
- Do not consult with physicians or other health workers on behalf of the client.
- Do not discuss other clients' problems.
- Do not lift the client. This takes skill and training as well as strength.
- Do not undermine the client's confidence in others who help.
- Do not criticize or give advice on housekeeping or other conditions in the home.
- Do not give money to the client, and do not accept money or gifts of substance. Remember, you are a volunteer.
- Do not be discouraged or frustrated if your client is slow to develop an interest in you.
- Do not get emotionally involved. Try to be objective, but not callous or tough.

Guidelines of this nature serve a valid purpose in helping to make the interaction between volunteer and client viable. They establish a structure within which volunteers can conduct themselves with confidence. In turn, clients develop trust. It then becomes possible for an effective relationship to develop. Training of the volunteers in the VVN program, essential to validating the guidelines and also to eliminating poor candidates, consists of open group discussions led by the program coordinator. There is a didactic quality to the subjects under discussion, which include the process of getting old, attitudes of the homebound elderly and the volunteer's reaction, developing relationships, medical problems of the elderly, and understanding the end of life. The groups serve purposes beyond the simple transmission of information. Volunteers have the opportunity to ask questions, express concerns, and share in development of mutual support. Their stereotypes and clichéd attitudes toward older people may be displayed, and corrected by others in the group.

Over the years, the coordinators have been the key factor in making the VVN viable. They get to know every volunteer visitor and aged client, maintain records, and conduct training programs and meetings; they are responsible to the board of directors for the organization's daily activities.

CURRENT STATUS OF VOLUNTEER PROGRAMS

Federal and state government and foundations have promoted the formation of volunteer programs. On the federal level, the Domestic Volunteer Services Act authorizes the Senior Companion Program and the Retired Senior Volunteer Program, both administered by ACTION. In addition, funds available under Title III of the Older Americans Act (see chapter 2) can be used to support certain forms of volunteer activity, including information and referral services, transportation, escort, and advocacy. Section 2176 of Public Law 97-35, which was passed in 1981, permitted waivers to the states for expansion of in-home services that in part could be offered through volunteer programs.

An example of a state-sponsored volunteer program is that in the state of Washington.[70] In 1981 the state legislature cut $27 million from the paid chore program, which offered paid workers to low-income elderly people who needed help to stay safely at home. As a substitute, later in 1981 the legislature allocated slightly more than $1 million for the development of statewide volunteer chore services. Catholic Community Services of Seattle, in cooperation with the Church Council of Greater Seattle, received part of these funds to establish a Voluntary Chore Ministry. Through this process it became possible to give staff assistance, insurance coverage, and mileage reimbursement to volunteers in local religious congregations who wished to do chore services for the aged.

The ministry staff provides support, counsel, and training for the contact persons at each congregation, by telephone, personal contact, and monthly meetings. The staff members see themselves as facilitators and enablers of the ministry of each local congregation. The actual service to each client is offered in the name of the congregation. By 1986, there were more than ninety-five congregations involved, representing fifteen denominations. In the prior year, through volunteers, 45,000 hours of house cleaning, laundry, shopping, moving, yard work, and home repairs were completed. A monthly average of 513 volunteers was available to meet the needs of the 1,839 referrals received. An average of 495 frail elderly people were on the roster each month.

The private sector has a lengthy history of work with volunteers. Some major organizations depend on volunteer workers to carry out virtually all of their functions. The American Red Cross, for example, utilizes more than 9 million such persons in a given year. Of these, about 1.5 million are service volunteers, and one-third of these, or about 500,-000 individuals, are involved in health-related programs. They share in services at neighborhood clinics and hospitals, help handicapped people move about, prepare and deliver meals for homebound people, and teach cardiopulmonary resuscitation and first aid. Health professionals who volunteer with the Red Cross offer courses in nutrition, health care, home nursing, and care of the aged. This example illustrates the size and potential of the volunteer pool available to the long-term care spectrum.

Foundations have chosen to spend some of their funds on development of volunteer programs. The Robert Wood Johnson Foundation, for instance, funded a study in 1982 to test the feasibility of using senior volunteers in long-term care.[71] It then followed with funding for a demonstration effort, called Project HELP (Homebound Elderly Linked with Peers), to explore the use of older people, who were reimbursed for costs, as integral parts of service programs.

Project HELP ran for twenty-one months, according to a detailed summary prepared by researcher Deborah Hillman,[72] ending in September 1985. It tested the feasibility of using older volunteers as caregivers to aged homebound people who needed companionship and assistance with simple, routine tasks. The project was administered by the New York City Department for the Aging, and served to: (1) determine the availability of older volunteers to assist in the delivery of services to aged people in their homes; (2) examine rates of retention and turnover of volunteers; (3) ascertain the most needed functions for volunteers who serve the frail elderly and the supports needed to sustain the volunteers themselves; (4) identify time and task configurations acceptable to senior volunteers, worthwhile for clients, and cost effective for the program; (5) determine whether the use of volunteers reduces per-client service costs and permits increased client load for paraprofessionals; and (6) explore future funding mechanisms to support senior volunteer home aides.

The study also documented the development and operation of the program, and evaluated its impact on volunteers and clients.

The New York City Department for the Aging chose two voluntary city agencies to host the program. Volunteer recruitment was pursued through presentations about Project HELP at senior centers, libraries, and other community organizations. It soon became evident that overcoming the resistance of community organizations to the project's search for volunteers was a challenge. Some local groups already providing services and advocacy for the elderly were concerned that this program might be an attempt to reduce paid home care services by using volunteers. Other volunteer groups were anxious about issues of supply and control, the competition for the volunteer base of healthy older persons. These issues were overcome through repeated review of project goals with all concerned.

Recruitment of clients was also difficult. This was due primarily to matters of client suitability and acceptance, and to issues of safety for the volunteers asked to consider visiting in geographical areas presumed risky. Ultimately an adequate base of clients was established through the community contacts used in the volunteer recruitment phase.

During the course of the project three volunteer training programs were held. Each took fifteen hours over a three-day period. Once trained, volunteers were matched with clients, and visiting began. Program supervision by paid staff of the two host agencies consisted of telephone contact, monthly in-service training sessions for the volunteers, and interim client assessments.

To cover associated out-of-pocket costs, volunteers were reimbursed at the rate of $3 per two-hour visit. Although they consistently said that this payment was not a major motive for their participation, program staff felt it to be an important ingredient. Volunteers also got support through enthusiastic staff involvement, shared friendships and interaction, and appreciation from their clients.

During the first twelve months Project HELP recruited, trained, and matched thirty-five volunteers. Three others left the program during training, and seven more just before matching. Five were asked to leave the program because of evident personal problems, poor language skills, and/or ambivalence. The subsequent attrition rate of volunteers remained below 9 percent, considered low for a volunteer program of this nature.

During this twelve-month period 116 clients were assessed for service and 77 matched with volunteers, who generally visited for two hours each week. The most common activities cited were companionship and conversation in the form of reminiscence. Reading, exercise, preparation of snacks, light shopping, and letter writing were noted frequently as well. To avoid duplicating services of paid paraprofessional staff, and for the sake of safety, volunteers were not allowed to perform such tasks as bathing, lifting, and clothes washing.

Cost analysis revealed that administrative overhead was expensive in Project HELP and operating costs were low. The average cost for a volunteer visit was $49.18 if training expenses were included ($33.74 if they were excluded). Expenses per hour of visiting, including and excluding training, respectively, were $21.59 and $14.82 for administrative costs and $2.99 and $2.05 for operating costs. These figures suggest that it might be more economical to develop similar programs within a preexisting home care agency. Cost factors aside, Project HELP was generally viewed as a positive experience. The study showed that older volunteers who wish to work with their homebound peers can be found and that they are competent; that with supervision the dropout rate will be low; and that a program of this nature can be an effective adjunct to the home care system. The volunteers supplemented and supported the paraprofessionals, and no evidence was noted during the project that paid services decreased.

ADVANTAGES AND DISADVANTAGES OF VOLUNTEER PROGRAMS

Among the hypothetical benefits of using volunteers in long term care programs is that costs will be lowered, as volunteer services will substitute for those offered by others at market rates. This point recognizes that, as the number of older people and the costs of their care increase, every means to shave expenses will be sought. If volunteers can be incorporated into staff of existing agencies and institutions for the aged, paid employees can focus on patients with the more complex needs and thus be used with greater efficiency.

Some volunteers may be able to offer flexible hours of service and therefore be available when paid staff is in relatively short supply, as on weekends or evenings. Some may have a few hours to offer, and thus able to help an older person for short periods at crucial times such as at meals, dressing, or retiring to bed. Paid employees, dependent on a full day of work, are rarely available for this sort of coverage.

There are programmatic costs for work with volunteers as well. Recruiting, training, and supervision require a paid management staff and the preparation of written guides and manuals. Expenses can be significant, as the results of Project HELP indicate. A further disadvantage of dependence on unpaid personnel is their inherent unreliability in many instances. Turnover consumes staff time and disappoints clients who have learned to rely on a specific volunteer.

Volunteer competition with existing paid paraprofessionals is a potential problem as well. Many tasks overlap. Examples include money management, reality orientation, feeding, hygiene, and dressing. Establishing quality control over the work of volunteers is a further concern, particularly difficult to handle because much of the service takes place in the privacy of the client's home.

While it has virtues, an emphasis on engaging volunteers who are themselves elderly brings with it negative aspects as well. A restriction that bars younger persons deprives them of an opportunity to learn about the elderly, to break down stereotypes. There is, after all, a significant value in promoting contact between generations. In addition, there exist inherent restrictions on the tasks that older volunteers can be expected to perform. Programs that use only elderly persons must take their physical limitations into consideration, and thus perhaps they may fail to address adequately the full range of client needs.

Finally, there are legal, regulatory, financing, and insurance considerations. These include program liability for actions of the volunteers, the rationale for payment of stipends, sources of reimbursement, and conflicts with unions. Certified home health care agencies and long term care institutions cite lack of liability insurance for volunteers as a reason for excluding them. This explanation may be a screen that masks the larger issue of union opposition.

The development of formal volunteer programs requires money and effort. To recruit, train, and retain volunteers, and to find meaningful work for them, are troublesome tasks, difficult to implement. However, if the process is successful, the range of rewards for the recipients of service, the larger community, and the volunteers themselves is significant.

CONCLUSION

As Cantor[73] emphasizes, the social support system, is an amalgam of informal help from family and friends and formal services from large organizations. These may be run by government or the voluntary sector, and offer both paid and volunteer assistance. There exists a balance among these systems, the network of natural supports, and the formal program structure. This balance should be understood and respected.

There is always the danger, in periods of presumed limited resources, that the informal care system . . . will be offered as a viable alternative to community-based services. Such an approach would not only destroy the balance between informal and formal but would result in a serious reduction in care for older people. Only when both systems are in place and functioning at optimum levels will the increasing number of elderly be assured the long term care they need and desire.[74]

PART FOUR

AUGMENTING THE LONG TERM CARE SYSTEM

Chapter 9

Day Care, Foster Care, Hospice, and Respite

In the fall of 1983, Jackson Gumb, director of the Adult Care Home Program of the Kansas Department of Social Security, testified before the United States Senate Subcommittee on Health of the Senate Finance Committee.[1] He reported that the state of Kansas was serving 453 persons through fourteen different service programs in an effort to delay or avoid institutional placement. He estimated that, as a result, Kansas was saving $65,000 a month. Gumb's testimony, highlighting a phenomenon that is spreading slowly across the country, revealed that in some instances the government was willing to pay for an array of services in order to enable the elderly and disabled to remain in their own communities. The results in Kansas during the next three years offered encouragement. By August of 1986, 894 individuals were enrolled, saving the state an estimated $2 million a year.[2]

A number of other important community-based services have been developed in recent years that allow frail older people and their families to cope with chronic illness without requiring nursing home care. The concepts are not necessarily new. Foster care and day care have been used extensively for other populations, and the hospice dates back to medieval Europe; but their applications to the needs of elderly people and the slowly increasing support of such services by federal and state funds has opened a new era in long term care.

This discussion covers four major programs: adult day care, adult foster care, hospice, and respite care. We consider them to be essential components of the long term care spectrum designed to serve the elderly by providing a more appropriate match of services to need.

ADULT DAY CARE

In some ways, the purpose of adult day care is quite similar to that of child day care. Such programs can be useful for working couples willing to care for an elderly parent who needs some form of supervision.[3] Adult day care can also respond to a need for planned therapy or learning activities— better nutrition, for example.[4] But adult day care obviously differs from child care in important ways. It "is a blend of psychosocial and health services that may exist in a variety of balances. What is essential is that the two services exist together for the two needs cannot be separated."[5]

PURPOSE

Adult day care emphasizes both achievement and a continued effort to retain and enhance independence. For many frail elderly people, adult day care enables them to live at home, to retain community contacts.[6] In *Adult Day Care—A Practical Guide,* edited by Carol Lium O'Brien of Boston College School of Nursing, former Congressman Robert F. Drinan says that the purpose of adult day care is "to encourage the elderly to maintain their physical level of functioning and to promote a renewed interest in life through a variety of social and emotional support services."[7] The book further identifies more specific achievements of adult day care: to provide health supervision, offer support with activities of daily living, and help frail older persons as they relate to a variety of community services.

Some centers focus on health aspects, specializing in rehabilitation.[8] In recent years, others have been created specifically for victims of Alzheimer's disease.[9] A report published in the *PRIDE Institute Journal of Long Term Home Health Care* noted that of 346 adult day care centers surveyed, all had some demented participants. While only 5 percent of such centers primarily served these individuals, almost 20 percent indicated that at least one-half to three-quarters of their patients suffered from dementia.[10] In these specialized instances, day care may be an integral form of respite for family members attempting to care for these complex patients.[11]

Because adult day care is provided in a group setting, it can offer extensive services and meet an array of needs. It incorporates aspects as disparate as the social center and the day hospital. In many respects, it is similar to the nursing home. But it maintains a critical distinction: The adult day care center strives to help patients live in their own homes. It does not supplant the independent housing functon.[12]

THE HISTORY OF ADULT DAY CARE

Current adult day care centers have their roots in psychiatric day hospitals established prior to World War II. In 1933 a psychiatric day hospital was established in Moscow. Twelve years later Adams House began operation in Boston, Massachusetts, to decrease the use of hospitals for psychiatric care.[13]

Like many other forms of community-based long term care, adult day care really developed in England. In 1952 the Cowley Royal Hospital in Oxford established the first geriatric day hospital. It provided therapy and social activities, and allowed patients to be discharged from acute care beds while continuing to receive needed services and support.[14]

The original English day centers were cost-saving options for a postwar country trying to respond to the needs of an aging population. In 1971 the British began to distinguish between the day hospital, for those people at greater risk, and the day center, developed for frail eldery people who required less attention. As part of Britain's National Health Service, day care has continued to grow and remains important in the schema of services to elderly people. In fact, "Britain is the leader of the adult day care movement, with the oldest and most extensive system of day care services. On any weekday, it has been estimated that 40,000 people attend 1,000 day care centers for the elderly."[15]

THE GROWTH OF DAY CARE IN THE UNITED STATES

Although other models of community treatment were tested after the Adams House experiment, no real growth occurred until the 1960s. President Kennedy's interest in the care of the mentally ill and his emphasis on deinstitutionalization created an impetus for other creative models.[16] There was no real public initiative to investigate the cost effectiveness or value of adult day care, however, for another decade. In 1972 Congress authorized the Department of Health, Education and Welfare (HEW) to study alternatives to nursing home care. The language of Public Law 92-603, Section 222, specifically requested the department to evaluate cost and quality issues regarding Medicare and Medicaid reimbursement for adult day care.[17]

As a result of this legislation, several demonstration programs were initiated to provide day care, homemaker services, and, in some instances, both. In addition, in 1974 HEW began a study of ten of the eighteen known adult day care centers operating in the United States. Besides studying cost efficiency, these evaluations were to review the quality of health maintenance and rehabilitation offered to the population at risk of institutionalization, the frail elderly.[18]

ADULT DAY CARE COMES OF AGE

The results of these studies have been controversial. Costs of care for the experimental population often exceeded costs for the control groups. However, William G. Weissert, Director of the Program on Aging at the University of North Carolina, and his associates studied six demonstration sites and found that rates of institutionalization were reduced while contentment, mental functioning, and social activity remained the same or improved.[19] A common judgment was that program targeting of its participants was associated with cost effectiveness. That is, for elderly people who would never consider nursing home care, adult day care became an added-on cost. For people truly at risk of institutional placement who lacked other support systems, day care could save money.

In spite of the difficulties experienced by the demonstration programs, the popularity of adult day care continued to increase during the 1970s. By 1980, when Congress passed legislation making adult day care an allowable Medicaid expense, there were over six hundred centers in operation.[20] That same year, the National Council on Aging established a National Institute on Adult Day Care.[21] Of the six hundred centers, three hundred received money from Title XX Social Services funds, one hundred were Medicaid-reimbursed, and 120 were funded by the Older Americans Act. Adult day care had become a distinct, significant resource for elderly people with a wide range of health and personal needs.

PROGRAM COMPONENTS

To facilitate reports of his studies in the 1970s, Weissert identified two models of day care: Model I, or the day hospital model; and Model II, the multipurpose model. Model I was affiliated with a health care institution and had a strong health and rehabilitation orientation. Participants were dependent in at least one major activity of daily living and had some previous institutional care. Model II frequently was affiliated with a community service agency, and the programs had a stronger focus on social needs and meals. The participants had fewer dependencies or medical problems, needed some form of supervision, and were recruited mostly from the community.[22]

Another view distinguishes between psychosocial and medical-rehabilitation models. The two differ in staffing and activities: Rehabilitation services are available in the medical-rehabilitation model and a stronger counseling component is offered in the psychosocial model.[23] Other analysts use broader terms, such as medical and social, or separate these larger categories into three or four more specific groupings.[24] At issue, of course, is not the label but the particular services offered. It is important to realize that there are variations in types of services, depending on the center's sponsor or the needs that have been identified by the community.

The following services can be found at most adult day care centers: medical, nutritional, nursing, restorative (physical, occupational, speech therapy), social service, transportation, and clerical.[25]

Regulations may require that a minimum number of services be offered for licensing, but there are no limits to the potential combinations. Unlike many other forms of long term care, adult day care is noteworthy in its flexibility and ability to meet the needs of many individuals with different problems. For a definitive example, see the discussion of On Lok in chapter 6. The models that emphasize social interaction respond to the people with perhaps the simplest needs. Medical-rehabilitative adult day care centers, on the other hand, have been able to delay or avoid prolonged institutionalization for the very frail.

MODEL PROGRAMS

Four representative examples of adult day care centers will be discussed. They include the Harbor Area Adult Day Care Center in Costa Mesa, California; Menorah Park in Cleveland, Ohio; Birmingham (Alabama) Day Care for Adults; and the State of Florida Community Care for Elderly program.

In 1980 a resident of Costa Mesa, California, began searching for services for a mother-in-law with Alzheimer's disease. With the support of a nursing home, a neurologist from a local university, and other volunteer staff, a center was established in a local church. The program, called the Harbor Area Adult Day Care Center, has a work activity center much like a sheltered workshop, a recreational program, respite services, counseling, personal care, and socialization.[26] From 1980 to 1986 the program's annual budget grew from $35,000 to $360,000. Client fees of $23 per visit contributed $230,000, $36,000 comes from the California Department for Aging, and the remainder from charitable support. About eighty clients are registered and thirty to thirty-five are served each day. In 1985 the program moved to larger quarters and spawned a second unit, also a day care center, called Huntington Valley. The combined project is entitled the South Coast Institute for Applied Gerontology.*

Menorah Park in Cleveland, Ohio, is a nursing home that sponsors an adult day care program. Its goal is to assist people who wish to remain in the community, to prepare others for admission to its facility, or to help those on its waiting list cope while they remain at home. The prime interest of the program is care for moderately impaired patients with Alzheimer's disease, although others attend as well. The median length of stay is eighteen months, but clients have been active for as long as twelve years. Individuals routinely attend twice each week, and about 140 persons are on the active case roster. Two-thirds are provided transportation by the center's vans. Cost per client day at the Menorah Park Day Care Program for nondemented persons averages $34.25, including three meals and transportation. For Alzheimer's patients, cost is $45.00 per day. If necessary, fees can be adjusted.†

The Housing Authority of Birmingham, Alabama, operates two day care centers, and in 1986 provided assistance to about forty individuals daily.[27] The focus is on "frail, moderately handicapped or slightly confused persons 18 years old or older," but the majority are elderly. The usual referral derives from inability of the individual to manage alone, or family need. Clients must be certified as eligible by the Department of Pensions and Securities. No fee is charged if the client is income-eligible. A full-time caseworker is on staff. The program provides transportation to and from the centers, and also transports clients to appointments for medical care or social service counseling. A hot midday meal is included, and a substantial arts and crafts program is a major element of the program. Field trips, picnics, plays, and outside speakers complete the array of programs. Those with high priority for acceptance include older persons at point of discharge from nursing homes; those who live alone and are about to be institutionalized because they are unable to care for themselves; persons whose families need respite; and those who could be discharged from an institution if day care were available.

The state of Florida has supported adult day care services since 1973 through its Community Care for Elderly program. In 1980 the state began to license programs, and by mid-1981, 35 were in operation. Since then enormous growth has occurred, and by October 1986, 1,344 centers were functioning. The minimum age for participation is sixty years, and the median is near eighty. Seventy-five percent of the clients are women. Each center has at least two staff members, a director and an assistant. Day care

*Daniel Sands, Director, Harbor Area Adult Day Care Center, Costa Mesa, California. Personal communication, October 20, 1986.

†Joan Scharf, Director, Menorah Park Adult Day Health Center, Cleveland, Ohio. Personal communication, October 20, 1986.

is supported by contributions and client fees assessed on a sliding scale dependent on income, with a rate determined by a case manager. Most participants pay nothing.[*,28]

FUNDING ISSUES

In Great Britain, the day center or day hospital receives full funding through the government-sponsored National Health Service.[29] In the United States, this is not the case. The great variety of funding sources has substantially molded the development of adult day care services.

Title XX, or the Social Services Block Grant, supports some of the social components of adult day care. Medicaid (Title XIX) may fund some health service components. For example, when the Medicaid 2176 waiver program was introduced in 1981, many states agreed to allow reimbursement for adult day care for eligible participants. Various titles of the Older Americans Act have been used by states and localities to support adult day care, as in New York City and Florida. Revenue sharing, community organization funds, and private philanthropy have all been tapped by various centers in order to provide services for those who could not pay at least part of the daily rate. This irregular set of funding mechanisms has made financial management difficult. In addition, because the focus of each funding source varies, centers have had to balance certain demands and restrictions from the sources.[30] (See chapter 2 for further discussion of funding.)

Also at issue is the total lack of third-party reimbursement for some individuals. For those elderly people not eligible for services through Medicaid 2176 programs, adult day care can be financially unfeasible. Day care costs vary from as high as $60 to $70 per day to as little as $5, depending on the level of service offered.[31] While the monthly cost to attend an adult day care center may be far less than that for a nursing home bed, the elderly person may be eligible for full reimbursement in the latter case and for no financial assistance in the former.[32]

Few other forms of long term care have been scrutinized as carefully as adult day care services. Weissert's research raised considerable concern about the validity and value of adult day care. That analysis is important, both for the shortcomings it identifies and for the potential areas for financial savings upon which it did not focus.

Adult day care programs can attempt to achieve cost savings, focus on improved outcomes of participants, or seek to provide a better quality of life.[33] Even in Weissert's rather negative study, success was attained in

---

*Merrick W. Collier, Senior Human Services Program Specialist, State of Florida Community Care for Elderly Program. Personal communication, October 20, 1986.

some of these objectives. For example, a significant component of the experimental group retained or improved its functional ability, compared to the control group.[34] The experimental group maintained a generally higher level of contentment, mental functioning, and activity level, and death rates were statistically lower for certain subgroups. The rate of institutionalization was also lower. However, because a large percentage of the control group did not use any nursing home services, even in the absence of adult day care, Weissert concluded that adult day care was an add-on cost, not a substitution.

In some respects, he is correct. If the objective in providing adult day care is cost effectiveness, for some populations it is not the optimal solution. But Weissert's work also illustrates the variable nature of this analysis. For example, his initial study in 1974–75 involved the more social models of adult day care. Costs for these were lower than for the adult day care services studied in 1978–79, which were health-oriented.[35] Also, the populations considered were seriously disabled. A more appropriate focus might be persons only moderately disabled. Another factor is the availability of another person in the home at night, to help. Adult day care services are more successful at delaying or preventing institutionalization if a person is not left alone at all other times.[36] Finally, personal choice and cultural values have an impact. A study of adult day care services in Massachusetts revealed that about half the participants would have gone to a nursing home were it not for the program. Others would have refused, even if such services were deemed necessary by family or physician.[37]

By 1986 gerontology theorists had begun to notice the field of adult day care,[38] which appears to be a growing phenomenon. However, it remains poorly understood in regard to the population it serves, its possible structures, and the processes through which it operates. A major step toward better comprehension of adult day care may derive from a formal assessment of programs across the United States to be conducted by the Center for Health Services and Policy Research of Northwestern University.[39] Regardless of the results, however, it is clear that adult day care programs cannot serve all older persons. The needs of the elderly are too varied and the nature of the programs too diverse.

FOSTER CARE

Only in recent years has attention been focused on creating a structured form of foster care for frail elderly persons. As a first step in the development, analysts have attempted to identify its availability. Multiple names have been used: adult foster home, personal care home, and family care home.[40] In other instances, foster care occurs without a formal name. It is merely the logical response in a community, an informal adoption of an older person in need.[41] In addition, because no standards have existed, it has been difficult to eliminate inappropriate variations. The services cannot be traced by any specific funding source, and a variety of government entities may sponsor or oversee foster care services.[42]

Realizing that such confusion could be corrected only if a standard was introduced, states are now beginning to define the identifying features of adult foster care. In 1978 a study was conducted describing a geriatric foster care program in Illinois. That report provided the following definition for geriatric foster care:

the programmatic use of a private residence for the care of a nonrelated elderly person who requires supervision and/or assistance with the essentials of daily life such as feeding or personal hygiene. Geriatric foster care is considered among the least restrictive housing options available and helps older persons remain a part of the community while availing themselves of needed supportive services.[43]

Furthermore, geriatric or adult foster care is differentiated from adult domiciliary care by the personalized matching process that foster care involves. Client needs and family characteristics are taken into consideration in a foster care placement.[44] Domiciliary placements frequently depend on space availability or proximity to other family members.

PROGRAM DESCRIPTION

In spite of the impetus the foster care movement received in the 1960s, advances have been slow. A few programs have been developed by departments of mental health and general social service agencies. In most instances the same key components have been included: board and care, familylike environment, professional supports, and some form of supervision.[45] However, emphases among programs have differed. Studies have revealed differences in the ages of the populations,[46] and variations in the degree of supervision provided by the sponsoring agency.[47] The following program descriptions illustrate some of these differences. They also reflect the slow but growing interest in adult foster care as a method of responding to the particular needs of frail older persons.

Washington State Family Homes Project

The state of Washington applied for and received funding from HEW to operate a three-year foster home demonstration. In September 1968 programs were started in two sites. A third was added in 1969. By October 1971, with a statewide program in place, there were 560 homes licensed for foster care placement and 449 active placements.⁴⁸

The project had aims and goals to meet its definition both as a research project and for ongoing service. Project issues included proving acceptability of foster care as a concept and extending available services to adults in the state. On a second level, foster care was to promote a delay of institutionalization and offer a discharge alternative for persons leaving nursing homes. Within those four areas, specific points concerning the feasibility and desirability of the program design were also to be considered, such as cost, staffing, and training needs.

Participants in the Washington project were referred from various sources: 27 percent from their own homes, 13 percent from a relative's home, 16 percent from a nursing home (skilled), 18 percent from a mental institution or corrections facility, and 7 percent from a nursing facility (intermediate). Of the 1,641 referrals received from 1969 to 1971, 540 were placed and just over 200 were still in foster homes at the end of the demonstration. Of the other 340 participants, 35 percent had been able to return to their own homes, 6 percent had died, and 35 percent were in a nursing home or mental institution. Participants were accepted who required supervision, had motivation and limited nursing needs, and were sufficiently emotionally stable to adapt to the foster care environment. Drug or alcohol abuse, incontinence, or serious behavior problems normally precluded placement.

The Washington State project was considered successful. Homes were found and appropriate clients could be identified. Placements were considered beneficial, and comparison of program costs with costs of alternative forms of care proved foster care to be cost effective. The monthly cost per client, with state staff included, averaged $349, in 1971 dollars.

The Johns Hopkins Hospital Community Care Project

In 1978 Johns Hopkins Hospital, through its Social Work Department, initiated a foster care program for older adults in Baltimore. The Robert Wood Johnson Foundation provided funding for four years, with the goal of learning whether such a project was feasible, able to meet the needs of the elderly and of the hosts, and financially sound.⁴⁹ Frail elderly candidates were found on the inpatient units of the hospital and placed in foster homes if all standards were met. A control group was discharged to nursing homes.

To conduct the foster care component, Johns Hopkins employed a full-time nurse, a part-time social worker and secretary, and provided office space and guidance. From 1978 through 1982, all costs were covered by grant funds. In the postgrant years the hospital has attempted to break even on staff expenses through private philanthropic support, but by 1986 it recognized that the project was running at a financial loss.*

From the start, elderly tenants and sponsoring families were thoroughly screened for selection. A matching process then took place, following which the hospital provided training to the family members responsible for caregiving. The nurse and social worker were responsible for making regular visits to the home, to assure safety and quality of service.

The monthly costs of foster placement, consisting of fees given to the sponsoring families, have remained at about $400 a month. Of this, $35 is provided by Medicaid as a case management fee. The remainder is the responsibility of the elderly tenants, derived from their Supplemental Security Income (SSI) checks or personal funds.

The program was maintaining a total of twenty-five persons in foster care by the fall of 1986† and was not attempting to recruit new referrals, because funds for expansion were lacking. The intent was simply to keep stable the existing placements.

The Robert Wood Johnson Foundation and the hospital had originally hoped that the Maryland government would pick up a substantial part of the costs by allowing a long term care Medicaid waiver.[50] This goal has been thwarted by anxiety about cost at the state level. Despite this concern, the program appears to have been fiscally prudent. Johns Hopkins estimates its costs for staff support at $50,000 per year, or $2,000 per patient. Foster care families receive about $5,000 for each older person placed. The total of $7,000 yearly is modest if the alternative is nursing home placement.

The hospital's final report to the foundation noted:

This study shows that foster care can be a viable alternative to institutional care [nursing home care] for some frail elderly patients. It cannot serve all of those in need. Many people require too much care to be handled in a foster home. Others are not interested in this alternative. Thus it is not recommended that this be a replacement for institutional care. Instead it should be a part of a range of long term care services available to the elderly so that free choice and independence can be maximized. Caution is necessary in the development of similar programs as a highly trained and dedicated staff is absolutely necessary to prevent abuse in this type of program.[51]

North Dakota Foster Care

In 1983 North Dakota passed House Bill 1314 "to provide state funding for community alternatives to institutional care on behalf of elderly and

---

*P. J. Volland, Director of the project, personal communication, October 23, 1986.
†Ibid.

disabled persons."[52] The bill established two forms of services, family home care for related providers and recipients and adult foster care for unrelated persons. Payments were to be made available if the individual seeking care was eligible for Medicaid services and qualified for entry into a nursing home.[53] Subsequent to the 1983 legislation, amendments were developed to ease the access of potential recipients to foster care. The state legislature has continued to refine the program, and in 1987 further streamlining was anticipated.*

The program is paid through state Medicaid funds to either the individual or the provider. Services offered must include room, board, supervision, and personal care. Where possible, remedial services that can support the elderly or disabled person at a maximum level of functioning are encouraged.[54] By making payments directly to the provider, the state can keep intact any supplemental income allowed the recipient, within constraints applied to living arrangement standards.

In addition to this specific program, some forms of adult day care have been identified in South Carolina, Iowa, Michigan, Nebraska, and Hawaii. The latter state has two levels of homes, determined by the client's needs, and three levels of payment, determined by the services provided.[55]

UNRESOLVED ISSUES

The system of adult foster care is far less developed than adult day care. Where it exists, funding is sharply limited or absent. Some states, such as North Dakota, make Medicaid funds available. Others use Title XX funding. In New York State, an addition is made to SSI. Participants are expected to pay the providers through these monies and/or pensions, Social Security, and veterans benefits.

Funding is an issue. So too is the question of regulation. During the 1970s states began to license or at least certify homes. However, licensure can create problems. When Illinois instituted a licensing process, homes that could not comply were closed and residents who did not meet the needed criteria were released.[56] Even with licensing, the comprehensiveness of care varies, resulting in unintentional health and safety hazards. Another area of concern is the degree of family environment that actually exists in foster homes.[57]

Finally, the issue of training and support must be considered. Most foster caretakers are female. In New York a study indicated that over 90 percent were women, 11 percent of whom were still employed. Fifty percent had worked in the health field.[58] Money is frequently a motivation

*Marlowe Kro, Administrator, Home and Community Service Division, Aging Service, Bismark, North Dakota. Personal communication, October 22, 1986.

for participation; 56 percent of the home care sponsors in Washington indicated finances as the most significant reason for their participation.[59] The sponsoring agency therefore has an important role in overseeing the transition of the client into the home, supervising the delivery of services, and working with both the provider and the client throughout the placement. There is a need for increased social work involvement in the development of adult foster care. Social workers can help to expand foster care and improve the public's attitude about the concept.[60]

Adult foster care involves a multitude of concerns that in many instances must be managed by a single caretaker. Medical, legal, financial, social, and psychological issues arise in the operation of an adult foster care program.[61] It may be a positive value that adult foster care has not been systematized. As a result, however, it is difficult to develop funding sources and actually manage a program that retains its homelike environment. Adult foster care will never serve a large number of people, but for those frail elderly individuals who can adopt to the environment of another person's home, it offers a humane and caring possibility.

HOSPICE CARE

Of all the new long term care options, hospice has probably received the most publicity and public attention. Prior to the introduction of a hospice benefit within the Medicare program in 1983, studies and reports were prepared at state and local levels. Because considerable information describes hospice services and programs, this discussion focuses on the philosophy of hospice and a brief historical review of its development.

HOSPICE: A CONCEPT OF CARING

"If hospice can remove the fear of suffering, the fear of being dependent, the fear of being a burden, and the fear of loneliness and isolation, the time will come when death is no longer feared. Death will become what it really is, the natural end of life."[62] This statement, offered by Dr. Josefina B. Magno, a past executive director of the National Hospice Organization, gives us an understanding of what hospice represents and what motivates those who provide hospice care.

The hospice concept has several distinctive characteristics: Care is given to those who are dying; a patient and family members are cared for as a unit; great attention is taken to assure that the patient is as comfortable and free of pain as possible; and care is provided by a multidisciplinary team, often including volunteers.[63] As Sister Anne Munley, Director of Apostolic Planning for the congregation of the Immaculate Heart of Mary [Scranton, Pennsylvania] has described it, "The hospice approach creates a context where it is possible for one to live while dying."[64]

The hospice concept can be practiced in any setting: a patient's home, a free-standing community hospice, or as a part of a nursing home or hospital. The important issues are the attention to pain control and the fact that the patient is dying. When all forms of treatment have failed and the family can no longer continue alone, then hospice must support the last months of living in as much comfort as is possible.[65]

The pure hospice concept does not describe an eligible person. There are no dates and times that denote eligibility. Nor does hospice connote an argument against the use of technological equipment. When curing is still possible, then hospice supports its use. In many cases technology can help alleviate pain.[66] But at a certain point in a battle against a terminal illness, the value of the remaining days must be evaluated. At that juncture, the emphasis switches and palliation becomes the uppermost task, a principle that distinguishes hospice from other forms of care.

HOSPICE MODELS AND SERVICES

Most hospice care fits into one of the following categories: (1) free-standing, providing inpatient and home care services; (2) services delivered by a home health agency; (3) hospital-based hospice units; (4) roving hospice teams within hospitals; and (5) hospital and medical school–affiliated programs.[67] About half of the United States hospice programs in 1983 were hospital-based. Hospices in Great Britain are more often free-standing programs.[68]

Hospice programs include social-psychological care, case management, and help with activities of daily living.[69] These services are provided by a multidisciplinary team, including the patient, family members, nurse, physician, and others; and a major focus is on the control of pain. Ninety-five percent of hospice patients have cancer, and 60 percent are sixty-four years of age or older.[70]

CONTROVERSIES ABOUT HOSPICE

Once federal reimbursement developed, the role of hospice in the long term care spectrum should have become well established. However, numerous controversies have developed.

An initial issue with the federal legislation was the level of reimbursement allowed. Four levels of care were identified, at the following rates of reimbursement: general inpatient care—$271.00 per day; inpatient respite—$55.35 per day; continuous care—$358.67 per day; and routine home care—$46.25 per day. Many felt that hospice was being used simply as an inappropriate means to contain health care costs.[71] Fearing that service costs would outstrip reimbursement, few programs initially attempted to achieve certification. Finally, in the fall of 1984, Congress passed legislation increasing the allowable level of reimbursement for routine care to $53.17.[72]

Another cause for concern is the requirement that the patient and/or family members must make a choice between hospice care and other more traditional curative services, such as those provided in a hospital.[73] Critics of the legislation do not feel such exclusionary restrictions are necessary or appropriate.

In addition, as hospice authorities Elizabeth G. McNulty and Robert A. Holderby note in their 1983 book, *Hospice—A Caring Challenge,* hospice most appropriately defines a type of care rather than a specific institution.[74] If all health professionals were better prepared to care for dying patients, then hospice services could be integrated more easily into existing health care delivery systems.[75]

Finally, there are concerns that the new accrediting procedures will reduce hospice's flexibility to meet individual needs. Others believe that once the six-month prognosis is officially made, patients will lose the will to fight their illness.[76] Whether these fears are realized will not be known for some years.[77] Initial studies have shown some limits to cost savings but improved management of pain. Current concerns tend to focus on the formalization of hospice, not with the concept. Rare is the person who would disagree with Dr. Magno. People can die painlessly, people can die peacefully, and people can die with dignity.[78]

RESPITE

Respite is "short-term, intermittent, substitute care for impaired family members on behalf and in the absence of the family caregiver."[79] In the long term care system, respite provides that precise service for many family caregivers. It is not a single, specific program but rather a service provided in a variety of optional settings. In concept, it gives caretakers of patients the opportunity to respond to their own needs or take care of personal matters.[80]

The distinguishing features of respite are its flexibility (no set program structure) and the emphasis it places on relieving the caregiver, as opposed to a direct and limited concern with the patient.[81]

Respite care can be delivered at home or in an institutional setting. It can include homemaker or home health services for a few hours a day, use of a day care center for day-long coverage, or short term stays in a nursing home or hospital that provide such services.[82] The type of program chosen may depend on the resources available in the community, the caregiver's needs, or a combination. Because family members provide such a major portion of care for the frail elderly, respite care has become a cost-effective and necessary component of the long term care system. If family members can be encouraged to continue to provide ongoing care, then respite can be a significant deterrent to long term institutional placement.

PROGRAM PURPOSES

Caring for a chronically ill member can place a heavy burden on the family. Substantial physical work, notable strain and loss of social contacts can result. Anger and guilt are a common consequence, along with depression and a sense of being overwhelmed with responsibility.[83]

Respite can meet various objectives for the caregiver, the care recipient, and the community at large. In the latter case, the deterrent issue is important if the value of limited health care resources is to be maximized. Keeping a person appropriately out of an institution can save money. It also frees up the nursing home for a person who truly needs such care.

For the caregiver, respite can allow family members to retain a pattern of living and still respond to caregiving needs of a frail relative. This is particularly relevant as more women enter the work force.[84]

As the problem of elder abuse becomes more prevalent, respite has gained additional importance as well. A demonstration initiated in 1980 in New York State saw respite as a preventive measure against abuse.[85] Periods of respite can offer the caregiver the opportunity to step out of the pressured situation and regain the motivation to persevere.

The results of the New York demonstration stressed the importance of the caregivers' needs. Respite was seen most positively as a deterrent to nursing home placement when it was utilized for vacation or general relief. In fact, 38 percent of the respite services provided by the demonstration programs were requested to allow caregivers to take vacations.[86]

For the patient, respite can offer important services as well. First, it can allow the person to remain living at home. Respite care also offers an opportunity for a general status review by a health professional and an opportunity to develop recommendations that may improve the care of the frail older person. Health workers may also note important changes in that person's physical condition at an early stage and thus prevent deterioration.

In France, creative innovations have occurred: Respite is used as a means of readaptation after hospitalization. It is also available to frail elderly people during the winter if they do not have sufficient heat in their homes.[87]

HISTORY AND PROGRAM DEVELOPMENT

Respite does not share the rich history of the hospice movement, nor has it been a celebrated cause like day care. Yet we should recognize that each of those programs includes a respite component. One reason they have been successful is because they offer forms of respite for informal caregivers.

A report issued by New York State Senator Hugh T. Farley in 1981 identified five additional states where some type of respite service was available (Texas, Wisconsin, Florida, South Carolina, and Connecticut).[88] In Wisconsin the program was a joint demonstration initiated in 1978 by the University of Wisconsin and a veterans hospital located in Madison. Between June 1978 and September 1981, nineteen patients used respite forty-one times. As a result of the study, protocols were developed to respond to patient and staff needs in dealing with short-term hospitalization. It is interesting to note that respite patients' degree of functional ability was similar to that of the average nursing home resident.[89]

Two additional programs were early pioneers in respite and deserve comment. The Somerville/Cambridge (Massachusetts) Elder Services project and the Veterans Administration Nursing Home Care Unit project in Palo Alto, California, both started in 1979. The Massachusetts program trained paid visitors to serve as short term companions.[90] The Palo Alto project offered short term institutional care for chronically ill but medically stable honorably discharged veterans who ordinarily were cared for at home by an unpaid caregiver. After passing a home interview and a trial stay, respite could be obtained for up to two weeks every eight weeks on a first-come, first-served basis.[91] The VA program has been so successful that in 1983 the number of respite beds was increased. A day respite program opened in 1982 three days a week and was expanded to five days in 1984. A biweekly support group for caregivers is also sponsored by the VA, with respite services provided.[92]

The Senior Respite Care Program of Portland, Oregon, is a viable and growing project,[93] offering services since February 1984. Its primary purpose is to avoid premature or inappropriate institutional placement of disabled or impaired persons due to caregiver burnout or breakdown. The target population are patients with Alzheimer's or Parkinson's disease or stroke. Caregiver relief is emphasized, particularly for vulnerable, aging spouses living on fixed income and whose own health is failing.

Basic program policies include giving of respite in the home; ensuring that services are affordable to persons and families at all income levels;

providing payment, training, and supervision to all respite workers; and placing no limit on the number of times caregivers can receive respite but limiting the number of hours available each week, now set at sixteen. Current program hours are 8 A.M. to 5 P.M., Monday through Friday.

The function of the respite care provider is defined as supervised companionship. Workers assist with activities of daily living, such as feeding, walking, and toileting, but do not offer homemaking, personal care, or transportation services. Fees are charged on a sliding scale of $2.00 to $5.00 per hour, and employees are paid about $3.50 per hour plus transportation costs. The budget has nearly reached a break-even point. Staff turnover has been low. Eight of the eleven respite workers on staff in 1986 had been on the job for more than one year.

By its twenty-seventh month of operation, the program had served 139 families. The goal for the next two years is to be self-sustaining and serve 300 families.

The respite demonstration initiated in 1980 in New York State was sponsored by the Foundation for Long Term Care. Services were offered at five sites, such as nursing homes, for one year. The average patient was 81.6 years old and the average stay eighteen days. During the demonstration year, 134 participants received respite services.[94] Seventy-eight percent of the participants rated the experience as "very satisfactory," and 20 percent were "satisfied." Respite is an allowable cost within the New York State's Medicaid program, when providers are available.[95]

Other respite programs can be found associated with hospitals, area agencies on aging programs, and nursing homes. No single model prevails, nor have significant numbers of programs been initiated anywhere.

CONTROVERSIES ABOUT RESPITE

If respite is such an important companion to informal caregiving, it is difficult to understand why its development has been so limited. The form of respite that relies on day care has been stymied by the lack of sufficient funding available to develop and support day care in general. Even where Medicaid reimbursement is allowed, only a small number of programs are available.

Institutional respite faces a variety of problems closely aligned with the constant financial pressures of the health care system. It is difficult for a hospital or nursing home to keep beds free for sporadic use by respite clients. On the other hand, closely monitored certificate of need programs preclude institutions from adding a few beds for respite purposes. Also, there are the issues involving other patients, staff, and the respite client's own adaptability to a short term stay program.[96] A nursing home that is accustomed to low turnover has to revise its procedures if respite services are offered to patients for short periods.[97]

As the New York State demonstration illustrated, these are problems to resolve, not barriers to providing high-quality respite services. The lack of financing for respite services is a more serious deterrent to their development.

CONCLUSION

The variety of services that can be offered to elderly people living in the community is limitless. Although up to now the United States has been less creative than many European countries, new programs are constantly being reviewed and developed. For example, Montefiore Hospital in New York offers a special "after care" program that brings groups of six to eight patients by van to the hospital for medical, social, and laboratory services.[98] A VA hospital in Sepulveda, California, has established a "geriatric evaluation." A one-year follow-up revealed that patients were "less than half as likely" to seek nursing home care after an extensive medical evaluation and implementation of support services.[99] Others programs have used rehabilitative psychiatry to respond to the complex pressures of old age, poverty, and widowhood.[100] In 1986 new and aggressive approaches to care for homebound persons with neurological and/or dementing disorders were burgeoning.[101]

In 1983 Greg Arling and Willing J. McAuley of the Center on Aging at Virginia Commonwealth University described a study undertaken by the state of Virginia. Applicants for nursing home placement and their families were asked to identify factors that had led to the application for admission. Money was never mentioned as a primary cause. Over 40 percent of the applicants, generally family members, felt that the burden of providing care at home and emotional strain were the most significant problems. Need for social or recreational time for caregivers, time with spouse and children, and interference with work were other concerns.[102]

Adult day and foster care, hospice, and respite are important ingredients in the long term care spectrum because they respond to the very needs identified by these families. While some growth in these services has taken place in the last two decades, we are far from the point where all such services are available to everyone who can benefit.

Chapter 10

Housing

William Pitt said almost two hundred years ago that "the poorest man may in his cottage bid defiance to all the forces of the crown. It may be frail—its roof may shake—the wind may blow through it—the storm may enter—the rain may enter—but the king of England cannot enter!—all his force dares not cross the threshold of the ruined tenement."

In the seventeenth century Britain's Lord Coke declared that "a man's house is his castle. One's home is the safest refuge to everyone," a principle that forms a cornerstone of English common law. Despite the development of significant changes in moral standards and a much more intricate understanding of the universe, modern society remains committed to the idea of the sanctity of home.

Home reflects the integral characteristics of an individual, young or old. For elderly people, however, it holds special importance: "Home becomes a symbol of security for the old. To stay in one's own home means to hold on to self-hood, to maintain identity. In a world which has become increasingly impersonalized, home may be the only nurturing place where a person can find himself and *be* just what he wants to be at the moment."[1] As older people lose other important self-affirming values—job, friends, loved ones—home becomes "the last bastion of reality and competence."[2]

In this chapter we explore the issue of housing in relation to long term care. Housing options themselves may offer substantial pragmatic solutions to the problems of caring for the elderly. Many creative program models have already been developed.[3] In some cases these have prevented or delayed costly institutionalization.[4] In others they have created pleasant alternatives while community living remained possible. It is generally accepted in the field that the nursing home industry has been successful largely because these institutions solve a housing need, rather than a health or a home care problem.[5] "There are three general categories of need that should be addressed in developing an appropriate long term care delivery system. Most basic of these is the need for shelter. . . . There is a spectrum of living arrangements in which individuals can reside, do reside, or might reside.[6]

THE SIGNIFICANCE OF HOUSING IN A LONG TERM CARE SPECTRUM

Food and shelter are vital for physical existence. Shelter, however, as a component of our identity, bears additional value. To an extent we are defined by where we live. The old woman in a nursing home who says she lives in her chair or calls her room "her apartment"[7] may not be disoriented. Many are worried by the aging of their current homes, the costs of repairs and heating, property taxes, and condominium conversions. They fear loss of control over their environment and therefore their lives. We all need the reassurance of familiar surroundings. Many members of our population who are over sixty-five years of age are not sure where they will live when they are older.[8]

In 1953 the American Public Health Association published a report on housing. It is a fine summary of the housing problems of the elderly: "An increasing proportion of older people is expected to continue, to result in longer periods of retirement involving economic difficulties; more chronic disease and other disabilities; further sex disproportion; and more individual households and smaller families headed by older people. All these changes pose continuing financial, medical, social and housing problems."[9]

WHO ARE THE ELDERLY HOMEOWNERS?

The current elderly population is the first United States generation to reach retirement under Social Security. According to the 1980 U.S. Census, there are 83,527,000 households in the United States. Of that total, 10,379,000 are headed by individuals sixty-five to seventy-four years of age or more.[10] This represents 12.4 percent and 8.3 percent of all households, respectively. Most elderly persons own their homes, and between 70 percent and 80 percent of all elderly households are owner-occupied. Of those homes, as many as 86 percent no longer carry a mortgage obligation.[11] As Joshua Weiner of the Brookings Institution pointed out in 1986, "even among the poor, about two-thirds of low income elderly are homeowners."[12]

Studies conducted in Denmark reveal an interesting characteristic of older community residents. Elderly people were found to be more content than any other age group with their housing situations. Almost half had lived in the same place for twenty years or more.[13] In this country as well, despite the current growth of retirement communities in the Southwest and Florida, the vast majority of elderly Americans do not move. They remain in their homes or communities, surrounded by what is familiar. That familiarity may in part explain their contentment, even though many live in borderline or inadequate housing.

Although home ownership would appear to be a positive resolution of the shelter problem, it actually exacerbates the difficulties of some frail older persons. Many live in stock built between the two worlds wars, when housing construction and community design were less sophisticated.[14] Elderly people are more likely to live in housing with substandard heating and plumbing (7.8 percent versus 4.3 percent for the general population). For older adults residing in rural areas, that likelihood increases.[15] Two-thirds of all substandard housing is found in towns with populations between ten and twenty thousand.

The matter becomes more serious when income level is considered.[16] A study conducted in New York State revealed that older persons spent nearly one-third of their income on housing. For renters, the proportion is even higher[17] when costs for heating, repairs, and general maintenance are included.

What is being done to respond to the need of elderly persons for easy-to-maintain housing that addresses the changes in their lives while maintaining proper quality? Nationwide in 1980, 750,000 three-bedroom homes were built as compared to 75,000 to 85,000 smaller-sized townhouses or condominiums.[18] For many elderly people whose incomes are shrinking, the only option remains to stay and maintain their large and inadequately built homes in a phenomenon known as the "heat or eat" syndrome.[19]

ENVIRONMENT AND HOUSING

Factors and their relationships that explain the impact of the environment on the elderly include: (1) characteristics that distinguish aging residents from others and from each other; (2) aspects of their behavior and well-being that can be affected by the physical environment; (3) aspects of the physical environment that can affect their behavior and well-being; and (4) subdivisions of the physical environment.[20]

The relationship between environment and behavior and well-being moves in both directions. Just as the type of shelter for an older person affects mobility and confidence, so does the larger environment.[21]

In the strictest sense, the environment includes the physical surroundings in which a person lives. Neighborhood is obviously an important consideration. The definition, however, must be broadened to include socioeconomic factors such as marital status, presence of children, and health status.

PHYSICAL WELL-BEING

Health status affects living arrangements. Residents in congregate settings are generally noted to be in relatively poor health;[22] other studies reveal the same for individuals living with another.[23] These persons were usually less able to cope unassisted with the activities of daily living. A 1956 study of older people who suffered from major illness supports this point. Fifty percent of those questioned had changed their living arrangements following illness. Thirty-eight percent moved into someone else's home.[24]

For some elderly people, however, environmental changes may accelerate decline. Although the existence of transfer trauma remains a controversial issue, some studies have clearly revealed higher mortality among the aged who make major changes in their living arrangements than among those who remain in familiar surroundings.[25] Just as health status may influence a person's housing choice, change of living environment may affect health.

ECONOMIC WELL-BEING

Many older people move from their former homes because they can no longer manage the economic burden caused by physical and financial limitations. Older people who choose to share a home do so less for the emotional support than for health and financial reasons.[26] Cash costs of housing become a particular concern for homeowners, the largest percentage of older people. When income is limited, the costs of maintaining a home may become unacceptable.

FAMILY STATUS

The importance of the family in providing care for frail elderly people has been well documented[27] (see also chapter 8). While income is also a factor, the more children an elderly woman has, the more likely she is to be living with a relative.[28]

M. Powell Lawton, Director of Behavioral Research at the Philadelphia Geriatric Center, has noted that older individuals living together as couples tend to be part of the "younger old," those in their sixties and early seventies; and they tend to own and be more able to care for their homes. On the other hand, older people who live in a younger person's home have greater health needs. If the older person lives alone the housing is often poor, with housing of single older men often worse than that of single older women. In fact, Lawton discovered that housing conditions grew steadily worse for men who had never married, compared to those who had.[29]

Recent changes in living patterns have negatively affected the elderly. Whereas 58 percent of all single women (never married, divorced, separated, or widowed) lived with relatives in 1904, only 29 percent of all single women were living in the homes of family in 1970.[30] Children make a difference. The majority of older people who share housing live with their children.[31] Like so many other options, however, this becomes more taxing as the very old continue to grow in number and as their children themselves reach advanced age. In regard to those without children, gerontologist Anne Somers noted in 1985 that "already nearly 40 percent of the elderly live alone or with nonrelatives—a figure that inevitably will increase as the growing number and proportion of today's singles reach old age."[32]

COMMUNITY CHARACTERISTICS

Urban blight, crime, and gentrification are issues that older people must face as they try to remain independent. Each has implications for the ability of the elderly to cope physically, emotionally, and financially. Unfortunately, many of the elderly have been trapped in decaying inner cities. Stores, doctors, and other services are no longer available. With limited mobility and fear of the streets, simple tasks like grocery shopping or banking become difficult to accomplish. The deterioration of urban areas is often followed by an increase in crime. This is a particular problem for the elderly, who are often easy targets.[33] They become afraid to go out. They are unable to get the services they need and their lives begin to deteriorate.

Furthermore, many older people have limited assets. As they see their community decay, they witness the deterioration of their major holding, their home. A financial asset is declining in value at the same time that their capabilities to cope are decreasing. It is no surprise that older persons who express greater life satisfaction live in safer neighborhoods, regardless of their own health status.[34]

Studies have yielded diverse responses to life in the inner city. There are those who fear it and those who never consider leaving it. Certain benefits derive from a close-knit urban community that offers the necessary amenities. These benefits are, however, negatively influenced by urban congestion, crime, pollution, and noise.[35]

SOLUTIONS:
WHAT ELDERLY PEOPLE WANT

Housing has not been used constructively as a long term resource for elderly people, largely because few planners have asked older people what they want, what they think they will need. A letter that appeared in the 1984 book *Planning Your Retirement Housing* hits the target: "Housing planning for the elderly [is] unimaginative, stereotyped, and lacking in an understanding of the life-style requirements of older people."[36]

Studies of the elderly have indicated that most do not want to leave their communities, unless it is to achieve closer proximity to their families.[37] Foremost, they want to remain independent in their own homes. In a study of five thousand adult homeowners by the National Association of Home Builders, the ideal housing option after age sixty-five was identified as single-family detached by 50.3 percent; townhouse by 11.3 percent; condominium by 15.9 percent; and rent only by 0 percent. Another 22.5 percent were not certain of their choice.[38]

Many elderly people want neither to live with their children nor to share their homes, if finances and health permit independent living.[39] The problems arise when a move becomes necessary. Private homes are not possible for all.

Other types of housing have slowly become available in response to the needs of an older population. The Gerontological Society first discussed human factors to consider in the design of residential units for the elderly in 1978.[40] The society noted that, in addition to the community factors already discussed, access to transportation and services, building appearance, a lobby designed with places to sit, even the layout of units, the location of the elevator, and the number of units in a building can affect an older person's capacity to manage.[41] Other considerations are similar for all types of housing, such as designs that make a room functional for a person with visual or hearing limitations. Studies have identified both simple and complex methods of design,[42] including discussion of structural issues, color usage, the location of cabinets, and lighting. For older people, these simple considerations may determine whether continued independent living is possible or not.

In January 1979 the Federal National Mortgage Association convened Forum III. From a sampling of 1,500 retirees, 120 were chosen to discuss their housing needs. The group talked about inflation, independence, access, and the lack of suitable housing. Concepts of model housing were discussed; each room was considered, its shape and location within the unit described and its features noted. The proceedings indicated that retired persons need the same items in their homes as other segments of the population. The main difference is that retirees need them closer at hand and more immediately.[43]

Techniques for incorporating the concepts of elderly prospective tenants in new housing designs are being developed.[44] A program of this nature conducted by city planners Jack Nasar and Mitra Farokhpay in Columbus, Ohio, concentrated on obtaining information from residents in low-rent housing projects. High-priority activities—those that required particular attention in the environmental plan—were sleeping, watching television, preparing food, resting, and eating. Practical results of the analysis included recognition of the need for adjacencies. For example, the proximity of food preparation areas with resting space and the availability of an outside view and a dining area was a common request. Information of this nature can easily be converted into design configurations to create housing options more useful to older persons.[45]

THE HOUSING SPECTRUM

High-rise or low-rise, single unit or multiunit, rental or purchase are among many options in the "semantic tangle" of housing for the elderly. The variety is endless, and should be.[46] Elderly persons do not make a homogeneous group, and their needs are various. For some, housing should help support their capabilities and capacity to live independently. Others require supportive assistance but, for the most part, are still able to cope with the needs of daily life. A small but perhaps growing segment seeks a more protected environment, where health care and personal needs can be fulfilled as they develop.[47]

The 1981 White House Conference on Aging proceedings[48] illustrate that efforts are needed to strengthen the structure of existing homes, develop publicly subsidized housing, encourage more appropriate private housing construction, encompass a variety of service options that allow the maximum degree of independence, and maintain ties with the community and the informal support network. In this spectrum, repair and weatherization efforts, public housing, congregate housing, shared homes, retirement communities, and life care centers should be included.

A QUICK HISTORY
OF HOUSING FOR THE ELDERLY

The concepts of institutional care and community services can be traced to English poor laws. The almshouse is to some extent the forerunner of the nursing home. Many of our other systems of assistance also date back to the nineteenth century.[49]

Modern housing policy was established in Europe earlier than in the United States. In the 1940s some Scandinavian countries, the Netherlands, and England began actively to support the creation of housing facilities for elderly people.[50] Today we look to Denmark, Scotland, and England for models. Their housing allowances, sheltered housing programs, and network of health and social services are more extensively developed than ours. More important, however, is their adoption of a philosophy that promotes housing policy designed to serve the needs of their older people.

One of the first housing projects for the elderly was founded in 1922, in Orange Park, Florida. Moosehaven, sponsored by the Moose, a service organization, housed 374 people. The community included hospital and convalescent units and was run by an elected committee. Townhall meetings were convened to oversee the community's operations.[51] During the next fifteen years other facilities opened, including Ida B. Culver in Seattle, for teachers; Tompkins Square House in New York City; and numerous informal arrangements set up by lumbermen in Washington State or European refugees in New York.[52] These experiments were all privately built, organized, and designed to provide housing and, in most cases, services for older people.

In 1936 the New Jersey Housing Authority obtained federal assistance to develop a cottage colony in Millville.[53] It was located on land leased from the city and operated by an independent board. It marked the beginning of a new era in housing policy. In 1939, two years after the first federal housing act, New York State developed the Fort Greene Houses in Brooklyn. These were built under state housing law and included the first units for singles, including older persons. This is a noteworthy point because the elderly were not a significant element in early government housing plans. Public housing policy focused on the needs of families. About ten years later the City of Chicago Housing Authority had to relocate residents because of urban development. New units were provided for both single people and older couples.[54]

Federal housing policy continued to emphasize the needs of families, concentrating on insurance and assistance for home building. A title of the Housing Act of 1950 provided financing for cooperative housing, but most experiments were developed by nonprofit, charitable organizations. These included group homes and supported housing. Retirement centers also appeared, developed through conventional real estate methods.[55]

The first government-ordered set-aside program for the elderly was initiated by New York State in 1952. A minimum of 5 percent of all apartments in every state-aided housing project was to be designated for older people.[56] Shortly thereafter, a U.S. Senate report stated that need for housing of the elderly at a reasonable price was an important issue facing the country. The report advocated the inclusion of services as an important feature of any solution.[57] While it took more than a decade for the elderly to gain access to services in federally sponsored public housing, their needs have been an element in every housing act from the early 1960s to date.

We have already discussed a variety of government programs that assist or encourage the development of private housing options for older adults. Public housing facilities, rent subsidies, mortgage guarantees, and special loan arrangements are all made available to communities and private developers, both proprietary and not-for-profit. A 1969 provision allows the Federal Housing Administration to grant loans for purchase of mobile homes and land at mobile home parks.[58]

Federal policy originally regarded the person's ability to be physically independent as a necessity for residency. Housing advisors outside the government believed it important to extend that independence by providing supportive services. The Housing Act of 1970 emphasized the inclusion of space in public housing for the on-site delivery of services. The Housing and Community Development Act of 1974 provided approval for Housing Authorities to meet the special needs of residents in public housing through congregate services.[59]

Since then, housing policy has fluctuated in its relationship to the federal budget. The current view places increased responsibility on the private sector.[60] New considerations, such as tax exemptions for older people who sell their homes, have been approved. However, in general, under the Reagan administration, the federal government has significantly diminished its role in housing. The 1981 Budget and Reconciliation Act cut housing programs within the Department of Housing and Urban Development (HUD) and Farmers Home Administration (FmHA) by 60 percent. Expansion of the number of Section 8 certificates for subsidies was halted and tenants' shares of Section 8 rents increased from 25 to 30 percent of income. New construction and rehabilitation of units under Section 8 was halted in 1983 with the repeal of the authorizing statute.[61]

When the first new authorizations for housing programs in three years were passed in November 1983, a total of $9.9 billion was appropriated. This is a noteworthy sum, yet considerably less than the fiscal 1978 figure of $31.5 billion, the peak year.[62] These developments culminated in 1986 with a moratorium on new additions to the supply of subsidized housing.

RURAL HOUSING POLICY

For many years the housing support and repair programs made available to many older persons did not reach smaller towns and villages.[63] Conventional approaches were not practical, yet many elderly people in rural communities desperately needed better housing. In 1977 the Rural Policy Development Act became law, and in 1979 the Administration on Aging and the FmHA joined forces to establish congregate housing programs in rural areas. Nine projects were funded for a period of three years. An evaluation was prepared and a report by each project was to be submitted at the completion of its grant period.[64] Reports available in mid-1984 from four of the projects showed clear signs of success. Demonstrations in South Dakota, Iowa, New Mexico, and Virginia had achieved their objectives of providing housing and services to vulnerable elderly. In addition, the incidence of institutionalization had been minimal, although many residents were seventy-five years of age or older. While no plans exist to extend the demonstrations, the projects do provide models for public-private partnerships that could be replicated at state or local levels. Unfortunately, to date the federal government has not issued a final evaluation report on this project.

FINDING A SOLUTION

GOVERNMENT-SPONSORED HOUSING PROGRAMS

Publicly sponsored housing programs for the elderly fall into three broad areas: improvements to current housing, such as weatherization efforts; publicly assisted housing; and provision of subsidies for housing. Although the federal government has the major responsibility, state and local housing programs have also contributed substantially to the development of a housing spectrum for older people.

Home Improvement

The federal government, through a variety of agencies and activities, funds repairs and rehabilitation for the homes of elderly owners.[65] Some of the better known programs include the Department of Energy's Weatherization Program, Community Development Block Grant loans made available through HUD, and various home maintenance services funded through Title XX and the Older Americans Act and administered by the

Department of Health and Human Services. Repair assistance has also been provided through FmHA and other HUD-related grant and loan programs. Several projects are exclusive to the elderly. Others are open to all homeowners who meet need or income criteria.[66]

The extent of funding for many of the programs has varied considerably from administration to administration. The Comprehensive Employment and Training Act (CETA), for example, provided salaries for workers in many weatherization programs in the 1970s. In 1981 CETA was phased out. Weatherization was also targeted for elimination in fiscal 1984 but has continued to receive financial support through Congress.

The weatherization program has enabled many poor, rural elderly homeowners and some renters to remain at home, out of institutions. The following excerpt from a letter sent to the Senate Special Committee on Aging in April 1983, illustrates the value of such programs.

The handicapped and elderly poor occupy the lowest quality and the most energy inefficient houses in the nation. With an average income of $4,800 per year in [rural Arkansas] it is impossible for them to invest in energy conservation. . . . Without weatherization and a comfortable, energy efficient house to live in, the only other alternative available is a nursing home. . . . Without a doubt, it is the most cost-effective program Congress has ever devised.[67]

Through weatherization, homes can be insulated, storm windows installed, and other energy-conserving activities paid for by the federal government. Many of the other programs run by HUD, FmHA, and HHS provide loans or grants for similar activities. Some, however, also cover more substantial rehabilitation.[68] The weatherization program has improved the quality of homes and at the same time lowered the heating expenses of many elderly homeowners.

The Low-Income Home Energy Assistance Program must be noted as well. Financial assistance is made available to help low-income households cover energy costs. In recent years, this yearly one-shot payment has enabled many elderly people to meet their winter heating bills.[69] Congress appropriated $1.825 billion for this program in fiscal 1987.

Publicly Assisted Housing

Two types of domiciles fall within the domain of publicly assisted housing. The first, known simply as public housing, is financed and operated by the government. The other receives government assistance in its development but is operated privately. Various grant, loan, and mortgage guarantee programs fall into the latter category.

Public housing.   Public housing is one of the oldest forms of government activity in the housing area. However, federal housing projects were not originally designed to serve the elderly. In 1956 Congress mandated that public housing units be set aside for older people who might not have qualified under the general public housing guidelines. Now the largest number of elderly housing units in new construction is located in public housing[70] and the number of elderly persons so placed is sufficient to allow the development of relationships between persons.[71]

Public housing is run by local housing authorities with federal assistance. Some states fund and operate their own housing projects, such as the Mitchell-Lama program in New York. The building and management is supervised by the state government, and ongoing maintenance is funded publicly as well. In some areas of the country, elderly persons make up about 40 percent of all tenants in public housing.[72] Income limits determine eligibility. Unlike many other housing programs, public housing tends to attract an ethnically mixed population. Housing authority management also varies; some units offer additional services to older tenants.

Provision of Subsidies for Housing

Grants and loans: Section 202 housing. HUD and the FmHA manage a variety of programs designed to promote the private development of housing for elderly people. HUD's Section 202 loan program is one of the best known.[73] Its purpose is to subsidize the construction and operation of rental housing for aged persons and the handicapped. Nonprofit agencies can obtain 100 percent mortgages for new structures or major reconstruction of multifamily buildings.

From 1959 through 1968, 335 projects with 45,000 units were developed. The program was highly successful. Units were filled quickly and the elderly found themselves in attractive, affordable housing. These projects escaped some of the financial difficulties that later programs faced due to capital flow shortages. Since 1968 the pace of growth has slowed. By 1984 an estimated 155,000 units of Section 202 housing for the elderly were in operation or under development. A probable explanation for the slow development has been the cost. All funding assistance is made at the start of a project,[74] requiring the government to budget large sums at a single time, rather than space them out over several years. In addition, the tenants must bear all increases created by rising operating costs. It is estimated that the average Section 202 unit is about 12 percent more expensive to build than a comparable unassisted unit.[75]

The Reagan administration's intent to reduce or eliminate subsidies for housing has not been vigorously applied to Section 202, because it has been argued that these tenants require specialized housing resources that proprietary builders cannot offer.[76] Instead, the administration has fostered cost containment through attempts to achieve "maximum efficiency at the most reasonable cost levels possible."[77]

In recent years, federal Section 202 housing policy has shifted away from construction. More emphasis has been placed on rehabilitation and use of the fair market. In the 1984 federal budget, funding was once again allotted for the construction of housing units for the elderly through the Section 202 program, after a lapse of several years. In more recent budgets, funds have been provided for the direct loan program of Section 202. According to the 1986 National Council on Aging, the need remains unfilled and it is recommended that forty thousand additional units each year be funded under this program.[78]

Rent subsidies: Section 8 program.   Rent subsidies have greatly enhanced the abilities of low-income and some elderly people to reside in housing of adequate quality. The Section 8 program was initiated in 1974[79] after most construction programs were suspended. It is administered by HUD. Through a mix of tax abatements, low-interest loans, and subsidized tenant rents, nonprofit sponsors develop low-income housing specifically for the disabled and people aged sixty-two and more.

Since each nonprofit sponsor administers its own Section 8 housing program, applicants must apply to the individual sponsors rather than through a central office. Landlords are paid the difference between the fair market rate and their tenant's calculated Section 8 rent, directly from HUD. Sponsors' admissions policies and procedures are governed by HUD regulations. Beyond this, they are free to design whatever support programs they feel are necessary for their residences, such as on-site social workers or congregate meals.

In an attempt to protect the public from discrimination or favoritism, nonprofit sponsors must follow the HUD-prescribed processes when filling new units. Sponsors must publicize the availability of applications by advertising through local and regional newspapers and radio announcements. All eligible applications received by the cut-off date are collected, and a lottery is used to fill the available units. Remaining applications are then placed on a waiting list in order of date received. Waiting lists are generally long. Sponsors often stop accepting applications after a list reaches five years in length.

The Section 8 program has been used to entice developers into the housing market by virtually assuring 100 percent occupancy. It is also used in tandem with programs like HUD's Section 202 to lower both the costs of construction and the ongoing costs, or rent, for tenants. Income eligibility for Section 8 tenants is based on a federally mandated guideline maximum of 80 percent of the area median.[80] In New York City in 1986, for instance, the income limit was $17,400 for a family of two.[81] Problems of bureaucratic enforcement may be at issue in individual circumstances. Eligibility regulations for maximum income and rent are an example, as noted in this 1974 case report from a long term home health care program:

TM is an eighty-four-year-old ex-government official living in a privately-sponsored, middle-income building, paying $267 monthly for rent of a one-bedroom apartment. He has diabetes, is blind, with a below-knee amputation on the right, and partial loss of the left foot. He lives a bed-wheelchair existence.

His assets dwindled, because total income was $312, and expenses $377 per month. When he had less than $1,000 left in the bank, we applied for rent relief under Section 8 but were stymied by the regulation that the maximum limit for Section 8 on a one-bedroom unit is $225.

The patient, with confidence that he could deal with the bureaucracy by telephone himself, because of his political savvy and background, decided to challenge the ruling. A doctor's note in the chart records that: TM told me yesterday that he had a conversation with somebody at the housing office. The man on the phone said the rent was too high. TM said to him: "You tell me how I can find an apartment for $225 or less which includes utilities, in Manhattan, considering that I'm blind and have a double amputation." The answer was: "That's *your* problem."[82]

HOUSING OPTIONS FOR THE FRAIL ELDERLY

The programs that have developed in response to the long term care needs of older persons in frail health are as heterogeneous as the elderly themselves. Some are supported by state and local governments, some by private initiative. Some are simple, some complex. Some offer minimal support services; others provide care for life. The programs are packaged variably across the country; regional flavors are and should be preserved. The programs summarized in the next sections are part of a burgeoning field.

Home Equity Conversion

As already discussed, the majority of older persons in this country are homeowners, and their homes are often their most valuable possessions. The concept of home equity conversion enables homeowners to remain in their current houses and to collect income from the value of this asset.[*,83] The concept may be particularly attractive to an aged individual who has substantial health care costs and might otherwise sell the home under a conventional method to tap its value.[84] (See also chapter 2.)

Senior Citizen's Housing

"Senior citizen's housing" is a euphemism to indicate housing options that have historically provided an informal network of support for elderly residents but in most instances offer little formal program assistance. Senior citizen's housing includes such alternatives as long term hotel residences, apartments, and mobile homes.

*K. Scholen, personal communication, April 1987.

Mobile homes have become a serious alternative for older people. Known officially as manufactured houses, in part because so few are actually mobile, an older person or couple can enjoy private home ownership within a small community at a price lower than that of a constructed home. Many mobile home parks provide recreational facilities and organized social activities as well.[85] According to the 1980 Census, 10.2 million people resided in 3.8 million mobile homes. As many as 760,000 were thought to be owned by persons sixty-five years of age or more.[86]

Hotels offer a variety of usages. In major metropolitan areas, hotel dwelling is often synonymous with single-room-occupancy (SRO) units. These are often poorly run, crime-infested, low-income hotels. Yet in other areas of the country hotel living is an appropriate solution for those who can no longer manage a home or choose not to be burdened by the responsibilities of home ownership. In some communities in Iowa and upstate New York, for example, senior citizen's housing has been developed in hotels that are no longer financially successful. With the growth of motels and movement of the populace from the inner city, once-prosperous hotels have become liabilities. The buildings are structurally sound and often ideal for efficiencies or two-room suites. When they are located near restaurants, banks, and shopping, the apartments are appropriate for elderly persons who need a more manageable environment to remain independent.

Some of these apartments, built specifically for older tenants, offer services and thus fall into one of the more sophisticated categories like congregate housing. Others simply afford the older person a housing solution or an alternative to home ownership. These settings may offer no activities, or only minimal ones, such as daily hall checks to make certain no one has had an accident. In many such buildings, however, an informal support system develops, a spontaneous reaction from a population that senses its vulnerability and appreciates the importance of independence and the dignity that independence brings.

Shared Housing

Shared housing programs are various in nature: In peer homesharing, persons of the same age share housing costs; intergenerational homesharing involves people of different generations; and barter homesharing is defined as an exchange of services (for example, cooking, shopping, companionship during specified hours) for room and/or board or other financial remuneration.[87]

Proponents of homesharing emphasize the benefits for the elderly. These include reduced housing costs, companionship, security, and the presence of informal support. Homesharing promotes "independence through interdependence."[88] There are some negatives as well. Homesharing is not appropriate for all elderly people. It demands significant social, emotional, and adaptive skills. An older person already struggling with a chronic disability may find excessive the effort required to establish effective and intimate human contact with a stranger. Loss of privacy is another realistic concern.

Agencies that conduct homesharing programs match hosts who have appropriate homes they wish to share with people who want to live in someone else's home. The two basic forms are the referral model and the counseling model. Referral programs serve solely as housemate referral services. They screen prospective homesharers, check references, interview host and tenant separately for suitability of the match, and, finally, refer the host and tenant to each other. It is then their mutual task to negotiate the terms of the homesharing arrangement. Counseling programs are more involved in developing the original match and also help to sustain the result. Services include screening and counseling prospective homesharers regarding housing options, in-depth home interviews, home inspections, reference checks, facilitating introductions of prospective host and tenant, assisting in negotiating the homesharing contract or agreement, and follow-up assistance as needed.[89]

Staff members assess the reasons why prospective homesharers want to try shared living, personal preferences in such matters as smoking, taste in music, hobbies, financial and health status, and personality traits. It is a critical skill of the staff to evaluate adequately whether or not the proposed match will succeed. Often several trial periods of two to three days at a time will be recommended before the newly matched host and tenant negotiate a homesharing agreement. During the match-up period the host and the tenant reach a clear understanding about amount of rent and utilities cost, common living areas, prohibitions (such as entertaining), and the nature of assistance or service they may each offer the other.

There are no standard age or income restrictions for persons interested in homesharing. However, certain concrete requirements exist, as do some that vary with the personalities of the hosts and tenants.

1. Individuals receiving Supplemental Security Income or food stamps are poor candidates for homesharing. Under current regulations, they would lose these benefits.
2. A private bedroom must be available for the tenant.
3. Agency personnel strive to assure that a potential host and tenant have acceptable interpersonal capabilities. Candidates who are alcoholics, drug users, or mentally ill are poor candidates for homesharing.

Both parties are responsible for meeting the terms of the homesharing agreement. Either can request the sponsoring agency to help resolve difficulties. Conflict can sometimes be resolved by renegotiating the agreement, but occasionally there may be no alternative to disbanding the match. For those elderly tenants with no options, homesharing may therefore be a risky step. If the match fails, the tenant may have no home.

Congregate Housing

Congregate housing is characterized by the combination of housing and services it often offers, but there are many definitions. At a minimum, congregate housing must by definition include at least a medical/nursing service, personal care, or housekeeping.[90] Other definitions are more complex and add a patchwork of services, such as physical and other therapies, counseling, and transportation.[91]

Two other qualities are characteristic of congregate housing. First, although now funded on a small scale by the federal government, congregate housing is not by definition a federal program and the services are not generally funded directly through the federal government.[92] Second, a major distinction is the voluntary nature of the service package. Although some sponsors are beginning to include meals in the monthly payment (for health and social reasons, they say), most services are optional, to be used purely by choice. This point distinguishes congregate housing from most domiciliary care facilities. It is also a criterion highly regarded in relation to the resident's own sense of independence.[93]

Congregate housing appeals to a cross-section of the elderly population. Various income levels and most ethnic groups have shared in such projects. Only the black elderly appear to be underrepresented, even in the public congregate housing sites. Tenants in congregate housing tend to be older than age seventy-five (although most move in at a younger age), predominantly female, and are usually physically active, although their health status is poorer than the national average for the elderly.[94] A study to determine preferences in retirement housing of middle- to high-income elderly people revealed a large segment (91 percent) interested in facilities that were age-segregated and offered basic services.[95] Congregate housing is attractive because it responds to the anticipated physical decline of an older person. It affords active, mobile aged people the freedom desired. At the same time, it makes needed services available as they grow older and more frail.[96]

With the help of government agencies like the Administration on Aging and FmHA, congregate housing is spreading to rural areas, where such assistance is desperately needed for elderly people.[97] In urban areas congregate housing is developing independently, on a nonprofit basis, as well as through proprietary ventures that extend into the condominium and cooperative fields. The nature of development funding, such as the HUD Section 202 program, however, strongly favors the nonprofit sector.[98] It is not possible to say how many total units exist through both public and private initiatives.

Availability of services is the major factor that sets congregate housing apart from senior citizen housing projects or other apartment complexes that provide only shelter. The types of services a sponsor can offer are flexible. A universal interest is access to health care, although high-income tenants tend to place more emphasis on both this and on housekeeping assistance. Meal services are more important for those elderly people in poorer health. Good security is in high demand, according to one survey of high-income elderly. The presence in the neighborhood of grocery stores, cleaners, and transportation is also important.[99]

Opponents of congregate housing have argued that the availability of this service package encourages dependency. Yet studies do not support that contention.[100] Instead, providers and gerontologists see congregate housing as an effective mechanism for the delivery of care that encourages independence. Its flexible nature, providing only those services requested to those who need them, makes it more advantageous than institutional programs. In addition, it allows early detection of some problems, which can help delay the need for more costly care. Congregate housing offers a practical balance between dependence and independence.[101]

There are some potential problems, nevertheless. For instance, as the residents become older, the proportion who need services will increase.[102] Cost is a significant factor, and the greater the services offered, the higher the cost. Many operators are inexperienced in the financial planning required to develop successfully a congregate housing project. Location and design also become strategic matters if the right population is to be attracted.[103] When the facility begins to operate at a deficit, the operator is faced, often reluctantly, with the need to raise costs, cut services, or go bankrupt. In spite of these drawbacks, there are probably far more elderly people interested in congregate housing than there are facilities currently available.

Some of the earliest efforts were developed in Maryland. Two of the better known are the Sheltered Housing Program and the Group Home Project. Funded with private, municipal, and county assistance, the programs offer a range of homemaker services and meals to tenants in apartment complexes.

In 1978 New York State established Enriched Housing, a program tailored after the Maryland and private group living experiments. The program utilizes the SSI benefit (see chapter 2). The federal SSI benefit is supplemented by state funds to pay for the higher costs of domiciliary care. Enriched Housing is reimbursed at this higher rate. Local nonprofit agencies secure housing in apartment buildings and small family dwellings. These may include efficiency and one-bedroom units as well as larger units with several separate bedrooms. Program participants generally need some assistance with daily living but do not require twenty-four hour or medical supervision. Through SSI, or a person's own funding,[104] the agency pays the rent; provides homemaker, personal care, and social services; and helps arrange transportation and recreation.[105] By 1986, fifty-one programs operated by twenty-five approved sponsors, including local housing authorities, religious organizations, and a voluntary hospital, had developed places for 420 residents.* A high level of satisfaction has been noted.[106]

In 1975 the New Jersey Society of Architects began a program called Architects Housing, on land donated by the City of Trenton. Mortgage funds came from the state housing finance agency. The purpose was to allow architects to build housing for the elderly and handicapped based on the tenants' ideas of "what housing ought to be."[107] The Franklin County (Ohio) Commissioners and Office on Aging also sponsor familylike living arrangements through county subsidies.[108]

Private initiatives include a project in St. Louis developed by a local union at a cost of $20 million. It includes two residence buildings, offices, shops, and a park. A Kansas City, Missouri, program offers private quarters. All residents have certain housekeeping responsibilities. In San Francisco and Washington, D.C., Jewish services agencies operate housing projects for the elderly with meals, housekeeping, and social services provided.[109] An ambitious project recently opened in eastern Fairfax County, Virginia. Mount Vernon House is a seventy-two-acre development, with subsidized housing, doctors' offices, a mental health and public health clinic, and a skilled nursing unit drawn together. It took a private developer ten years to complete.[110] The important features include the availability of some types of supportive services and the flexibility and independence that the environment offers the tenant.

As the emphasis away from institutional care continues and as the number of elderly grows larger, the role of congregate housing will be enhanced. The coming years will probably bring new relationships among hospitals, nursing homes, and congregate housing programs as well as an extension of the current public and private sponsorships of congregate housing facilities.

Life Care

For many elderly people who can afford to relocate, the life care or retirement center has become an attractive and secure response to both housing and long term care needs.[111] In its purest sense, life care centers are one form of a retirement community.[112] Some of the examples discussed earlier, such as congregate housing, are sometimes referred to as

---

*M. McMahon, personal communication, November 7, 1986. M. McMahon is affiliated with the Enriched Housing Program, New York State Dept. of Social Services, Albany.

retirement communities, a term that at times denotes any living arrangement reserved for older people. On the other hand, some would argue that retirement centers resemble life care but do not include medical facilities. In addition, retirement communities vary in their housing structure. Some offer rental units; others provide equity ownership that can be sold or inherited. This is not possible with life care.[113]

Life care is commonly defined as a concept that combines separate apartments and skilled nursing facilities on the premises. There is an entrance fee and monthly payment.[114] Life care includes occupancy rights but not property ownership. The entrance fee, which can be quite large, is usually not refundable after a trial period, although many communities are now making small refunds upon the death of an occupant or when a unit has been reoccupied.[115]

Although life care centers are not a new concept, probably close to half of the facilities have been built in the past twenty years. The American Association of Homes for the Aging estimated in the fall of 1986 that there were six hundred continuing care (life care) communities in the United States.* Some buildings have vacancies. Others, like the Quaker-affiliated Kendal-Crosslands communities, have extensive waiting lists. In all, up to 250,000 adults reside in life care centers.[116] One of the oldest is Claremont Manor in California, built in 1953 by Methodist clergymen with an investment of $5,000 to $7,500. Others include Rossmoor's Leisure World in Maryland, John Knox Village in Texas, and the Ohio Presbyterian Home.[117]

A study prepared in 1982 by *Lifecare Industry*, a trade publication, revealed that life care residents came from middle- to upper-middle-income groups. The average age at entrance was between seventy-seven and seventy-eight, and the average age of a resident was between eighty-one and eighty-two. Most residents had been homeowners in the same local area.[118]

The entrance fee rates may range from about $30,000 to $150,000; the average one-bedroom unit fee is $60,000. Monthly costs vary as well, from as low as $200 to as much as $2,500. The average monthly range is approximately $600 to $1,800,†[119] depending in part on the extent of services offered.

In a life care center, each resident or couple has an independent unit, an apartment or small cottage. Many such communities have a central dining room, and most offer some organized activities and recreational facilities. Life care communities provide on-site skilled nursing care, often in a

---

*M. Webb, policy analyst, American Association of Homes for the Aging. Personal communication, November 6, 1986.
†Ibid.

separate building. Usually a resident is allowed short stays in the skilled wing without losing the private unit. If a physician ultimately determines that independent living will no longer be possible, the resident stays in the skilled wing and the unit may be sold to a new occupant. Policies concerning additional costs for skilled care vary from center to center. In most cases, the basic monthly fee covers board and care in the skilled wing. Other facilities, although less frequently, are Medicare-certified. Skilled nursing homes are also in a strong position to sponsor life care because of their existing skilled beds.

Life care requires a sophisticated balance between housing development and health care. It involves certain assumptions about longevity and degree of impairment as well as mortgages and other financial developments. Poor planning can have a disastrous effect on the financial stability of a life care center. Communities must be built in an area where there is a strong market. Sufficient funds from entry fees must be placed in escrow to cover special management costs and to ensure cash flow following the principle of pooled risk to support a lifetime of care.[120] Most centers have been successful in establishing financial plans that take these factors into consideration.[121] A few, like Pacific Homes in California and Fiddler's Woods in Philadelphia, have not.[122]

The financial base of a life care project rests in seed money put up by the developers, entry fees, and construction loans. This money must cover all costs for development, plus a cash reserve. Monthly fees should be sufficient for daily operations. If these fees are too low or a cash reserve is not maintained, the center may become insolvent as the population ages and new entry fees arrive less frequently.[123]

To ensure that potential residents are safeguarded from projects that are poorly managed, intentionally or unintentionally, many states are establishing life care regulations.[124] Various mechanisms are used, through the states' departments of insurance, social services, securities commissions, and public health. Among the regulations are those requiring full financial disclosure to residents. This allows the prospective buyer to verify that construction funds are being used properly and are not eroded by consultants', accountants', and other professionals' fees. Laws requiring escrow accounts and defined financial reserves, regulating contract and advertising, and setting procedures for takeover are also being established. Among the leaders in this area are Florida, California, Colorado, Illinois, Maryland, Massachusetts, Michigan, and New York.[125]

In spite of its problematic history, life care is growing. Development slowed in the early 1980s when interest rates climbed but picked up in 1983 when the rates lowered. Life Care Services, Inc., a major operator, had one center underway in September 1982. A year later, four new centers were being built.[126] By 1986 it was evident that proprietary interests were engaged.[127] However, life care's growth could be affected by the current tax law revisions that limit the industrial development bonding authority of state and local governments. Most life care communities are established as tax-exempt projects to be eligible for tax-exempt revenue bonds.[128] It is unclear what effects a cap on industrial development bonds might have on the future of life care. The implications of the 1986 tax revisions may be significant.

CONCLUSION

No single housing choice is sufficient, no one model always appropriate for the aged. Older persons, just like members of any other age group, have various interests, needs, and capabilities.

Housing plans for the elderly require creativity. Penn South housing in Manhattan, developed by the International Ladies Garment Workers Union in 1961 as a nonprofit cooperative, is home to about six thousand five hundred persons. Because of real estate tax subsidies allowed during the original construction, housing costs have stayed low, and tenants have largely remained in place.[129] By 1986 it was evident that many were frail, disabled, isolated, and in need of help. Management of Penn South succeeded in obtaining a substantial philanthropic grant to employ social workers and nurses for guidance, obtaining benefits, and offering basic health services. This is an effective and caring response to the aging-in phenomenon. A college in Michigan was losing money because of declining enrollment. Older members of the community needed housing at a reasonable price. In a perfect match of resources, the college changed an unused dormitory into housing for the elderly.[130] And a rural hospital in Wisconsin constructed supervised living apartments for the aged in conjunction with a more traditional nursing home, to meet expressed needs of local older persons.[131] Other communities have converted elementary schools or are building small units on larger properties.[132] Many older people are willing to adapt to the resources available in the locality; they simply need to be given a chance.

We are starting to recognize the fragile relationship between shelter and well-being. Greater sophistication and sensitivity is shown in the design of special units or the refurbishing of older homes to make daily living less strenuous. However, exceptions to this attitude still exist. Note, for example, the Clarksville, Texas, judge who arbitrarily relocated twenty-six tenants from two housing projects in order to facilitate racial integration. The goal may have been honorable, but many older residents were forced to tear up their roots as the price.[133] In this case, all the principles relating to the housing needs of older persons were broken.

The essential element for success in developing housing for the elderly is understanding the importance that home plays in an older person's life. "We shape our buildings and then our buildings shape us."[134] Our buildings shape us, and thus they control our independence, our dignity, our freedom. This point is especially valid for the aged. Home is a container for daily activities, a storehouse of experience and memory. Older persons depend on their homes for emotional as well as physical shelter.[135]

Chapter 11

The Nursing Home

As more people become candidates for admission to a nursing home, the character of those institutions increases in importance. Those fortunate enough to avoid such placement themselves will be likely to witness the admission of a family member or friend to such a facility. The pressure of increasing demand for space compels us to study every conceivable facet of nursing homes, from projections of future bed needs to sophisticated dissections of current utilization patterns. Analyses of staffing, medical care standards, informed consent and living wills, government regulation, family participation in health care decisions, and novel uses of beds, such as for respite care and day care centers, is now underway. Improved health professional training programs, legislative initiatives, third-party reimbursement mechanisms, and environmental design research are being developed.

Recent progress in the provision of good-quality care in the nursing home has been gratifying when the history of the past forty years is reviewed. There are now many excellent nursing home programs to emulate, while in the past there were few. As nursing home residents become more dependent, due to advancing age and frailty, new issues surrounding staff morale, family involvement, death and dying, and nontraditional medical management methods are emerging.

An Institute of Medicine expert committee on nursing home regulation submitted a report in 1986 intended to respond to these matters.[1] It recommended changes in policies and procedures designed to improve the quality of care for residents. The impetus for this project grew from reaction to proposals of the Health Care Financing Administration[2] in 1985 that made certain nursing home inspection, compliance, and certification procedures less rigid. Consumer advocacy groups disputed the wisdom of the change, and the expert committee report resulted. Key recommendations include:

1. *Assessment.* A nurse should be available for accurate assessment of each resident on admission and when indicated thereafter.
2. *Quality of life* should be emphasized in the care of each resident.
3. *Quality of care* should be high, and meet physical, mental, and psychosocial needs of each person.
4. *Residents' rights* should be understood by all.
5. *Physical and environmental qualities* of the home should be acceptable, and include attention to temperature, humidity, lighting, and noise.
6. *A full-time social worker* should be employed by all facilities of one hundred or more beds.
7. *Surveys* should be surprise visits, not planned ones.
8. *Standard surveys* should rely on matters of life quality, measured by such things as poor outcomes.
9. *Quality assessment* in surveys "should rely heavily on interviews with, and observation of, residents and staff, and only secondarily on 'paper compliance' such as chart reviews, official policies and procedure manuals. . . ."
10. *Compliance with standards* should be enforced by sanctions, including ban on admissions, civil fines, emergency authority to close facilities, and receivership.
11. *Ombudsman programs* should be strengthened.

A federal government response to these recommendations is to follow.

Finance and reimbursement issues shaped the initial growth of the nursing home industry and continue to evolve. Any new cost-containment laws and regulations will affect the function of these facilities. If, for example, reimbursement were to follow the Diagnosis Related Group method now required of hospitals, the nursing home population would change and some current patients would no longer be eligible or sufficiently profitable to continue to receive care. The impact of these new developments must be carefully studied; the institutional stress they may create could adversely affect residents.

It is easy to deal with abstractions away from the battlefield of beds. We must require that we picture the patients, each with a private history of illness, stress, loss, family, strength, dignity, and destiny. The real measure of success or failure in nursing home life seems to center on the qualitative relationships between the patient and significant other persons, usually an aide, but occasionally the floor nurse or even the doctor. Although the quality of care usually correlates with the general ambiance and standards of the home, good care can occur in the dingiest of settings and can often elude accurate measurement and consideration.

While most of us have some idea of what nursing is, the definition of "home" in the institutional context is more elusive. We derive pleasure from such sentiments as "anywhere I hang my hat is home," "home is where the heart is," or "home, home on the range"; they all seem to suggest a state of mind that provides salubrious security and comfort. But when an older person retreats deeply into mental isolation, the comforting aspects of home decline; freedom from pain and the indignity of helplessness and protection from self-injury take precedence and may possibly be better achieved in a group environment such as a nursing home.

This discussion focuses primarily on skilled nursing facilities (SNFs) with some reference to intermediate care facilities (ICFs), also known as health-related facilities (HRFs). SNFs provide twenty-four-hour nursing services, regular medical supervision, and daily rehabilitation therapy on an inpatient basis. They must meet a variety of health, safety, and other requirements mandated by law and regulation.

An ICF is licensed under state law to provide, on a regular basis, health-related care and services to individuals who do not require the degree of care and treatment that a hospital or SNF is designed to provide. Yet because of their mental or physical conditions, patients in ICFs require care and services above room and board that can be provided only through institutional facilities.[3]

These definitions leave the states considerable leeway for interpretation. They were sharpened in 1972 in response to the need for standards that would legally qualify care providers for federal reimbursement through the amendments to the Medicare and Medicaid provisions of the Social Security Act.

The federal government defines long term care as:

those services designed to provide diagnostic, preventive, therapeutic, rehabilitative, supportive, and maintenance services for individuals who have chronic physical and/or mental impairments in a variety of institutional and noninstitutional health settings, including the home, with the goal of promoting the optimal level of physical, social, and psychological functioning.[4]

This definition explicitly states that SNFs are not the exclusive providers of such services.

HISTORY

In colonial times, the options for an ailing elderly person were limited to the charitable acts of immediate family or when isolated, to neighbors, religious organizations, or some form of public housing. The earliest public houses included social outcasts, the chronically ill, and the insane, all grouped together by virtue of poverty and disenfranchisement rather than age. Public houses probably more closely resemble present-day shelters for the homeless than modern nursing homes. Any preferential treatment of the elderly most likely occurred by chance.

Florence Nightingale's descriptions of English nursing homes in the nineteenth-century highlight a unique blending of home and hospital, domestic concerns juxtaposed with health care for the chronically ill and dying.[5] Nightingale describes the inappropriate placement of certain patients by family who brought them to the nursing home for the wrong reasons, with promises that they would take their elderly relative back home.

In her review of the history of treatment of the elderly, historian Carole Haber[6] points out that by the late nineteenth century there were sufficient numbers of elderly in the public houses of the United States to require creation of separate homes for the aged. Surveys during the late part of that century showed the national almshouse population was 160,006, with 69,106 (43 percent) over age sixty. Because public funds, then as now, flowed to institutions rather than directly to the residents, the elderly in general were often wrongly placed when family ties or financial independence was lost. There were few options. To compound the problem, it served the system well that these facilities not be too pleasant lest the more functional elderly seek asylum before their time. The homes then were perceived by the population at large as choices of last resort. This image has persisted, and today many candidates for admission retain feelings of dread when mention is made of "a home."

The period between the turn of the century and the advent of the Social Security Act of 1935 proved definitively the inadequacy of the almshouse and the poorhouse system.[7] In 1923 more than half of the almshouse residents were age sixty-five and over. Another 20 percent were between fifty-five and sixty-five. Most were seriously disabled. At that time fifty thousand persons, or less than 1 percent of those over sixty-five, lived in almshouses, and about the same number lived in charitable private homes for the aged. Another one hundred thousand over-sixty-five-year-olds resided in mental hospitals.[8]

The passage of the Social Security Act allowed public money to flow directly into the hands of the elderly who could use it as needed to pay for board in a proprietary home. Expansion of the proprietary homes occurred then, as did, perhaps expectedly, entrepreneurial abuses. Some of these were dealt with by the 1950 amendments to the Social Security Act, which: (1) removed the prohibition on payments to residents of public medical facilities, in recognition of the shortage of institutional beds and of the growing dissatisfaction with private nursing homes; (2) permitted the use of federal funds to match direct payments made by state and local agencies to parties other than beneficiaries, such as health services suppliers; and (3) required the states that made payments to residents of public institutions or to vendors to establish a program for the licensing of nursing homes.[9]

Through the provisions of the Hill-Burton program (The Hospital Survey and Construction Act) as amended in 1954, federal funds went directly into the construction of nursing homes. A 1954 public health service survey stated that 60,000 beds in total were in existence. By 1975 the program had provided funds for the construction of 41,168 new beds.[10] The Federal Housing Administration (FHA) Section 232 of the Housing Act of 1959 and later amendments in 1968 provided additional impetus to the construction of new and the improvement of existing nursing homes.

On the heels of the 1960 Kerr-Mills amendment to the Social Security Act, which provided medical assistance to the aged, came the Medicare and Medicaid programs. Prior to the implementation of these programs, the total national expenditure for nursing home care amounted to $1.3 billion. In 1965 only about 36 percent ($449 million) of the bill for nursing home care was paid through public sources, primarily state and local governments. Insurance coverage for nursing home services was rare. The remainder was financed almost wholly out-of-pocket. Medicare initially limited the provision of reimbursible medical services to one hundred posthospitalization days. Subsequent amendments further limited reimbursement in the nursing home area to the point where Medicare now plays a minor role in the total nursing home bill. On January 1, 1966, the Medicaid amendment to the Social Security Act, Title XIX, became effective. This in essence shifted half the fiscal responsibility for nursing home care onto the states.

Medicare and Medicaid demanded substantial regulation and modification. The Miller amendments of 1969–70 permitted some SNFs to be reclassified as ICFs and in many instances allowed funds to flow into substandard homes, many with SNF-level patients. The Social Security Amendments of 1972 (PL 92-603) defined SNF and ICF and set minimal standards. Inspections would certify compliance and result in reimbursement on a cost-related basis. The amendments limited federal payments for certain capital expenditures, authorized 100 percent federal reimbursements for survey and inspection costs of new SNFs and ICFs, permitted waiver of requirement for registered professional nurses at rural SNFs, and required disclosure of ownership of ICFs and the independent review of ICF payments.

In 1977 the Medicaid-Medicare Anti-Fraud and Abuse Amendments (PL 95-142) were passed. The Omnibus Reconciliation Act of 1980 (PL 96-499) increased the period during which Medicare beneficiaries could be transferred to a nursing home after discharge from a hospital; approved new alternatives to decertification of long term care facilities; authorized rural hospitals to enter into "swing bed" agreements, which permitted the use of hospital beds for long term care; and changed reimbursement rates under Medicaid for SNFs and ICFs.

By 1981 the nation spent a total of $24.2 billion on nursing homes. The public share was $13.6 billion. Federal funds made up $7.5 billion, with state and local government sharing the remainder. Of the $13.6 billion, $12 billion was spent through the Medicaid program. Nursing home costs accounted for 40 percent of the total Medicaid expenditures for personal care in 1981.[11] By 1984 the percent of Medicaid funds so spent had risen to 49, or $14.8 billion.[12]

It is interesting to note how quickly the discussion of the evolution of nursing homes turns to methods of reimbursement. One hopes that the patient in the bed is not forgotten, but reality, even in the day-to-day operation of a home, presents a tug of war between quality of care and budgetary constraints. Questions such as whether another in-house physical therapist or another nurse's aide on night duty is needed arise constantly. The laws as written never seem to provide the right answer. The unique demands of each home and its patients often require specific solutions not covered in the usual state and federal guidelines.

THE NURSING HOME POPULATION

There exist many generalizations about the SNF population in the United States.[13] Most residents are elderly: 90 percent are over sixty-five years of age, 40 percent are seventy-five to eighty years old, and 43 percent are over eighty-five. Many have functional limitations, including the inability to perform activities of daily living, such as eating, toileting, bathing, and dressing.[14] Many suffer chronic physical illness, such as cancer or digestive, blood, metabolic, genitourinary, bone, joint, or circulatory disease. Mental disorders such as dementia, chronic brain syndromes, and chronic alcoholism are also common. When able, residents often articulate an unfavorable judgment about the quality of life in the home.

The nursing home population is becoming older, and the patients are increasingly frail, mentally ill, being transferred to hospitals, and suffering from chronic illnesses and isolation. These conditions cause conflicts with nursing and personal care requirements, administrative headaches, and staff morale crises and consequent high turnover rates for employees on all levels.

As the nursing home population continues to age and evolve, several paradoxes remain. Among the population at large is an enormous number of extremely dependent persons managing on their own without professional support, while a significant number of nursing home residents, when closely scrutinized, could manage safely at home. This distortion is fortified by the reluctance of the welfare programs to recruit new beneficiaries and the generally irreversible path of an individual toward ever-increasing levels of dependence once institutionalized. With the advent of better assessment techniques, emphasis on in-home service, and the resumption of family support that occurs when relief services are available, undoubtedly the numbers of the truly frail in the nursing home will increase.

This goal, for good or ill, may become a practical reality. In 1986 a three-state trial of resource utilization groups was started. RUGS are a mechanism through which fiscal pressures are applied to make only the most disabled individuals placed in SNFs fully reimbursable.[15] (RUGS are discussed further in chapter 2.)

Patient satisfaction and quality of individual life in nursing homes are difficult to measure; examples abound where one patient seems content to survive with severe incapacity while another involutes with a trivial event, such as a lingering minor respiratory ailment with cough. One has only to walk down the halls of a nursing home and witness some residents standing and striding alongside others who are bound to wheelchairs to realize that the apparent enjoyment and well-being of each bears little relation to their ailments. While this variety of self-satisfaction characterizes any group at any state in life, it is more obvious in this setting. Here a person's whole world may be restricted to a few feet or a room; the surroundings are interchangeable and former stations in life voided. Yet a gamut of reactions exists. The behavior of each individual is unique and must be appreciated as such, as the following example illustrates:

Mr. B has been in a nursing home in New York for the past seven years. He can walk well, has had numerous self-limited illnesses, but can communicate only by nodding in various ways or growling at unwelcomed gestures toward him. Nevertheless, he has imprinted his new, albeit deformed, persona onto his environment so that aides, nurses, administrators, inspectors, students all relate to him in some way: some by ignoring him, some by teasing him, some by stroking him, and others by toiling to keep him clean, dressed, fed, and smiling. This last capability he retains, and though no one can tell if his smile means what it did prior to his disabling condition, it often inspires a smile in those who witness him. Examples of the negative side of his care include an episode of oversedation that caused him to suffer a near-fatal aspiration of food, an instance when an aide elicited his expression of disgruntlement for the amusement of others, and skin injury while sitting restrained in a geriatrics chair too long.

For each nursing home resident there exists a kind of balance sheet on which we can weigh the positive and negative aspects of many different facets of care, including medical services (are diagnoses properly sought and made?), family relationships (are the families fully involved, or is their participation limited to instances of abuse?), nursing issues (how much restraint is acceptable?), and moral and ethical issues (did the patient die with dignity?). All can be rated.

It must be stressed that this evaluation should not reflect a removal or sublimation of patients from active participation in life. Even though many patients are unable to make responsible decisions, they retain the capacity for suffering, pain, and pleasure on some level. They can frequently express their feelings through innovative, reprehensible, or self-assertive behavior, which can be used as a basis to grade their care.

The 1985 National Nursing Home Survey (NNHS) data base, portions of which were made available in early 1987, includes a thorough analysis of nursing staff cadres and function, degree and value of family involvement, health status of residents, and admission patterns.* Preliminary review of information related to discharge planning indicates that short-stay and long term nursing home residents differ significantly in number, health, and social characteristics. It has been noted as well that many persons who use nursing homes have multiple admissions over short time spans.[16] At this writing, the most recent fully analyzed NNHS was conducted in 1977.

An Urban Institute study[17] based on data drawn from the 1977 NNHS and the 1977 Health Interview Survey indicates that the need for assistance with activities of daily living is a frequent cause for institutionalization. These data are subject to question because of the great variability and self-reporting methods by which they were obtained, techniques known to distort the facts. Yet certain seemingly irrefutable truths emerge: Old age and living alone were the only sociodemographic characteristics significantly related to nursing home entry.[18] Other variables, such as marital status, sex, Medicaid eligibility, education, and relatives who live nearby are not as clearly related, if at all.[19]

The patient's length of stay is another vital part of the institutional picture. The 1977 NNHS found that, on one day in that year, 16 percent of the 1.3 million residents had lived five years or more in the nursing homes surveyed; 14.8 percent from three to five years; and 32.8 percent from one to three years. It would seem to follow that someone who lived for five years in a nursing home might have been hearty enough to survive at home, but that often turns out not to be so. The following case illustration by a physician is pertinent:

*Evelyn Mathis, Long Term Care Statistics Branch, Health Care Financing Administration, Washington, D.C. Personal communication, April 1987.

Mrs. J, a patient at a nursing home, lived a bed-to-chair existence with severe kyphosis, chronic obstructive pulmonary disease, and intermittent pulmonary edema. Although her appetite was good, she was barely able to maintain her frail body considerably below the estimated ideal body weight. On one occasion, she developed acute shortness of breath and cyanosis, and upon evaluation by the staff it was determined that she had aspirated some food. As it was her clearly stated wish not to be transferred to the hospital, she was treated in her room at the nursing home with suction, fluids, and oral antibiotics. Her vital signs faltered and it appeared that she had little chance for survival. My recollection of this today is that I had made some self-reassuring assessment that thank God she *was* so frail and therefore less likely to be deprived of much meaningful life. The patient survived. This same patient now resides in a new room, with new roommates (many have come and gone) and does not appear to have changed appreciably in eight years.

Many such individuals in nursing homes seem to defy the odds and survive for years despite incredible disability and dependency.

Although the median length of stay in the 1977 NNHS was seventy-nine days, those few who live much longer push the average up to 456 days. The population divides into two peaks on a length-of-residency curve: those of long stay (2.5 years) and those of short stay (1.8 months). Those who stayed longer were characteristically unmarried women diagnosed as demented and supported by Medicaid.[20] Short-stay patients may, for instance, have been recovering from hip surgery for six weeks or so and then were able to return home, their nursing home stay supported in great part by Medicare. (See chapter 2 for a discussion of Medicare limits on long term care.) Comparisons of the NNHS data from 1973–74 to 1977 amply demonstrated an increase in dependency in the nursing home population.[21]

In a study by demographers Korbin Liu and Kenneth G. Manton,[22] the population, admitted in 1976, again broke down into two widely divergent groups. While 14 percent remained in the nursing homes for more than three years, one-half of the patients were discharged in three months. The likelihood of being discharged alive was related to a short stay: 80 percent of the hip-fracture patients were discharged alive, 69 percent within ninety days of admission. Of bedfast patients, 72 percent died in the nursing home, 53 percent after a stay of ninety days or more. The patients with chronic brain syndrome utilized twice as many nursing home days as did patients with cancer, even though there were twice as many cancer patients. Rehabilitation potential is a major factor in the possibility of discharge home.

Further analysis of these and similar studies emphasizes the heterogeneous nature of nursing home residents.

TRANSFER TRAUMA

It is difficult to gauge the complex yet subtle impact of transfer trauma, the untoward effects on the elderly of change of surroundings.[23] Transfer trauma has been studied extensively; some conclusions minimize the effect and others depict grave results.[24] We find eloquent arguments, including the opinion of a Supreme Court Justice that " 'Transfer Trauma' does not exist and many informed researchers have concluded that this danger is unproved."[25] Yet the grim evidence in one study that only half of 639 aged persons remained alive one year after they changed their living arrangements cannot be ignored.[26] These transfer effects, however severe they ultimately seem, relate to the individual's susceptibility to and tolerance of stress. For the person entering a nursing home for the first time or transferring from one home to another, the risk will always be great if the staff does not orient and welcome him or her, or if family support, which has proven effective in the past, is not invoked at the appropriate time. These principles also apply to the return to the community or home.

Several studies conclude that many patients in nursing homes could be returned to a less restrictive level of care, with more independence and a better chance of survival.[27] One study concluded that the greater the choice the individual has in the relocation and the more predictable and controllable the new environment, the more positive the change will be.[28]

But severe barriers currently exist to the return of nursing home residents to the community or to lower levels of care.[29] These include fear of potential relocation trauma, possible family resistance, limited knowledge of the health care alternatives available in the community, lack of housing, and systemic fragmentation or a nonsystem for those trying to pull together all the elements necessary to make the discharged patient happy, healthy, and independent. The incidence of unnecessary nursing home placement might be reduced through better assessment of the patient when institutionalization is first contemplated, such as at hospital discharge, following a trauma or illness while still at home, or when the family becomes exhausted.[30]

There is another barrier to discharge. Soon after entry into the nursing home, a patient's personal financial resources evaporate. The hard-earned, preinflation dollars that the individual was able to save are spent quickly. This financial disincentive explains why so many extremely disabled people choose to remain at home: They would simply rather die at home than surrender their savings, the cherished legacy for their loved ones.

QUALITY OF LIFE
IN THE NURSING HOME

There are many measures by which a nursing home can be rated or graded. Because its mission is both a "home" and a place where skilled nursing and medical care must be provided, a nursing facility must satisfy a wide variety of health standards. It also must be a nice place to live and, for the majority of residents, to die.[31] The national and thus the institutional trend toward populations that are more frail and dependent, with larger numbers of severely mentally impaired patients, presents great problems for administrators who wish to provide the ambiance of a home with sufficient attention to softer services, such as social activities or communications groups. When overwhelmed with patients who need to be fed or are incontinent of urine and feces, little time and few resources are left for other interaction. The staff can become demoralized and turnover may be high.[32]

The ownership and management of nursing homes vary. Some are non-profit institutions sponsored by religious, charitable, or fraternal groups or run by government agencies at the federal, state, or local levels; others are private businesses operated for profit.

In 1985 there existed approximately fifteen thousand nursing homes in this country, holding about 1.5 million beds, certified for payment under the Medicare and Medicaid programs.[33] Based on 1982 figures, an additional one thousand nursing homes and perhaps seven thousand board and care homes were in business as well. These were not licensed for such reimbursement.[34] In that year over 1 million persons were employed in the nursing home industry.[35] Between 5 and 10 percent of such institutions are operated directly by government, and the remainder by charitable organizations, often under religious or denominational auspices.[36] The availability of each type of home varies widely throughout the country, and the correlation of quality with type of ownership is poor.

Thus in general terms, an individual home should be evaluated in accordance with the particular needs of the person who will reside there. Patient A has an active medical problem and would ideally go to an SNF that is noted for its strong medical and nursing staff and affiliation with a back-up hospital. Patient B, who is medically stable, will choose a different SNF because of its proximity to family, better ambience, or human mix. The finest food can be negated by the lack of staff to administer it properly. Or in the case of ethnic patients, if the food does not reflect their tastes it may not be well accepted.[37]

A nursing home checklist would include:

1. *Credentials.* The home and its administrator should be licensed by the state and certified to participate in the Medicare and Medicaid programs.
2. *Environment.* The home should be safe, clean, well lit.
3. *Workers* at all levels should be courteous, conscientious, properly certified and adequately paid, satisfied with their work, caring and warm toward the patients.
4. *Location.* A home near the families of most residents can optimize invaluable family input.
5. *Medical, dental,* and other consultative services should be available.
6. *Pharmaceutical services* should be well monitored and every effort made to reduce polypharmacy, the overuse of medications often seen in institutions.[38]

   In this regard, it is essential to understand the analogy, developed by Professor Howard Waxman and associates,[39] between a drug-addicted individual and medication misuse by an institution. Waxman argues that "institutions themselves become addicted to prescribing drugs." The internal politics of some nursing homes press for the use of sedating agents in order to make patients inert, a response to a demand at all levels of staffing. "There is abundant evidence that psychotropic medication use in nursing homes is less for the relief of patients' symptoms than for behavior control and staff utility."[40]
7. *Rehabilitation services* should include full-time physical, occupational, and speech therapy. A strong *social service department* aids patients with such issues as consent, apprising the family of changes in the resident's care or condition, and mediation of the common painful and frustrating incidents that can surround institutional life.

While all these points are essential, the quality and organization of the nursing home's administration deserves special consideration by prospective residents and their families.

ADMINISTRATION AND ORGANIZATION

Administrative teamwork can be as simple or as complex as the occupants of the various offices make it. Different homes require different talents at different times. The elements that most often promote the delivery of high-quality care are good community support and attention to the morale and dignity of the entire nursing home staff, regardless of the formal organizational structures. When any member of the care team is demeaned or sidestepped in important concerns of the patient, the mission fails.

Administrators' effectiveness is reflected in the harmony, code compliance, appearance, and morbidity of the patients in relation to safety, cleanliness, and attention to common medical challenges such as infection or bedsores. Administrators must provide the reagents for success and must make any changes necessary to further the best interests of the home and the residents. Labor relations issues are demanding, and an administrator's credentials should demonstrate ability in this field.

In addition, administrators must be attuned to reimbursement, costs, capital development, loan sources, community support, investors, and be able to interact synergistically with the board of directors, often in times of strained relationships and panic. It may be hard to find one administrator with all these skills who can attend to patients' needs and wants. Fiscal considerations must be balanced with the delivery of costly services. The board of directors must place the administration of the home in the hands of its choice and have the courage to replace the administrator when the need is agreed upon, but not meddle.

The nursing service is the next most vital area of the organization. While it may be argued that medical care is more central, the hierarchical arrangement between physician and nurse becomes secondary to the importance of the individual roles when they are clearly defined.[41] Despite today's changing perception of the nursing mission, the credo of nursing is well represented in nursing homes.

Nursing is primarily assisting the individual (sick or well) in the performance of those activities contributing to health, or its recovery (or to a peaceful death) that he would perform unaided if he had the necessary strength, will, or knowledge. It is likewise the unique contribution of nursing to help the individual to be independent of such assistance as soon as possible.[42]

If the nursing home is considered to be a home or household, then the nurse is at its head. The nursing staff—whether a few registered nurses in a small nursing home or the floor nurses in larger homes—must set an example for the junior staff and approach daily patient incidents on an individual level with respect and understanding.[43] The nurse's goal must be to preserve the patient's dignity and allow the most enduring element, love, to grow between staff and patients. The nurse must provide effective in-service education to aides, practical nurses, and in some instances volunteers and other personnel. In addition, as the professional person with the most direct patient contact, the vital observations the nurse reports to the physician can often determine whether a condition is fatal or reversible. For these skills to receive the emphasis that they demand, nursing fundamentals have been expanded to adapt to the special instances of the aged patient.

The nurse constantly draws both from training in the traditional medical sciences, and from sociology, psychology, and gerontology. Research has identified crucial interventions by nursing in transfer trauma; decubitus ulcer management; care of various appliances such as Foley catheters, colostomy bags, and suprapubic tubes; communications skills; and functional enhancement. When a patient goes to the hospital from the nursing home, the nursing home nurse's observations and notations are crucial to minimize transfer trauma. The nurse's description of patients and their premorbid status enable hospital receiving personnel to comprehend and respond in a way that can make the transfer experience less terrifying and humiliating.[44]

The relationship between the nurse and the physician may be marred by overlapping roles, widely divergent incomes, sexual stereotypes, and the shifting body of medical knowledge and practice methods. Nursing decisions have, in the eyes of some, been undervalued and excessively deferential to those of the doctor. Physicians spend relatively brief periods of time in the nursing home compared to the amount spent by the nurse.

On the basis of these inequities, it has been argued that practitioner capabilities should accrue to the nurse by further training and experience, leaving a consultative status for the physician.[45] However, since physician availability has increased in many areas, redirecting the physician to spend more time on site is perhaps a more logical approach. This will be promoted by the current emphasis on geriatric training in medical schools and may ultimately improve medical care in the nursing home. Notwithstanding, the health needs of patients in the nursing home are great and the work tests the skills of all concerned.

Nurse's aides also play a significant role in providing care. Vladeck has written:

> Ninety percent of direct patient care in nursing homes is delivered by aides, a category that by law and usage implies no formal training or education. Just under half of all nursing home employees are aides. It is aides who rouse the patients in the morning, escort them to the bathroom and to meals, assist them in dressing, clean up after them, and as a general rule administer—illegally—at least some of their medication. When residents are incontinent, aides clean up after them. When residents cannot bathe themselves, aides assist them. When residents cannot speak or make themselves understood, aides must divine their meaning.[46]

At the core of any approach toward improving the nurse's aide experience is an institutionalized respect for the aides' work and support when the job threatens to overwhelm them. While the daily tasks may be inherently distasteful, an even greater problem may be the pain of witnessing the functional deterioration and death of their charges, without an appropriate vent for their feelings. As part of the care team, attention should be paid to the aides' observations and reports on the patients.[47]

Good spirit among the aides in the institution is invaluable for the delivery of high-quality care. During each tour of duty the aides must assist each other to lift, communicate, or cross-cover patients for the smooth performance of the day's chores. When superiors participate in the aides' work, it bolsters morale and also dignifies and underscores the aides' contribution to the home, as does a show of appreciation for a job well done.[48]

The relationship of aides with patients and their care demands innovative development.[49] At this time their job requirements and the methods by which they are trained are primitive. Only when substantive study is directed at friction points, such as dealing with the abusive or demented patient, will the suffering of the aides, who daily witness and endure these trying tasks, be alleviated.[50]

THE MEDICAL DIRECTOR

The enactment of federal legislation in 1974, partly in response to a 1970 epidemic of salmonella infection in a Maryland nursing home that led to thirty-six deaths, led to the requirement that a medical director be present in nursing homes.[51] When questioned, the facility's principal physician told the commission of inquiry that he had never been told what his responsibilities were.

Section 405-1122 of the Code of Federal Regulations as amended in 1974 requires those nursing homes participating in Medicare and Medicaid to appoint a medical director, who must hold a state license to practice medicine, to coordinate medical services.[52] The medical directors' positions may be full or part time, and they may serve as directors for more than one facility.[53] The number of hours they work is often unspecified. They usually report to the administrator. To this extent the medical director is a subordinate employee of the nursing home, paid by the nursing home.

The medical director's disciplinary power over staff physicians lies in the enforcement of by-laws relevant to health care standards that usually derive from state law. This translates in many instances into a "paper tiger" position because even in the acute care hospitals staff physicians are almost immune from actual disciplinary action. It is even more unlikely that staff doctors in a nursing home, with its traditional low-key atmosphere, will be touched by disciplinary action. This may change as the supply of doctors who wish to work in nursing homes increases and quality control improves.

During a search for a new medical director at the Village Nursing Home, a two hundred-bed nonprofit home in New York City, members of the search committee compiled a list of the medical director's responsibilities, drawn from other homes in the area and from the federal public health by-laws that govern nursing home regulations.[54] Among these responsibilities were the direction and coordination of the medical care in the home and the adequacy and appropriateness of the medical services provided to patients; the execution of resident care policies that reflect an awareness of and provisions for meeting their total needs; and collaboration with medical staff, specialty consultants, and/or other professional staff in the development of problem-related medical care guidelines and protocols (for example, urinary tract infection, and decubitus ulcers.).

Of particular note are the relationships among the medical director, the staff doctors, the administrator, and the board of directors. While the medical director's relationship with nursing is not uniform in all homes, a cooperative relationship is crucial for the successful provision of care. The nursing director and medical director may each be the best candidates for their jobs, but if they cannot work together, service delivery always suffers.

The tone of the home is set in part by the medical director's ability to relate to all its constituents. In-service education is an excellent forum for the medical director to demonstrate specific aspects of patient care and the proper way to refer to patients, and to highlight various aspects of the work at hand.

The medical director should be a gerontophile, not be put off by the infirmities of the aged, and must have the desire to establish close, warm, long term relationships with patients and staff. There should exist strong ties to local hospital staff as well.[55]

THE TEACHING NURSING HOME

In 1981 Dr. Robert Butler[56] exhorted the American medical establishment to address the obvious deficiency of suitably trained and deployed geriatrics experts. The nursing home in his model would be located on the campus of an academic medical center and would tap the permanent faculty in medicine, dentistry, nursing, and social sciences. In addition, regular rounds, lectures, required courses, research, and interdisciplinary activity would stress excellence in service as well as provide hard research data in a long-neglected area. The nursing home would be a hub for outreach services into the community, including home care, nutritional and family counseling, information and referral for health, transportation, housing, and other social services. Physician education would be enhanced.[57]

To date, the largest obstacle to the implementation of this model has been lack of money. In addition, serious concerns have been raised about what might result if the teaching nursing home model grew too quickly.[58] These concerns include fear that too great an emphasis on the institutionalized elderly in these settings might create a distorted picture of the nation's dependent elderly; the predominance of debilitated and demented patients might dampen rather than stimulate student enthusiasm; excessive attention might be drawn to the high-tech solutions of today's acute care hospital models to the financial detriment of the homes; and the nurse, whose presence is indispensible to the mission of the homes, might be bypassed in this revision.

The nursing student's experience in the study of geriatric nursing is often positive[59] and frequently appeals to the idealism that abounds among students in the helping professions, so much so that geriatric nursing is gaining on the popularity of the intensive care unit in career choices. Several foundations have supported work in this area. The Robert Wood Johnson Foundation has funded eleven programs to establish clinical affiliations between nursing schools and nursing homes.[60] The W. K. Kellogg Foundation has provided grants to facilitate the training of geriatric nurse practitioners so that they can play a major part in providing nursing home care. The Beverly Foundation has enabled three medical schools to offer teaching nursing home programs that focus on the training of physicians and other nursing home employees.[61] A consequence of study in these areas may be a change in the current finance patterns for nursing home services. If only a single patient returns to the community and is maintained at half the cost of the nursing home stay, and is replaced by a patient awaiting placement in a hospital at three times the nursing home expense, we would see a benefit. What difference does it make if these same nursing home beds are going to be filled anyway? The real gainer is the patient for whom appropriate placement means proper surroundings and care.

QUESTIONS OF ETHICS

The nursing home, as a domicile for many different patients who interface with professionals, lay persons, students, families, and each other, is a natural pool for the evolution of ethical challenge.[62] As the nursing home becomes the focus of study, the ethical issues of privacy, informed consent,[63] exposure to disease, preservation of dignity, rights of disclosure, restraints (pharmacological and mechanical), access to comprehensive (expensive) medical technology, and the right to choose the conditions of life and death must be addressed.[64] The public nature of the institution renders public the issues surrounding the activities within.

Merely probing these issues is not enough. The methods employed in the ethical studies must ensure that all conclusions are themselves ethically drawn and do not subject the patients to needless intrusion wrongfully justified by erroneous data.[65] The Village Nursing Home in New York, for example, opened these discussions with the help of an ethicist, interviewed nurses, physicians, social workers, aides, families, and drew up rough guidelines for practice in areas of decisions about resuscitation and transfer to hospital. We shall look at some of these issues more closely.

A recent Supreme Court ruling illustrates an important issue that will probably be argued in different ways in the future. Patients in a New York nursing home brought suit because they were transferred from skilled nursing facilities to lower levels of care based on doctors' evaluations. At issue was the fine distinction between what constitutes a purely medical decision and what becomes a decision of medical and financial expediency.[66] The court ruled in this case that the doctors' decisions were medical in nature and therefore not under the jurisdiction of state action.

How shall we deploy limited and expensive new technology? The answer is perhaps obvious when the question is whether it really makes sense to perform a coronary bypass operation on a severely demented Alzheimer's disease patient who is refractory to medical treatment. It is a more subtle matter in the decision to carry out renal dialysis in an alert, extremely care-intensive patient who has become severely distressed with symptoms of uremia and who suffers from several other chronic illnesses. Other issues under discussion are whether or when to give orders not to resuscitate, not to treat, and not to hospitalize.[67] Still, the consequences of survival are worthy of emphasis here,[68] especially when both the high costs of the intensive care unit and also the additional expense of the remaining nursing home years are considered.

No issue has been dissected more completely than the conduct and responsibility of caregivers at the time of death.[69] Most of us agree that the process of dying should occur at the right time, in properly dignified surroundings, according to the wishes of the patient, the family, the physician, and under the legal guidelines of the institution itself. Nevertheless, exceptions occur and lawsuits follow.

Many excellent books and articles are available to guide helping professionals in their approach to the dying patient.[70] Newspaper attention to scandal and court cases is also broad and well documented.[71] But the literature often complicates rather than aids the process of finding what course to take in an individual instance. Too often those who work with a dying patient see reversals and suffering that are surprising and upsetting. Assistance and understanding must be cultivated and enlisted from the caring team, including the patients, their families, and clergy, to determine the wishes of the individual or the family, no matter how difficult this may be.

We must become aware of the high-tech options that may come into play in a highly mechanized intensive care unit. It is difficult to clarify a discussion of modern heroic measures for elderly patients without frightening them into outright refusal. And yet there are numerous examples of patients who arrived in the hospital's intensive care unit moribund, and survived despite horrendous incursions and indignities, enjoyed many functional, useful days and years, but have sworn never to go through such an experience again. At times, simply raising the question of whether or not to resuscitate with the patient or the family produces great anguish and pain, with no appreciable good effect.

Terminally ill patients may be indistinguishable from those who will go on living for years. Even where advanced cancer, cardiac disease, or decubitus ulceration is present, prognoses remain indeterminate. It is for this reason that proper development of patient care in the nursing home setting requires teamwork. The most satisfying instances of allowing residents to succumb to their medical problems are those in which the patients were well assimilated into the nursing home. Families were acquainted with the staff and had individual relationships with aides, nurses, physicians and others.

Mrs. F entered a nursing home at the age of eighty-eight. Her family requested and paid for the services of an extra nurse and for specially prepared foods. She was totally dependent, her movement was limited to bed-to-chair activity, and she was virtually mute except for rare utterances of "yes" or "no." She moved all extremities, and a complete neurological medical evaluation revealed no obvious reversible cause for this high degree of dependency. Her condition stabilized, and because of her native strength and loving family, she lived on in this manner for several years. When she began to decline and grow more frail the constant presence of the family permitted much discussion about her values, wishes, and preferred surroundings. The family, heavily involved emotionally and financially, had spent thousands of dollars. They were desperate for support in allowing their mother to die, despite their earlier wish that everything be done to save her. They needed the assurance that everything had been done, that prolongation of the dying phase of mother's life contradicted all reasonable judgment. They could now accept this because of the long period of adjustment they had had. They witnessed many other families in the same situation. They had built trust in the staff and in the physician. When death finally came to Mrs. F, they were relieved and grateful and accepted the event with resolve and with a feeling of completeness. They seemed enriched rather than emptied by the experience.

This bonding of family and staff and the witnessing of the prior death of other patients is of deep value in preparing for the eventual death of the individual in question.

Illuminating insights develop when care team family members and patients try to decide by consensus what are the most important features of care, and then supply it. These features can be simply the restoration of comfort and serenity to death, with special application of modern technology, to relieve pain or facilitate function. In this way the patient is enabled to attain spiritual fulfillment, and the family is protected from destructive self-reproach and impoverishment.

Dr. R. H. Fisher[72] states:

> Proper care of dying elderly patients requires excellent symptom control, judicious use of investigations, and no unwarranted treatments. . . . If such care is given, there is less need for specialized units, which are staff-intensive and costly. In addition, the relocation of elderly patients during terminal illness, away from a familiar environment and familiar staff, is contrary to good management. It is preferable for the same staff to remain with the patients through the terminal phase.

Other suggestions, such as those involving in-service education[73] and specialist consultations for palliation of particular problems, are advanced with the view that the matter of dying patients be removed from the isolated realm of responsibilities of each individual person who works in the nursing home. The field of hospice care has provided crucial information relevant to dying and has returned this issue to the mainstream of modern conscience.

Often these matters are not discussed until too late, resulting in undue burden to all those involved. Lack of communication prior to crisis often results, for instance, in sending the patient to the hospital or in litigation, because the family wished that more be done and the physicians had issued a do-not-resuscitate order. When the decision is deferred, the physician must decide how much pain and suffering the patient bears and then convey the information to the family, along with a recommendation. When physician and family disagree on the course of action, consultation with a committee can remove the burden from both parties, who may be overwhelmed by the full magnitude of these decisions. It must be emphasized again that these considerations differ from case to case, and each must be carefully weighed.

The practice of these principles is often burdensome, especially to institutions that have functioned for years with an ad-hoc or unspoken code of ethics. The impersonal bond between the institutional physician and nurse does nothing to alleviate the patient and family's worst suspicions and fears. The increasing frailty of the average resident and the frequency of transfer to the hospital often eliminates the time for reflection necessary to make such decisions, even though many of us today are more familiar with these issues through media coverage and education. Only through research at the academic level and frank discussion and trial in the institutions will each person's demise approach the ideal. This approach may reduce many of those sad, empty departures by death that nursing home staffs have witnessed.

Still, to use the experience of the Chelsea-Village Program[74] at St. Vincent's Hospital in New York, the picture is further confused by the many examples of patients who, despite all the assessment scales showing that they are qualified for nursing home placement, carry on at home for life at less expense and to their apparent satisfaction. This sort of patient decision is a challenge to the imagination of planners, legislators, and families. Before decisions are made to place people in long term care institutions, we must remember that a patient frequently requires more intense levels of care for a while and then may return to a stable lower level of care, after the threatening factors are addressed.

The question of whether more nursing homes or better home care is needed seems to be answered by considering the mounting numbers of the frail and very old. Even a slight increase in the percentages of those severely impaired in today's nursing homes will have serious impact on the current quality of nursing home care. Professionals in the homes would have to prepare for an even more depressing and alienating experience. The dilemma of David Hilfiker,[75] a practicing primary care physician, will continue to weigh on all of those who care for these individuals:

Finally, and most important, it is simply too difficult to define all the varieties of illness, suffering, prognosis, and treatment with sufficient precision for the definitions to be of much help in the actual situation. A physician may know, for instance, that the patient does not want to be "kept alive" "unnecessarily" "if I'm a vegetable" and there is "no hope of improvement." The real-life situation is, unfortunately, much more complex. What constitutes keeping a person alive? Is it giving him a warm room and regular meals rather than allowing him to lie at home paralyzed and with no heat? Is it giving him an intravenous infusion? Routine antibiotics? And what quality of life constitutes "being a vegetable"? Furthermore, in real life there is rarely any certainty about prognosis. Improvement may be unlikely, but it is often possible. So, even in the best case, in which a self-aware person had talked with his physician or made out a recent Living Will,[76] the complexities of the actual situation would probably render those efforts of little practical use to the physician. And because of his debilities or the seriousness of his acute illness, the patient himself is rarely fully available to the physician at the needed moment.

Chapter 12

Trends and Forecasts

The long term care spectrum for the elderly in this country will develop only if the need is understood. Concerned people, including the interested general public, elected and appointed officials at all levels of government, planners and analysts, and older people and their families, must be engaged in the process. The force of consensus is required, in order for the necessary resources to be applied during this era of intense and conflicting demand for use of limited funds.

How can the necessary spirit and drive be generated? A reminder of the demographic imperative is indicated. We must understand, and combat as well, the negative feelings that exist in our country toward persons who are old and the idea of old age. Here, education of the young is necessary. Training in the health professions must include a solid information base in gerontology. Equally important is early career training that takes students to places where older people live and where practical application of techniques and ideals is realized.

Money is needed to develop and conduct the service programs that make up the spectrum. Funds must derive from a broad variety of bases; and new sources must be generated. The various and competing elements that make up government must be asked, must be expected and required, to work together for the common good. Medicare shall talk to Medicaid. The Health Care Financing Administration and the Area Offices on Aging will shake hands. Through coherent long-range planning—to the extent that this is possible in our country—and through trial and error if necessary, a long term care policy must be elaborated that will serve the broad needs of our population. Policy must then be enshrined in legislation.

THE DEMOGRAPHIC IMPERATIVE

Dramatic changes in the numbers of older people in our country, and in their relative proportion, continue to take place.[1] Note that:

- From 1900 to 1950 our gross population doubled in number while those age sixty-five and older quadrupled.
- From 1950 to 1980, the elderly portion of our population increased by 100 percent, twice the pace of the general populace.
- Between 1980 and 2020, while the total number of people in the United States is expected to grow by 30 percent, the number of elderly will, again, grow by 100 percent.

In terms of proportionate change, 4 percent of the population was sixty-five and older in 1900; and by 2020, this figure will grow to more than 29 percent. People now eighty-five and over, called the old-old or the very old, "are currently the fastest growing age group in the U.S. population. This group represented only 0.2 percent of the total population in 1900, but increased to 1.0 percent in 1980; by 2020, they are projected to be 2.4 percent of the population, and nearly 14 percent of the elderly population [up from about 9 percent in 1980]."[2] The implications of this growth in numbers of extremely old people are noteworthy. It is these people who pack our nursing homes now; who occupy beds in acute care hospitals because no effective plan for discharge exists; or who are sent home prematurely, only to fail at home or be readmitted, because assistance is not available.

If we are interested in prudent use of resources and humane concern about our fellows and ourselves, we ignore these demographic projections at our peril. If we base our judgment on the current use of resources and on the anticipated changes in the makeup of our population, the recognition that there will be a major growth in demand for all forms of long term care services for the elderly is inescapable. Unless a coherent long term care spectrum is created, a virtual doubling of the nursing home stock by the year 2000 will be required. This would serve merely to warehouse the same proportionate number of people as at present: 5 percent of the population age sixty-five and over and 9.5 percent of the very old.[3] The dollar costs to build and maintain these institutions are an impossibility. The social costs of incarcerating all these people, many against their will, is beyond measure.

For every resident of a nursing home, there now exist about twice as many people living in the community with similar needs for help.[4] Some are fortunate. They have funds, judgment, and ability to find and pay for the assistance they require. Others live with or are cared for by family members and/or friends. The cost to these helpers in personal time, energy, and money may be enormous,[5] but is often offered willingly, as a matter of felt duty. Many family members of the next younger generation are themselves reaching advanced age. This must be expected when we are considering the system of care for people in their late eighties.[6] Other old people, in significant but unknown numbers, vulnerable because of their advanced age,[7] suffer alone without effective assistance. They require special understanding of physiological, psychological, and pathological need.[8]

ATTITUDES ABOUT AGING

Our nation's ability to establish a long term care spectrum for the aged will depend in large part on the attitudes of those in the position to develop and pay for it. These people include the larger general public who pay taxes and who elect our government and the individuals in legislatures and executive offices themselves. The views they hold toward old people, toward their own aging process and mortality, are critical factors in the process.

Deeply held cultural attitudes about the meaning of age and death are potent forces. Fear of becoming old, or even of appearing old, are realistic in our culture. Many, although not all, old people are poor. Some are ignored. Others are abandoned. Even among the wealthy and successful, unhappiness may prevail. The writer Garson Kanin has given us the following anecdote about W. Somerset Maugham. Maugham had a severe stammer and generally avoided public speaking. The Garrick Club held a dinner to celebrate his eightieth birthday, however, and he felt the need to make remarks in acknowledgment. Maugham was introduced, began with the customary salutations, and then said, "There are many virtues in growing old." Here he paused. At first the audience thought he had stopped for effect. As the pause continued, it appeared that he was overcome by his stammer. Finally concern grew that he had become ill and was unable to speak. Maugham stretched out the pause to the maximum and, at last, said, "I'm just . . . trying . . . to think what they are!"[9]

We are now attempting to deal with problems of funding Social Security and Medicare. One consequence of the recent public debate on these matters is a recrudesence of pejorative views toward older people. These thoughts focus on the idea that the elderly are getting a free ride, that they are simply another welfare group. There are complaints that, in large cities, their living costs are subsidized because many live in rent-controlled apartments. It is correct that some older people have ample funds, and reason demands that they provide largely for themselves in terms of dollar costs of care. However, as is true of every demographic group in our country, enormous diversity exists among the aged.

There has been a notable decrease in the poverty rate of older people. The rate in 1959 was 35 percent. Twenty-five years later, in 1984, it had fallen to 12.4 percent. The latter figure places the elderly in a position superior to the population in general, because the poverty rate for the country at large in 1984 was 14.4 percent.[10] Note that the cut-off dollar figure here, the estimated poverty threshold for people sixty-five years of age and more, was $4,979 income per year; for two-person families with head of household that age or more the figure was $6,282. As O'Shaughnessy and her associates indicate, however, this presentation obscures marked distinctions among subgroups of the elderly. Particular note must be made of the fact that the overall rate is skewed by the markedly high index of poverty among children.

There are specific groups among the elderly that are at substantially greater risk of poverty. Poverty rates increase sharply with age; in 1980, the rates varied from 13.6 percent among those 65 to 69 to 27.3 percent among those 85 and over. Women have rates that are two to three times as high as men; women 85 and over had poverty rates of 34.1 percent compared to 17.2 percent among men. Finally, elderly who live alone have much higher rates than do persons living with a spouse or with children.[11]

The group particularly at risk of institutional placement is made up of very old and isolated people, usually women. The poverty rate figures offer an explanation. These data are ominous as well in regard to the potential of costs for long term care. The demographic growth of the very old in the next several decades evidently will increase substantially the numbers of people who are both aged and poor. This is probably true despite the fact that the upcoming cohort of the old-old seems to be somewhat better prepared financially than their predecessors.[12] For many elderly people, especially women, Social Security and payments from other government programs make up from 85 to 95 percent of total income. The current broad concern about the federal budget deficit and the various devices suggested for its control are threatening to the borderline financial stability of these individuals.

TRAINING IN GERONTOLOGY

Curricula should be developed and promoted in schools of medicine, nursing, social work, and health care administration that provide appropriate information about the health and social needs of older people. The education of people in the health professions is a complex and lengthy process. Proficiency in technical skills is a clear essential. Beyond this, it is appropriate that young people entering these fields develop the capacity to function at a high level, often under stressful conditions, and yet maintain sensitivity and concern for the welfare of their patients.[13]

The population of old and very old people in our country is increasing, and the health care services they need must be given in noninstitutional settings much of the time. As a result, while we develop the spectrum of long term care programs, we must examine the methods through which student training is conducted. In recent years a moderate amount of attention has been directed toward the teaching of gerontology in professional schools, but it is rare that students have practical application of these lessons. For instance, while about 80 percent of medical schools offer some sort of didactic education in geriatric fields for their students, only 43 percent include a home health care experience, and this is often of an elective rather than a mandatory nature.[14]

Many residency training programs in internal medicine and primary care provide programs for house officers (interns and resident physicians) that are well balanced between inpatient acute care services and traditional ambulatory care settings. (The latter may be defined as outpatient departments and emergency rooms of hospitals.) Few such programs provide resident doctors with experience in treating the elderly in community settings, such as nursing homes or patient's homes. This sort of exposure, however, is of substantial educational value, and policies promoting such experiences in postgraduate medical education should be developed.

Young physicians must respond to the clinical challenges homebound patients present by recognizing the complex needs of chronically ill elderly people. Without this experience residents may complete their training with no understanding of the patient's life as a human being, beyond the walls of the clinic or hospital ward. When residents are properly trained, a startling realization of the richness of each individual's life emerges, and with it a greater sensitivity to the nonmedical elements in successful management of sick people and their illnesses.

Advanced training for nurses is equally valuable and should be encouraged. A focus on education of nurses in the field of geriatric practice is especially pertinent. In 1985 there were thirty-five geriatric nurse practitioner training programs,[15] a modest number considering the potential need. As in other health care areas, nurses must have the necessary clinical skills and the requisite sensitivity for work with the frail aged as well.[16]

In home health care programs, for instance, where the complexities of patient need may be marked, the multidisciplinary team approach has proven essential.[17] Health care students should be introduced to the concept of teamwork while in training. In this setting students of each discipline learn the values and strengths of the others, lessons of permanent career value.

POLICY

Policy issues must be addressed in order for us to begin developing a coherent national plan of long term care for the elderly. Among these issues are: (1) access to services for those who need help (including establishment of eligibility standards, innovative financing models, housing, transportation, discharge planning and case management systems, and sufficient money resources); and (2) allocation of resources, and financing and management for each of the program elements on the long term care spectrum, followed by program development.

ACCESS TO SERVICES

ELIGIBILITY

Medicaid is the largest payer of long term care costs, largely for nursing home beds; but variations in eligibility between the states are notable. Medicare eligibility, while essentially universal for all people age sixty-five, is not an effective force in long term care.

Eligibility should be defined as well by the personal financial resources of the individual at risk, and perhaps the family. It is theoretically feasible to purchase any sort of care, if a program exists in the local area. Nursing homes, paraprofessional assistance, visiting nurse services, even home visits from a physician are available. The challenge here is the program design, the orchestration of the necessary services. The older people who need help are, by the very nature of their disabilities, often not able to accept the challenge of their own case management. For the elderly who lack family or friends to help, even ample money may be useless. It is more common to find that the person who needs assistance has only modest amounts of money available. It is in these instances that long term care insurance, or a reverse annuity on a house, might generate the needed personal funds to help an elderly individual avoid placement in a nursing home as an expensive ward of the state.

INNOVATIVE FINANCING MODELS

New financial resources will become necessary for care of the elderly. Since, for the measurable future, government money will not be available, the private sector must be tapped. Here, ingenuity and innovation may pay off. For instance, many commercial companies are developing long term care insurance policies. Reverse annuities and home equity conversion plans are under test. Life care retirement centers serve to protect some older people from harsh decisions.

HOUSING AND TRANSPORTATION

The fate of an elderly frail individual, when long term care services are needed, may be determined by arbitrary matters such as the structure or location of the home. For instance, if the person at risk lives in an apartment on an upper floor of a walk-up building, someone else will be needed for matters as simple as obtaining food. If, on the other hand, the individual concerned happens to live on the ground floor or in an elevator building, arranging for independence at home is a simpler matter.

In sparsely populated areas, or locations where public transportation is not available, sustaining a safe existence outside of an institution may depend on a kind friend with a car. Otherwise, the degree of isolation that occurs may ultimately prove too risky for a continued life at home.

DISCHARGE PLANNING

Effective use of elements on the long term care spectrum is dependent on personnel equipped with needed information.[18] Within hospitals, the task of defining for each elderly patient the available resources for care falls to discharge planners. Usually this task in a formal sense is the responsibility of staff social workers, although any appropriately trained person can serve. A considerable problem remains: the mind-set of many discharge planners that the quick, easy solution for most frail elderly patients is a nursing home referral. It is a common event for a hospitalized older patient to be transferred to a long term care institution without substantive discussion. The job of the discharge planning section of any acute care hospital in the late 1980s is to move people out. Otherwise, under the Diagnostic Related Group regulations, the hospital faces financial risk.

As a matter of policy, new approaches are required. An acceptable solution will be to train discharge planners as case managers.[19] The field of case management concentrates on helping people to negotiate systems and to overcome obstacles.[20]

FINANCIAL RESOURCES

When individuals have access to sufficient private funds, service choices will be broad. For people who must depend on Medicaid, however, a no-frills set of options exists in most instances. Thus care is not distributed equally. Prospective payment systems such as that promulgated under the DRG legislation do not bar people from purchasing health care services with their own funds, beyond the allowances provided by government. Furthermore, as Professor Lester Thurow of Massachusetts Institute of Technology indicates:

There will be a market for those able and willing to pay more for health care. But markets exist to distribute goods and services in accordance with the distribution of income. Since the top 20 percent of the population has 11 times as much income as the bottom 20 percent, any market system will end up providing at least 11 times as much health care to the top 20 percent as to the bottom 20 percent.[21]

When money is sparse, decisions about the fate of individuals lie in the hands of the government. The result is often an enforced nursing home placement. In some instances the only other option for those who wish to remain in their own homes is a borderline or dangerous life situation, because basic necessities may be hard to obtain.

ALLOCATION OF RESOURCES

A reasonable ideal for any form of government is the prudent use of available resources for the general good, with concern for the wishes of individuals.[22] This applies to the long term care spectrum as follows:

1. The family, friends, and neighbors of the frail older person at risk should be encouraged and assisted. Their involvement is likely to be

loving and caring, often untainted by financial consideration, and of a humane value beyond what dollars can provide.

2. Government regulations should be appropriate to the situation. Overregulation is expensive and wasteful of resources because employment of unnecessary personnel results. Also, overregulation impedes coherent and timely action. Government regulations should be limited to assurance of financial probity and patient safety.

3. Local initiative should be stressed. Tapping the zeal of energetic people in the community is useful. Voluntary agencies can initiate programs that make up parts of the long term care spectrum. Organizations of friendly visiting neighbors, Meals-on-Wheels, day care centers, and telephone reassurance efforts make an impact. Minimal amounts of money are often adequate for this sort of project, and can be obtained from modest fund drives and local philanthropic organizations. As demand grows, additional resources for those programs that remain viable can be sought from local and regional government in the form of grants. As long as bureaucratization is avoided, there is a reasonable chance that the focus of the effort will remain the patient in need rather than the organization giving the service.

A critical missing element in much of the country is a central source of information about available resources for the frail elderly. Without this, even if excellent and diverse programs for the aged exist, they will often not be used, and resources thus will be allocated poorly. Local initiatives to establish centralized information and referral services at well-known and trusted community agencies should be encouraged.

PROGRAM DEVELOPMENT

Government at various levels, and in association with local voluntary groups, should work toward a coordinated development of service programs for older people. These services should be designed to encourage the elderly to maintain maximum feasible independence. At the same time, we should seek the goal of prudent use of resources, so that the least costly appropriate form of care is used and that those who most need help are aided.[23]

PARAPROFESSIONAL SERVICES

Homemaker, home health aide, and housekeeper assistance should be available to the frail elderly. Access to these personnel must be based on proven need, or the costs will become excessive. On the other hand, if need for help is truly present, it must be arranged in a timely fashion. The design for service must therefore be flexible.

Innovative methods of deploying paraprofessional staff are important, in terms of dollar savings and effective use of personnel hours. For instance, in areas where patients are clustered, one worker could effectively care for the basic needs of a number of older people in a given day. This would require the courage of agency employers and government regulators to be creative, and in particular to alter the current policy, which often requires a minimum four-hour shift.

RESPITE CARE

Respite services are designed to give relief to families who have accepted the basic responsibility for an older relative. The term respite is defined broadly. It may in practice mean that the older patient is placed temporarily in a nursing home while the family takes a desperately needed vacation, or it may imply the placement of paid staff within the home on a temporary basis.

The value of respite care as a means of preserving the stability of a structure that allows older people to maintain a life in their own homes has been established through demonstration programs. A study of the results reveals that complexities exist, however. For instance, it must be carefully planned that chronic care institutions in the local area will have respite care beds set aside and available when needed. At the same time, these beds must be constantly used, or the financial status of the institution will suffer. The implication is that a year-round respite program must exist, one that will guarantee the use of a given number of beds at all times and that will work through preplanning and by appointment. Furthermore, the means for payment of the patient's brief stay must be established. Should this be through the person's Medicare entitlements, which already exist, or through a temporary draw on the state's Medicaid funds? Should the patient or family pay the costs personally? Perhaps respite care should be paid for by cost-sharing among various levels of government, private insurors, and individuals. Decisions of this nature can be made coherently only when all parties, particularly including federal and state governments, are willing to join in program planning and implementation.

ADULT DAY CARE

Proof of the value for day care services remains unclear. Certainly in some individual situations, placement of the older person at risk in a safe place for the day while family members work is important. More demonstrations of how such programs can be conducted, paid for, and made usable by sufficient numbers of older people are required. Among the considerations is a safe, efficient, and inexpensive means of transportation to and from the day care center for elderly persons, who may be frail and/or confused.

FOSTER CARE

Foster care services offer a logical opportunity for isolated older people who cannot maintain their own homes to stay out of institutions. Government policies should encourage this development, particularly for the elderly who are frail and physically handicapped, who need a degree of straightforward observation to make certain that they are safe, take their medications, and eat adequately, and yet who are stable enough to remain free.

Development of foster care in its proper place on the spectrum will require cooperation between government agencies and local groups. The means for finding and screening individual foster homes, observing the success of placements, and paying the costs all must be planned. The example—the merits and the problems—of child foster care programs should be studied in the planning process, but the assumption of replicability should be avoided.

HOSPICE

The hospice movement in this country is now well advanced. The spirit behind this effort, the humane concern for the physical and spiritual welfare of people who are dying, is laudable and generally accepted. Definitions of hospice care are diverse, and range from specific physical settings, called hospices, where people are brought to die, to programs that consist only of trained staff members. These people go to wherever the patient is—the home, the hospital—to give appropriate help.

Hospice is the only significant new Medicare entitlement of the last six years, but the financial and programmatic restrictions are sufficiently severe that they handicap growth. Considering the anxieties that exist about

Medicare viability, these restrictions are understandable but not necessarily wise. A natural consortium of interests can be gathered about hospice and what it represents. The participants include spiritual leaders of the movement, advocates of the rights of the elderly and the dying, guardians of the public purse, institutions such as hospitals and nursing homes, and insurance companies. In order to fulfill the prospects of hospice care as part of the spectrum of services for the aged, these forces must gather and make the national case for deployment of more substantial resources and less arbitrary entry regulations.

Dollar savings are important, and well-used hospice services save on the costs of inpatient care for dying people. Other values of at least equal weight exist, and must be considered. These relate to the feelings, the emotions of the dying person and family members. There often develops between patient and loved ones a cruel conspiracy of silence about the fact of approaching death.[24] The patient usually understands that death is near but cannot mention it to anyone because it is a "dirty secret." The family members are afraid to talk about it. Yet it is almost always true that people are relieved and feel better if the subjects of death and dying can be discussed with sensitivity, freely and openly. At the least, finding the means to help patients express their feelings and emotions is valuable. The skill and experience of hospice team members can be used for this purpose:

AD was a seventy-year old woman dying of cancer, being cared for by her husband and her son at home. The bed was moved into the large kitchen, where she would be in the heart of all family activities. Dear relatives and friends visited regularly, but the patient's impending death was never discussed. On the day of the [program team's] last visit Mrs. D's poodle was nearby. After the doctor and nurse had finished examining the patient, the social worker picked up the dog and sat by her bedside. Mrs. D patted the dog and started to weep. She said, "I'm feeling very lonesome. I just hate to be leaving my family behind. They look so sad. Thank you for letting me cry and for letting me talk."[25]

CERTIFIED HOME CARE AGENCIES

Certified home care programs operate broadly around the country, based largely in hospitals or visiting nurse agencies. Reimbursement for the care they provide, limited in nature and time, derives from Medicare, Medicaid, Blue Cross plans, and occasionally self-payment. Public policy will be served by reasonable expansion of certified home care programs into parts of the country where they are lacking. Health maintenance organizations may become involved. However, the attitude of HMOs to date toward home care is equivocal. HMO entrepreneurs both fear engagement with the frail elderly because of the financial risk and at the same time perceive involvement as a marketing opportunity. Where the gage will fall is hard to judge.[26]

LONG TERM HOME HEALTH CARE

Programs designed to bring health care services to homebound frail elderly people serve to help them remain independent at home for lengthy periods of time. In many instances, patients enrolled in these programs would otherwise have failed and died alone, or have been forced into institutions. Because Medicare was designed and is regulated as an insurance program for the care of older people who are acutely ill, it does not meet their health care needs when problems become prolonged or chronic. As a consequence, older people who need help must either devour their assets (the "spend-down" phenomenon) in order to become Medicaid-eligible or depend on others, usually their children, to pay the costs of service.

The common fate of many frail elderly persons is placement in a nursing home. Most long term care funds are used for this sort of institutional care. The dolorous consequences include massive costs; older people deprived of their independence and ability to control their own life decisions; and a bankrupt policy, because the numbers of older people are growing, and caring for them by building more nursing homes raises dollar and social costs beyond counting.

Health care at home is preferable. When the costs of maintaining people at home through the few long term home health care programs that now exist are compared with those of institutional placement, it is evident that the former is often less expensive. Government, at state and national levels, should use its leverage, and to a reasonable degree its funds, for the development and support of such efforts. New York State, through its Nursing Home Without Walls program, has created a replicable example for the nation. Local hospitals are logical sponsors of these efforts.[27]

While government begins to move from long term home health care policy planning to implementation, it should at the same time maintain a wary eye toward expansion plans for nursing homes and other institutions of chronic care. Over time, home health care programs will prove themselves fiscally sound to government only if costs of nursing homes are held in check. One approach toward maintaining a proper balance will be to require that any geographical area or institution that wishes to expand the number of chronic care beds provide evidence that an effective long term home health care program is in place. Further, the program should be large enough to care for all local elderly people who wish help and are appropriate candidates. Nursing homes should be reserved, if possible, for people who need twenty-four-hour-a-day observation and are willing to be so placed.

INSTITUTIONAL SERVICES

Nursing homes (skilled nursing facilities), health-related facilities, and other institutional resources must exist. They are necessary in order to meet the essential health care needs and the requirements for physical protection of the most disabled or demented members of the frail elderly population. As the demographic imperative imposes itself upon our country, a strong thrust will develop to increase the bricks-and-mortar component of long term care, the institutions. Government, through its control of funds and the certificate of need process, can resist. Uncontrolled expansion of these resources is fiscally unsound. It is also an inhumane, uncaring method of responding to the long term care needs of the elderly. Institutional placement is quite properly perceived by many as simply the warehousing of older people.

In the spectrum of long term care services for the elderly, institutions have their place. It is the place of last resort.

LEGISLATION

Policies of excellence can be formulated, but in order for them to be realized they must be legislated. Changes in law designed to increase emphasis on long term care must take place at both national and state levels. Appropriate means for legislative decisions to be fulfilled must be provided as well. Examples exist in which nonelected civil servants have blunted the effect of legislation by writing obstructive regulations.[28]

Medicare revision is the key to creation of the long term care spectrum. Virtually all older people in our country have Medicare entitlements to coverage of major health-related needs associated with acute illness. We must recognize both that long term, chronic health problems are handled poorly by Medicare as it is now formulated and that the need for help with these matters has become imperative. The people served by Medicare have changed in number and need since the original legislation of 1964. A change in policy designed to meet the requirements of the older and more disabled population of the late twentieth century is a logical and practical necessity.

However, in the field of long term care for the aged major obstacles interfere with immediate federal legislative solutions to the issues under discussion here. The current mind-set in Washington tends to produce negative legislation. The focus of attention is the massive federal deficit and its untoward consequences to the economic life of the country, and the resulting climate is cold to innovation and to long term thinking.

The important Catastrophic Health Insurance legislation proposed in 1986 by Otis R. Bowen, Secretary of Health and Human Services, and as amended by congress in 1987,[29] characterizes this point. The goal of Secretary Bowen's plan is to protect against the expense of catastrophic illness, and older persons in the United States particularly need this protection. However, the proposal is designed solely to insure against the catastrophic expenses of those under treatment in acute care hospital beds for prolonged periods. The design is significant because it uses the Medicare program as the mechanism through which coverage will be provided.

While a laudable first step, it does not go far enough. Benefits will accrue only to those persons, small in number, who must stay in hospitals for lengthy periods of time. The proposal fails to respond to the demographic imperative of the aging in this country and the need for additional amendment of the Medicare law to insure against the much more common catastrophic costs of care for chronic disease. Arbitrary regulations now bar persons entitled to Medicare from long term services through devices such as the skilled nursing[30] and intermittent care requirements. These regulations illogically apply for costs of care only if the disease requires attention intermittently and that those with prolonged illness do not need skilled care. This makes no sense. The catastrophic health care problems of the elderly demand skilled care over the long term.[31]

The aphorism "timing is everything" is pertinent. Now may be the wrong moment to propose new and significant Medicare entitlements. If we want to prepare ourselves for future opportunities, however, we must understand the following points:

1. We are moving through a political cycle that began in the late 1970s. For several years prior to Ronald Reagan's election as our thirty-ninth president, the focus on health policy in Congress had shifted away from enacting new programs and toward legislating cutbacks.[32] It was during Jimmy Carter's presidency, for instance, that Congress developed an initiative to control the growth in hospital expenditures. Prior to that, a variety of health planning and oversight groups were established. They were designed to limit federal capital expenditures for health facilities and decrease hospitalizations deemed unnecessary by government planners. These developments were forerunners

of the present DRG regulations. More recently, harsh emphasis has been placed on threats to the fiscal viability of the Medicare Trust Fund. As a consequence, cuts in Medicare expenditures and increases in co-payments have been instituted.

2. As the lawyer and consultant Earl Collier has emphasized,[33] this political cycle will extend through the Reagan presidency and well into the following term. The next president, whoever he or she may be, will require several years to establish priorities. So will Congress. Thus we must anticipate a period of thinking and planning that will extend into the mid-1990s before the political timing might be right for action in the Medicare area. "There's an inertia about events that can't easily be reversed."[34]

3. We are also in the midst of a planning and evaluation cycle. It is a bit more than twenty years since the advent of Medicare and Medicaid. These insurance/entitlement programs were major forces for change in the way that health care was supported. The results of two decades must be studied, analyzed, and the programs themselves ultimately altered, to reflect the lessons learned. The study period may take a decade, thus paralleling the political cycle.

4. The timing of the national mood must be considered as well. Legislators respond to voters, and at present voters are not pressing for change in the field of long term care with sufficient energy to produce results. The spirit of twenty years ago, with its emphasis on social programs, has been replaced by one of concern for the economy. The mood may change as increasing numbers of older persons need help, as the impact of DRGs becomes more evident, and as the consequences impinge in an onerous manner on the daily lives of families.

Proper timing for change in national policy toward long term care also demands a clearly formulated set of goals. At this moment, concerned people seek a consensus about program development for the aged. However, "there is no current stated policy that anyone can espouse. There is a little conversation about this and about that, but not much coherence in conceptual discussions, and beyond that very little knowledge. . . . It is going to take awhile for models to be devised. From the viewpoint of influencing legislation these models are essential."[35]

Legislators want to develop programs that work. Lessons from previous models, or those now in existence, thus have great value. At the same time, we must recognize that our various layers of government have a complex puzzle to solve: the fiscal conflict between Washington and the states in regard to who pays for long term care. To date, Medicare remains an acute care program, one of little use in handling the long term requirement of the frail elderly. In some states Medicaid has been the legislative vehicle for carrying out chronic care needs, but in these situations only the most impoverished are eligible for services. In other states no action has been taken. As the crisis becomes ever more acute, which level of government will get stuck with the bill for long term care? Who will pay for the poor?[36] This conflict is the major axis around which the long term care policy debate has revolved. In order to halt the circular discussion and move toward solutions, creative and aggressive policy leadership is required.[37] Several strong and innovative legislators have made the initial moves.

THE COURSE OF FEDERAL LEGISLATION

In the mid-1970s our sense of the meaning of long term care for the aged began to change. Earlier the term had been "essentially a euphemism for nursing home care."[38] Recognition that nursing homes were often disgraceful warehouses for the elderly, the nursing home scandals, the evidence that increasing numbers of older people in the population needed help, the onerous costs of institutional placement, all led to a search for alternatives in care for the frail elderly. The first long term home health care programs were developed in the early and middle years of that decade, and they helped to establish the validity of choices for older people.

Concerns about humane care were preeminent for the innovators in the field and for the aged who sought to remain at home. For people in government, particularly those responsible for controlling expenditure of tax monies, the impact of long term care programs on state and federal budgets was the first consideration. It was during the early 1970s that Medicaid became significantly utilized for long term care, particularly nursing home payments for the elderly. Before this, Medicaid had been thought of primarily as a welfare program for poor families with children. The fact that government was in the long term care business caught the country by surprise. In parallel, it became clear that Medicare, the program that the public naively thought appropriate for covering health-related needs of older people, would not support long term care costs.

With this background, the first relevant federal legislative moves took place seeking remedies for these programmatic and payment enigmas. Considerable energy and initiative has been put forth in Congress since 1975 in attempts to enact long term care legislation. Efforts directed toward establishment of home health care services stand as a paradigm.

NATIONAL HOME HEALTH CARE ACT OF 1975

Four major home health care bills were introduced in the 94th Congress.[39] Of these, the National Home Health Care Act of 1975 stands out. It concentrated on Medicare reform and contained a legislative concept inherited by the major proposals of later years. This would have permitted Medicare reimbursement to hospital-based long term home health care programs, as an alternative to institutional care, if such payments were not otherwise covered by Medicare. This bill incorporated the critical factors necessary for national development of long term home health care services for the frail elderly: (1) Medicare pays; (2) programs are based in hospitals; (3) programs are genuine alternatives to institutional placement; and (4) eligible services are beyond those already permitted.

The author of this legislation was then-Representative Edward I. Koch (Dem-NY). The National Home Health Care Act of 1975 was followed by that of 1976, and of 1977. Then Mr. Koch was elected Mayor of New York City. His legislative proposal did not succeed in reaching the floor of the House for a vote. However, the principle was now recognized.

In 1980, during the 96th Congress, Orrin G. Hatch, the junior senator from Utah, known as a conservative Republican, established himself as a key proponent of home care with his Community Home Health Services Act (S.3211). In a revised form, this legislation was presented to the 97th Congress, in 1981.

THE COMMUNITY HOME HEALTH
SERVICES ACT OF 1981 (S.234)

In the 97th Congress, Senator Hatch became Chairman of the Senate Labor and Human Resources Committee. The leverage available to him in this position allowed the opportunity for development of and action on a long term home health care bill close to the ideal.[40] S.234 in its final form included an emphasis on expanding home health services under Medicare (and Medicaid as well) with an explicit focus on chronicity of care[41] and an altered definition of home health services, to include nursing for chronic conditions, thus eliminating the strangling limitation on service under Medicare of the Skilled Nursing Requirement; the services of a homemaker when medically required; and transportation when essential.

The theme of S.234 is the hospital base for home health care programs. The language of the key paragraph is taken virtually intact from the 1975 Koch bill, and its parentage has been acknowledged by Senator Hatch.[42] We repeat this paragraph for the benefit of legislators of the mid-to-late

1990s who may find it valuable when timing is right for successful proposal of long term home health care legislation:

> Section 4.(a) Section 1861(m) of the Social Security Act is amended . . . "Notwithstanding any other provisions of this title, the term 'home health services' includes [without regard to any of the preceding provisions of this subsection] any professional health services provided in an individual's home by a nonprofit hospital or by members of its staff acting as such [including its physicians, nurses, social workers, therapists, technicians, home health aides, homemakers, housekeepers, dietitians, and other personnel] as an alternative to institutional care, if such services do not qualify for payment [as outpatient hospital services or otherwise] under the other provisions of this title; . . ."[43]

The fate of S.234 is worth following. On December 15, 1981, Hatch's committee reported the bill favorably to the Senate. This was, and remains to date, the only long term home health care legislation to be moved past the committee level. As the senator pointed out at the time, however, "the remaining obstacles in this legislative home stretch include pre-Senate floor approval by my colleague, Chairman Bob Dole of the Finance Committee, and of course House action."[44] Death at the hands of the Finance Committee was, in fact, the fate of S.234. It was the victim of turf battles over control of Medicare and of genuine uncertainty about the ultimate cost of the proposal. The timing was wrong.

THE RECEDING TIDE (S.1181)

From the moment this legislation failed in 1982, the tide has receded. While Hatch has continued to propose long term home health care legislation in each congressional session, the strength and value of his bills has become increasingly attenuated. Yet each has had worthy qualities. In order to bypass the strangling effect of the Finance Committee, the latest Hatch bills (Home and Community Based Services for the Elderly Act of 1985, introduced May 21, 1985, and Home and Community Based Services Act of 1987, introduced April 8, 1987) omit any attempt at Medicare reform. Their intent, instead, is to authorize grants to the states for the purposes of: (1) coordinating all community and state services now provided through a complex maze of programs; (2) identifying ways of assisting the elderly at risk of institutional placement, so that they may remain at home; (3) educating the public and professional communities about available services; (4) encouraging the involvement of families, voluntary, religious and community organizations in the issue; (5) providing basic home-based services of paraprofessionals and certain therapists; and (6) developing analyses about cost-effective methods in the field of home health care for the Secretary of Health and Human Services.

If the 1987 bill were to become law, these laudable goals would be funded at $100 million per year for the fifty states. These are nice but pared-down concepts. The suggested funds are so paltry as to be of questionable impact. In effect, this bill, passage of which appears unlikely, simply keeps the concept of long term home health care alive in Washington.

OTHER LEGISLATIVE DEVELOPMENTS

Two other interesting legislative models, both of which have failed of enactment, are noteworthy. Senators Bob Packwood and Bill Bradley conceived a new component of the Social Security Act, a so-called Title XXI. Note that Medicare and Medicaid are Titles XVIII and XIX, respectively, and that Title XX of the Social Security Act covers certain services. Their proposal, introduced in 1981, would have established an entirely new long term service program for the frail elderly, home care expansion included.[45] The use of Medicare as a vehicle for this form of care would have been abandoned under the new Title XXI. The bill failed to move forward, in large part because its proposed solution to the problem was excessively complex. Further, through its failure to use Medicare as the base, the proposal lost the value of attachment to a familiar and comfortable program, broadly deemed to be effective.

Proposals that arose in 1982 for amending Medicare by creating a Part C have also foundered. Note that Parts A and B of Medicare cover a share of hospital costs and physician's fees, respectively. Proponents of a Part C would have removed home care and other components of the long term care system from the mainstream of Medicare. The death of this proposal may in part have been due to its association, in one of its formulations, with proprietary nursing home chains.

We are still spinning in place. It has not been possible to amend the basic Medicare law in favor of long term care programs. On the other hand, efforts to develop such programs through legislative means that are broadly seen as distorted (Title XXI and Part C are examples) have failed as well.

The Koch bill, and its acknowledged successor, the Hatch legislation, failed to become law. However, they have been responsible for significant movement in the area of long term care and for developments that have followed. Hatch's 1980 proposal (S.3211), the predecessor of his major landmark home health care legislation of the following year (S.234), had important impact on the Omnibus Reconciliation Act of 1980.[46] This act deleted the requirement that a patient must have been in the hospital for three days prior to eligibility for Medicare Part A home health benefits (such as they are) and erased the hundred-visit limit on skilled nursing visits to the home under both Parts A and B. Note that the word skilled remained a prerequisite.

The next development, the Tax Equity and Fiscal Responsibility Act [TEFRA] of 1982, began to establish limits on costs for certified home health agencies. The design was to minimize the costs of such programs based in hospitals; the result, however, was to stimulate hospitals to discharge patients sooner, thus enhancing the importance of home care. TEFRA also required the development of a prospective payment system for the future, which we now know as the DRG system. As Yale epidemiologist Kyle Grazier points out, this "constitutes perhaps the most influential legislation to date for both home health care and hospital-based health care in America."[47]

The prospective payment system [PPS] mandated by TEFRA was placed into law through the Social Security Amendments of 1983, as Public Law 98-21. The PPS reimburses hospitals on the basis of patient diagnosis rather than length of hospital stay. Thus the inevitable urgency on the part of hospitals to discharge patients expeditiously and the concomitant need for development of resources for care of sick people outside the institution. Home health care would seem to be the logical answer, but we remain stymied by fear of new costs. In the meantime evidence grows that Medicare patients are being sent home from acute care hospitals more quickly and in a poorer state of health than before the DRG system was initiated.[48]

New models of payment for home care services are being considered, once again to control costs. A prospective method of reimbursement may develop, following the same motives as in-hospital DRGs: limit services to inhibit expenditures.

Will a home care PPS work better than the current retrospective payment-per-service method? There are competing factors. First, the demographic imperative will exert continuing pressure for more help at home. Second, reverse forces designed to inhibit costs will press for less payment per unit of care and for rigid restrictions on nature and number of services given. A PPS may control well for the second set of factors, but it cannot halt the number of older people newly in need.[49] Further, a PPS for home care will inevitably throw out of the system people who continue to need help, just as does the in-hospital DRG process today.

FINANCING
THE LONG TERM CARE SPECTRUM

Incoherence in national long term care policy is particularly obvious in its relationship to money. The means of paying for services are characterized by overlaps and gaps, redundancy, and confusion. Reference to federal programs makes the point. More than eighty programs emanate from Washington that offer some kind of long term care assistance. These range from direct cash support, to provision of food or other goods, to specific services.[50]

Among these many federal programs, six are considered to be the major sources of long term care support: Medicare, Medicaid, the Social Services Block Grant, the Older Americans Act, the Supplemental Security Income Program, and the Veterans Administration. As O'Shaughnessy and her associates have recognized, however, "No one program . . . has been designed to support a full range of long term care services on a systematic basis."[51] The challenges an older person faces in order to understand the process are formidable. The variety of state, county, city, philanthropic, and proprietary services that may also be available add significantly to the thicket of difficulty that any person in need of help must negotiate.

Incoherent policy is expensive. As Anne Somers emphasizes, the costs of long term care services paid for by Medicare and Medicaid have increased significantly, with about two-thirds of the dollars spent on nursing homes.[52] Were there a more logical and flexible system, the available funds could be spent on less intense care for a significant proportion of the people now arbitrarily placed in institutions.

The very structure of law and regulation, and the hierarchical nature of the flow of authority from national to state to local government, seem to ordain rigidity. Policy analyst B. J. Curry Spitler makes the point:

> The federal level of government must relate to fifty state governments because many human service programs are passed to the states to be carried out. The Older Americans Act, Medicaid . . . and the social services provided through Title XX of the Social Security Act . . . are examples. . . . Further complicating the implementation and administration of human services programs are the arrangements made with counties or parishes [in the United States, there are approximately three thousand local governments].[53]

In regard to financing of the long term care spectrum, we find ourselves with two major problems. First, the massive current convolution of payment structure denies the simple and easy movement of an older person from one program to another as need requires. Second, we are in an era of funding cuts. Thus we seem to be refused the logical use of scarce Medicare dollars for appropriate chronic long term care services for the aged because of fear that a new demand will be created. If the federal budget is reduced, so will be spending on health care services, a development which characterizes a change in national viewpoint, as Thurow notes: "The federal government used to view health care as a social problem. Today it views it almost solely as a budget-deficit problem. The shift in perspectives is important. Social problems can be left to fester; budget-deficit problems require more immediate solution."[54]

To a degree, this is an overstatement. Social problems can stew for a while, but ultimately they come to a boil and demand attention. The consequences of the demographic imperative will in time be felt with irresistible pressure.

Dr. Hirsch S. Ruchlin of Cornell University Medical College indicated in 1982 that a search for new funding approaches for long term care was needed. National fiscal developments since that date make it increasingly uncertain that the federal government will continue to offer even the minimal dollar resources to sustain the present level of long term care services. "Thus, for pragmatic reasons if not philosophical ones, one must recognize that heavy reliance on public financing may no longer be a feasible or acceptable option."[55]

The current state of paralysis in planning and financing of a long term care spectrum for the country at large has occurred because of a rough balance in competing viewpoints rather than as a result of inattention. Here we assume that the demographic curve and the growth in nursing home costs are understood. One response to these points has been promotion of the concept that noninstitutional services are less costly and more humane than nursing homes. It follows, in this argument, that increased government monies devoted to these services would decrease the cost of long term care to the taxpayer by shrinking the need for highly expensive nursing home placements. The bias in government long term care policy favoring institutional services is indisputable. Medicare focuses its expenditures on acute care hospitals. Medicaid spends almost half its resources on nursing homes. Reversing this bias in favor of a more diverse set of long term care programs for the elderly has an attractive and logical budgetary appeal.

This rationale is disputed by those who argue that paying for more noninstitutional services would in fact add to the government's share of the costs. The concern here is that nursing home expenses would continue unabated, but that in addition uncounted numbers of older people now kept safely at home through the unpaid efforts of family and friends would seek government money for care if it became available.[56]

For this and other reasons, the need to establish diverse payment sources for long term care has become increasingly clear. Since government cannot support the necessary services, creative and entrepreneurial elements in the private sector will move in. The ultimate intent of current policy, with its fix upon budget rather than program, is to insist that those who can pay for their own needs do so. This is the means to economy in health care expenditures, because money spent by people out of their own pockets is money spent with prudence. "The goal is to make the patient the main cost container."[57] The proportion of older persons whose income places them below the poverty line is falling. Some elderly persons will have available funds to pay for the kind of long term care they want. As this fact has become clear, the mechanisms have been created to attract their money or to help them convert frozen funds into usable capital. Among relevant developments of recent years are life care retirement centers, reverse annuities, home equity conversion plans, and long term care insurance. For those who cannot pay, the government will probably continue to be the funder of last resort for the minimal essential services.

CONCLUSION

A few truisms will serve to summarize our views. Older people are people. They should have the opportunity to make their own major life decisions. Fulfillment of the innate desire of all individuals to be as free and independent as possible is a reasonable goal of social policy. Development of a long term care spectrum for the elderly is a rational means for the attainment of this goal. Whether dollar savings must inevitably accrue through this means is not clear, but they probably will if legislation and regulations are written with prudence. However, regardless of this point, it is certain that the demographic explosion of the old and very old requires the creation of such a spectrum of programs.

Here we stop because, to paraphrase Sir Arthur Conan Doyle: ". . . Those who have said all they have to say have invariably said too much."[58]

Notes

CHAPTER 1

1. Barberis, M. (1981). America's elderly: Policy implications. *Population Bulletin, 35*(4): 3–13.

2. Soldo, B. J. (1980). America's elderly in the 1980's. *Population Bulletin, 35*(4):3; and Brody, S. J., and Persily, N. A. (1984). *Hospitals and the aged: The new old market.* Rockville, MD: Aspen Systems.

3. Soldo, America's elderly in the 1980's.

4. U.S. Bureau of the Census. (1982). 1980 census and middle series estimates: Projections of the population of the United States, 1982–2050. *Current Population Reports,* ser. P-25, no. 922:11; Davis, K., and Rowland, D. (1986). *Medicare policy.* Baltimore, MD: Johns Hopkins Univ. Press; Rosenwaike, I., and Logue, B. (1985). *The extreme aged in America.* Westport, CT: Greenwood Press; and Vaupel, J. W., and Gowan, A. E. (1986). Passage to Methuselah: Some demographic consequences of continued progress against mortality. *Am J Pub Health, 76:*430–433.

5. Maddox, G. L. (1982). Challenges for health policy and planning. In R. H. Binstock, W. S. Chow, and J. H. Schulz (Eds.), *International perspectives on aging: Population and policy challenges* pp. 127–158. New York: United Nations Fund for Population Activities.

6. Uhlenberg, P. (1977). Changing structure of the older population of the USA during the twentieth century. *Gerontologist, 17:*197–202.

7. Weissert, W. G. (1985). Estimating the long term care population: Prevalence rates and selected characteristics. *Health Care Financing Rev, 6:*83–91.

8. Technical Committee: (1981). Social and health aspects of long term care [Executive Summary]. 1981 White House Conference on Aging.

9. Kane, R. L., and Kane, R. A. (1980). Alternatives to institutional care of the elderly: Beyond the dichotomy. *Gerontologist, 20:*249–259.

10. Kodner, D. L. (1982, Jan.). The integration of long term care funding by channeling demonstration projects: Brief review of concepts and some existing models. National Long Term Care Channeling Demonstration Program, Temple University Institute on Aging, Philadelphia, p.1.

11. U.S. Senate Special Committee on Aging. (1984, Feb.). Developments in aging: 1983. Washington, DC, p. 423; Public Law 96-499, The Omnibus Reconciliation Act of 1980; Public Law 97-335, The Omnibus Budget Reconciliation Act of 1981; Public Law 97-248, Tax Equity and Fiscal Responsibility Act of 1982 (TEFRA); Public Law 98-21, Social Security Amendments of 1983; Public Law 98-369, Deficit Reduction Act of 1984; and The Consolidated Omnibus Reconciliation Act of 1985 (COBRA).

12. Long Term Care Case Mix Reimbursement Program. (1985, April). *PRI reference manual: RUG II training project.* Albany, NY: New York State Dept. of Health.

13. U.S. Bureau of the Census. (1981). Population characteristics of the U.S.: Age, sex, race and Spanish origin of the population by regions, divisions and states. *Supplementary Reports, 1980 Census of the Population.* Washington, DC: U.S. Government Printing Office.

14. U.S. Bureau of the Census, 1980 census and middle series estimates; and Weissert, Estimating the long-term care population.

15. U.S. Bureau of the Census. (1982, October). ser. P-25, no. 917, 1977, estimated, and ser. P-25, no. 922, Middle Series Projections.

16. National Center for Health Statistics. National nursing home survey, 1977; *American Medical News, 27*(14):20; and Brickfield, C. F. (1985). Long term care financing solutions are needed now. *Am Health Care Assn J, 11*:11–15.

17. Brickner, P. W. (1978). *Home health care for the aged.* New York: Appleton-Century-Crofts, p. 24.

18. Rosenwaike and Logue, *The extreme aged in America;* and Schneider, E., and Brody, J. A. (1983). Aging, natural death, and the compression of morbidity: Another view. *NEJM, 309:-*854–856.

19. Federal Council on Aging. (1981). *The need for long term care: Information and issues.* Washington, DC: U.S. Dept. of Health and Human Services, Office of Human Development Services.

20. Katz, S., Branch, L. G., Branson, M. H., et al. (1983). Active life expectancy. *NEJM, 309:*1218–1224.

21. Chelsea-Village Program, Dept. of Community Medicine. (1983, 1987). *Ten-year report* [1983] and *Fourteen-year report* [1987]. New York: St. Vincent's Hospital and Medical Center.

22. Feifel, H. (1971). The meaning of death in American society: Implications for education. In B. R. Green and D. P. Irish (Eds.), *Death education: Preparation for living.* Cambridge, MA: Schenkman, p.7.

23. Brickner, *Long term home health care.*

24. *Taxonomy of long term care services.* (1983). St. Louis, MO: Catholic Hospital Association of the United States.

25. Fordham, C. (1983). Medical manpower issues: Health policy in action? *Ann Intern Med, 99:*400–401.

26. Steele, R. (1712, Oct. 12). *The Spectator,* no. 509.

27. Public Law 96-499, The Omnibus Reconciliation Act of 1980; Public Law 97-335, The Omnibus Budget Reconciliation Act of 1981; Public Law 97-248, Tax Equity and Fiscal Responsibility Act of 1982 (TEFRA); Public Law 98-21, Deficit Reduction Act of 1984; and the Consolidated Omnibus Reconciliation Act of 1985 (COBRA).

28. Haber, C., (1983). *Beyond sixty-five.* New York: Cambridge Univ. Press, p. 3.

29. Spiegel, A. D., and Domanowski, G. F. (1983). Beginnings of home health care: A brief history. *PRIDE Inst J, 2*(3):28.

30. Moynihan, D. P. (1981, Apr. 2). Remarks on S. 861. *Congressional Record, 127:*54, 97th Cong., 1st sess., S. 3356.

31. Health and Welfare Division, Metropolitan Life Insurance Company. (N.D.). *Lillian D. Wald: Pioneer in public health nursing.* New York: Metropolitan Life Insurance Co., pp. 1–2.

32. Steward, J. E. (1979). *Home health care.* St. Louis, MO: C. V. Mosby; Buhler-Wilkerson, K. (1985). Public health nursing: In sickness or in health? *Am J Pub Health, 75:*1155–1161; and Roberts, D. E., and Heinrich, J. (1985). Public health nursing comes of age. *Am J Pub Health, 75:*1162–1172.

33. Steward, *Home health care;* and Clark, L. L. (1981). *History of homemaker/home health aide services.* New York: National HomeCaring Council.

34. Salzman, H., Langendorf, R., and Ravenna, P. (1987). Home health care [Michael Reese Hospital, Chicago] [Letter to the editor]. *NEJM, 106:*168; Cohen, C., Kessler, D., King, L., and Eisdorfer C. (1983). The Montefiore-Einstein health care complex. In S. J. Brody and N. A. Persily (Eds.), *Hospitals and the aged.* Rockville, MD: Aspen Systems, pp. 137–147; and Levenson, D. (1981). Martin Cherkasky at Montefiore. *Montefiore Medicine, 2:*47.

35. Cherkasky, M. (1947, May). Hospital service goes home. *Modern Hospital.*

36. Ibid.

37. Cherkasky, M. (1981). Hospital service goes home. *Colloquium, 1*(2):6–7.

38. Part 765 10 NYCRR, Laws of New York State—Approval and Licensure of Home Care Services Agencies.

39. Chelsea-Village Program, *Fourteen-year report.*

40. Fox, P. D. (1983). Quote from p. 29. Long term care: A bird's eye view. *PRIDE Inst J, 2*(1):23–30.

41. Stevens, R., and Stevens, R. (1974). *Welfare medicine in America: A case study of Medicaid.* New York: Free Press; and Vladeck, B. C. (1980). *Unloving care.* New York: Basic Books.

42. Aiken, L. H., and Bays K. D. (1984). The Medicare debate—round one. *NEJM, 311:* 1196–1200; and Dept. of Health and Human Services report to the President. (1986, Nov. 19). *Catastrophic illness expenses.* Washington, DC.

43. Vladeck, B. C. (1983). Two steps forward, one back: The changing agenda of long term care reform. *PRIDE Inst J, 2*(3):3–9.

44. Hoffman, J. C., and Mangiaracina, A. J. (1984). *Report on Management Office selected issues, No. IX—Federal health care costs.* Washington, DC: President's Private Sector Survey on Cost Control.

45. Wehr, E. (1984, Feb. 25). National health policy sought for organ transplants. *Congressional Quarterly,* pp. 453–458; and Leaf, A. (1984). The doctor's dilemma—and society's too. *NEJM, 310:*718–721.

46. Committee on Labor and Human Resources, U.S. Senate. (1982, Dec. 7). *Report to the chairman: The elderly should benefit from expanded home health care but increasing these services will not insure cost reductions.* Washington, DC: General Accounting Office/IPE-83-1, p. iv.

47. Vladeck, *Unloving Care.*

48. PL 97-248, Tax Equity and Fiscal Responsibility Act of 1982 (TEFRA).

49. Diamond, L. M., and Berman, D. E. (1981). The social/health maintenance organization: A single entry, prepaid, long-term-care delivery system. In J. J. Callahan and S. Wallack (Eds.), *Reforming the long term care system.* (Lexington, MA: Lexington Books), pp. 185–217; Governor's Long Range Medicaid Planning Committee. (1982, March). *The feasibility of developing and operating social/health maintenance organizations in New York State.* Albany: New York State Health Planning Commission; Greenberg, J., and Lentz, W. N. (1983, Nov. 16). *The Social/ Health Maintenance organization: Its role in the long term care system.* Paper presented at the annual meeting of the American Public Health Association, Dallas, TX; Greenberg, J. N., Lentz, W. N., and Abrahams, R. (1987). The national social health maintenance organization demonstration. In N. Goldfield and S. B. Goldsmith (Eds.), *Alternative delivery systems* (pp. 33–57). Rockville, MD: Aspen; Harrington, C., Newcomer, R., and Newacheck, P. (1983, Apr.). *Prepaid long term care plans: A policy option for California's Medi-Cal program.* Berkeley: Institute of Governmental Studies, Univ. of California; Kodner, D. L. (1981). Who's a S/HMO: A look at Metropolitan Jewish Geriatric Center and its plans to develop a social/health maintenance operation. *Home Health Svcs Quart, 2*(4):57–68; Schneider, D. (1981). *Policy analysis of coordinative integrative services: The Social/HMO.* Albany: New York State Health Planning Commission; SHMOs: A new experiment in health care. (1986, Sept.). *The Internist,* p. 20; and Winn, S., and McCaffrey, K. (1978). *Issues in the development of a prepaid system of long term care services.* Seattle: Batelle Research Center.

50. Lipsman, R. (1983). Editor's perspective. *PRIDE Inst J, 2*(1):2.

51. Wallack, S. (1983). New dollars for long term care: Proceedings from the PRIDE Institute conference, December 1982. *PRIDE Inst J, 2*(2):21–29.

52. Fullerton, W. (1982). Finding the money and paying for long-term care services. In J. Meltzer, F. Farrow, and H. Richman (Eds.), *Policy options in long term care.* Chicago: Univ. of Chicago Press, pp. 182–208.

53. Scholen, K. (1983). Financing home care with home equity. *PRIDE Inst J, 2*(2):43–45; and Kenny, K., and Belling, B. (1987). Home equity conversion: A counseling model. *Gerontologist, 27:9–12.*

54. Lichtig, L. K. (1981). New Jersey Evaluation of ICD-9-CM DRG's. Trenton: New Jersey State Dept. of Health, pp. 1–3; English, J. T., Sharfstein, S. S., Scherl, D. J., et al. (1986). Diagnosis-Related Groups and general hospital psychiatry: The APA study. *Am J Psychiatry, 143*(2):131–139; Iglehart, J. K. (1983). Medicare begins prospective payment of hospitals. *NEJM, 308:*1428–1432; Interim final rule, Medicare program. (1983). Prospective payments for Medicare inpatient hospital services, interim final rule with comment period. *Federal Register, 48:*39752–890; Pettengill, J., and Vertrees, J. (1982). Reliability and validity in hospital case-mix measurement. *Health Care Financ Rev, 4:*101–128; Schweiker, R. S. (1983). *Report to Congress: Hospital prospective payment for Medicare.* Washington, DC: U.S. Dept. of Health and Human Services; Vladeck, B. C. (1984). Medicare hospital payment by diagnosis-related groups. *Ann Intern Med, 100:*576–591; Wennberg, J. E., McPherson, K., and Caper, P. (1984). Will payment on Diagnosis-Related Groups control hospital costs? *NEJM, 311:*295–300; and Lewis, M. A., Lenke, B., Leal-Sotello, M., et al. (1987). The initial effects of the prospective payment system on nursing home patients. *Am J Public Health, 77:*819–821.

55. Lind, S. E. (1984). Transferring the terminally ill. *NEJM, 311:*1181–1182.

56. Gornick, M., Greenberg, J. N., Eggers, P. W., et al. (1985, Dec.). *Twenty years of Medicare and Medicaid. Health Care Financing Review: 1985 Annual Supplement.* Baltimore, MD: Health Care Financing Administration; and Greenberg, G. (1987). Historical perspective and the current national picture. *PRIDE Inst J 6(1):*4–6.

57. Markson, E. W., Steel, K., and Kane, E. (1983). Administratively necessary days: More than an administrative problem. *Gerontologist, 23:*486–492; McCormack, J. J. (1987). The place of extended care in the health system. In B. C. Vladeck and G. J. Alfano (Eds.), *Medicare and extended care.* pp. 45–52. Owings Mills, MD: National Health Publ.; PRIDE Institute, Department of Community Medicine. (1982). *Hospital overstay survey report.* New York: St. Vincent's Hospital and Medical Center; and Robbins, F. D. (1982). A study of discharge delays in Rhode Island hospitals. *PRIDE Inst J, 1*(1):8.

58. American Association of Professional Standards Review Organizations (Quality Assurance). (1980). *Long term care one-day census.* Bethesda, MD: American Assn. of Professional Standards Review Organizations.

59. Markson, Steel, and Kane, Administratively necessary days.

60. *Potential Effects of a Proposed Amendment to Medicaid's Nursing Home Reimbursement Requirements.* Washington, DC: General Accounting Office/HRD-80-1, October 15, 1979, p. 7; and Feder, J., and Scanlon, W. (1981, Nov.). *Medicare and Medicaid patients' access to skilled nursing facilities.* Washington, DC: Urban Institute, pp. 29–30.

61. Kramer, M., Pollack, E. S., and Redick, R. W. (1972). *Mental disorders/suicide.* Cambridge, MA: Harvard Univ. Press.; Talbott, J. A. (1984). Psychiatry's agenda for the '80s. *JAMA, 251:*2250; U.S. Dept. of Health, Education and Welfare. *State trends in resident patients: State and County Mental Hospitals In-patient Services, 1967–73.* Statistical Note 113, no. [ADM] 75-158; and Dept. of Housing and Urban Development. (1983, Feb.). *Report to the Congress. Report of federal efforts to respond to the shelter and basic living needs of chronically mentally ill individuals.* Washington, DC: Dept. of Health and Human Services.

62. Portnoi, V. A. (1979). Sounding board: A health care system for the elderly. *NEJM, 300:*1387–1390.

63. Gottesman, L. E. (1974). Nursing home performance as related to resident traits, ownership, size and source of payment. *Am J Pub Health, 64:*269–276.

64. Special Committee on Aging, U.S. Senate. (1971). *Alternatives to nursing home care: A proposal.* Washington, DC: Government Printing Office.

65. U.S. Bureau of the Census. (1978, June). *Current Population Reports,* ser. P-23, no. 69. Washington, DC: Government Printing Office.

66. Technical Committee, Social and health aspects of long term care.

67. Willging, P. R. (1986). The unresolved dilemma: Institutional vs. home care. In T. C. Fox (Ed.), *Long term care and the law* (p. 328). Owings Mills, MD: National Health Publishing.

68. Campion, E. W., Bang, A., and May, M. I. (1983). Why acute-care hospitals must undertake long-term care. *NEJM, 308:*71–75.

69. Allison-Cooke, S. (1982). Deinstitutionalizing nursing home patients: Potential versus impediments. *Gerontologist, 22:*404–408; Borup, J. H. (1982). The effects of varying degrees of interinstitutional environmental change on long-term care patients. *Gerontologist, 22:*409–417; Borup, J. H., Gallego, D. T., and Heffernan, P. G. (1980). Relocation: Its effect on health, functioning and mortality. *Gerontologist, 20:*468–479; and Bourestom, N., and Pastalan, L. (1981). The effects of relocation on the elderly. *Gerontologist, 21:*4–7.

70. Johnson, K. G. (1983). Home placement and confounding variables. *J Am Geriatrics Soc, 31:*570; Chaffee, M. L. (1987). Volunteer chore ministry. *PRIDE Inst J* 6(2): in press; and Scharer, L. K. (1984, June). Volunteerism in long-term care: An overview. In P. H. Feinstein and J. N. Gornick (Eds.), *Long term care financing and delivery systems: Exploring some alternatives.* Washington, DC: Dept. of Health and Human Services, Health Care Financing Administration, Pub. no. 03174.

71. Dronska, H. (1983). Focus: The role of case management in long term home health care: Introduction. *PRIDE Inst J,* 2(4):19–20. Quote from p. 20.

CHAPTER 2

1. Dept. of Health and Human Services report to the President. (1986, Nov. 19). *Catastrophic illness expenses.* Washington, DC; *Health insurance coverage against catastrophic illnesses, a proposed amendment to the Public Health Service Act.* (1987, Jan. 6). S.210, Title XXIII.

2. O'Shaughnessy, C., Price, R., and Griffith, J. (1985, Oct. 17). *Financing and delivery of long-term care services for the elderly,* (DOC. 85-1033 EPW). Washington, DC: Congressional Research Service, Library of Congress, p. ix.

3. Goldman, C. M., and McTernan, M. T. (1984). Financing the care of the elderly: Strategies for hospitals. In S. J. Brody and N. A. Persily (Eds.), *Hospitals and the Aged: The New Old Market.* pp. 89–109. Rockville, MD: Aspen Systems. Quote from pp. 89–90.

4. Sawyer, D., Ruther, M., Pagan-Bertucci, A., et al. (1983, Dec.). *The Medicare and Medicaid data book, 1983.* Baltimore, MD: U.S. Dept. of Health and Human Services, Health Care Financing Administration [HCFA], Office of Research and Demonstrations, pp. 80–81.

5. HCFA. (1983). HCFA program statistics. *Health Care Financing Review, 4:*127–132.

6. Bristow, L. R. (1985, Dec.). Contribution to symposium, Twenty years of Medicare and Medicaid. *Health Care Financing Review* (1985 Suppl.), pp. 63–67. Baltimore MD: HCFA. Quote from p. 63.

7. Public Law 99-177, Balanced Budget and Deficit Control Act of 1985. Also known as the Gramm-Rudman-Hollings Act.

8. O'Shaughnessy, Price, and Griffith, *Financing and delivery of long-term care services for the elderly;* and Office of the Actuary, HCFA. (1985, Aug.). *Health care financing program statistics: Analysis of state Medicaid program characteristics, 1984.* Baltimore, MD: U.S. Dept. of Health and Human Services.

9. House Select Committee on Aging. (1985, July). *America's elderly at risk.* (Pub. no. 99-508). Washington, DC.

10. U.S. General Accounting Office [GAO]. (1983, Oct. 21). Medicaid and nursing home care: Cost increases and the need for services are creating problems for the states and the elderly (GAO/IPE-84-1). Washington, DC.

11. U.S. GAO. (1983, June 15). Memorandum to Congressmen Waxman and Pepper. Ref. #B-196673, p. 3; and Tilly, J., and Brunner, D. (1987). Medicaid eligibility and its effect on the elderly. Washington, DC: American Association of Retired Persons.

12. U.S. GAO. (1983, Oct. 21). *Medicaid and nursing home care.* (GAO/IPE-84-1). Gaithersburg, MD.

13. Stevens, R., and Stevens, R. (1974). *Welfare medicine in America: A case study of Medicaid.* New York: Free Press; and Gould, D. A. (1987). Extended care comes home. In B. C. Vladeck and G. J. Alfano (Eds.), *Medicare and extended care,* pp. 109–127. Owings Mills, MD: National Health Publ.

14. U.S. GAO, Medicaid and nursing home care.

15. Schimel, D. (1983). Patients awaiting placement. *Manhattan Medicine, 2:*7–9. Quote from p. 9.

16. National Governor's Association. (1984). *Governors' guide to health care cost containment strategies.* Washington, DC.

17. Maloney, T. W., and Blendon, R. J. (1982). Report on the forum. In R. J. Blendon and T. W. Maloney (Eds.), *New approaches to the Medicaid crisis.* New York: F and S Press.

18. Office of the Actuary, HCFA. Data from the Medicaid Statistics Branch. In *Health Care Financing Review* (1985 Suppl.), pp. 28–29. Baltimore, MD: HCFA.

19. Ibid.

20. Office of Financial and Actuarial Analysis, HCFA. (1984). *State Medicaid tables for fiscal year 1984.* Baltimore, MD: U.S. Dept. of Health and Human Services.

21. Rymer, M., Burwell, B., and Madigan, D. (1984, Oct.). Short-term evaluation of Medicaid: Selected issues. In HCFA, Office of Research and Demonstrations, *Grants and contract reports* (HCFA Pub. no. 03186). Washington, DC: U.S. Govt. Printing Office.

22. Office of the Actuary, HCFA. Data from the Medicaid Statistics Branch; and Gornick, M., Greenberg, J. N., Eggers, P. W., et al. (1985, Dec.). Contribution to symposium. *Health Care Financing Review,* pp. 13–59.

23. Long Term Care Case Mix Reimbursement Program. (1985, April). *PRI reference manual: RUG II training project.* Albany: N.Y. State Dept. of Health; and Axelrod D. (1986, Jan. 14). Letter regarding PRI. Albany, NY: N.Y. State Dept. of Health; and Nursing Home Community Coalition of NY State. (1987). RUGS—problems and recommendations.

24. Harrington, C., Estes, C. L., Lee, P. R., et al. (1986). Effects of state Medicaid policies on the aged. *Gerontologist, 26:*437–443.

25. Davis, K., and Rowland, D. (1986). *Medicare policy.* Baltimore, MD: Johns Hopkins Univ. Press.

26. Ibid.; and U.S. Bureau of the Census. (1980). *Census of population and housing.* Washington, DC: U.S. Government Printing Office; and Davis, K. and Butler, R.N. (1987). Old, Alone and Poor. Report of the Commonwealth Fund Commission on Elderly People Living Alone. New York.

27. Cohen, W. J. (1985, Dec.). Reflections on the enactment of Medicare and Medicaid. *Health Care Financing Review* (1985 Annual Suppl.), pp. 3–11.

28. Bristow, L. R. (1985, Dec.). Contribution to symposium, *Health Care Financing Review,* quote from p. 65.

29. Cohen, Reflections on the enactment of Medicare and Medicaid, p. 8.

30. O'Shaughnessy, Price, and Griffith, *Financing and delivery of long-term care services for the elderly,* p. 18.

31. Guterman, S., and Dobson, A. (1986). Impact of Medicare prospective payment system for hospitals. *Health Care Financing Review, 7:*97–114; and Kelly, J. T., Shea, M. A., and Ross, J. H. (1987). Implications of Medicare hospital utilization trends for long term home health care. *PRIDE Inst J 6*(2), in press.

32. Heinz, J. (1985, Nov. 12). Opening statement, Hearing on Medicare DRGs: The Government's Role in Ensuring Quality. Washington, DC: Senate Special Committee on Aging.

33. U.S. GAO. (1985, Feb. 21). *Information requirements for evaluating the impacts of Medicare prospective payment on post-hospital long-term care services: Preliminary report* (GAO/PEMD-85-8). Washington, DC; Anderson, G. F., and Steinberg, E. P. (1984). Hospital re-admissions in the Medicare population. *NEJM, 311:*1349–1353. HCFA. (N.D.). *An important message from Medicare.*

Dept. of Housing and Urban Development, Dept. of Health and Human Services; Stern, R. S., and Epstein, A. M. (1985). Institutional responses to prospective payment based on diagnosis-related groups: Implications for cost, quality and access. *NEJM, 312:*621–627; and Van Gelder, S., and Bernstein, J. (1986). Home health care in the era of hospital prospective payment: Some early evidence and thoughts about the future. *PRIDE Inst J, 5*(1):3–11.

34. Grazier, K. L. (1986). The impact of reimbursement policy of home health care. *PRIDE Inst J, 5*(1):12–16. Quote from p. 14.

35. Foley, W. (1987). Creating a prospective payment system for home health care. *PRIDE Inst J,* 6(2), in press; Newald, J. (1987, Feb. 20). Alternate Care. Ambulatory care payment system ready, waiting. *Hospitals,* p. 80.

36. Leader, S. (1986, Sept.). *Home health care benefits under Medicare.* Washington, DC: American Association of Retired Persons.

37. Bishop, C. E., and Stassen, M. (1986). Prospective reimbursement for home health care: Context for an evolving policy. *PRIDE Inst J, 5*(1):17–26.

38. Ibid.

39. Office of the Actuary, HCFA, *Health care financing program statistics;* and Rowland, D., and Gaus, C. R. Reducing eligibility and benefits: current policies and alternatives. In Blendon and Maloney, (Eds.), *New approaches to the Medicaid crisis,* pp. 19–46.

40. O'Shaughnessy, Price, and Griffith, *Financing and delivery of long-term care services for the elderly.*

41. Office of the Actuary, HCFA, *Health care financing program statistics.*

42. O'Shaughnessy, Price, and Griffith, *Financing and delivery of long-term services for the elderly.*

43. Davis and Rowland, *Medicare policy.*

44. Spiegel, A. D. (1983). *Home health care.* Owings Mills, MD: National Health Publishing.

45. O'Shaughnessy, Price, and Griffith, *Financing and delivery of long-term care services for the elderly,* pp. 29–30.

46. Administration on Aging. (1985, Sept. 10). Testimony before House Select Committee on Aging.

47. Goldman and McTernan, *Financing the care of the elderly.*

48. Heinz, Opening statement, Hearing on Medicaid DRGs; Van Gelder and Bernstein, Home health care in the era of hospital prospective payment; HCFA, *An important message from Medicare;* Jennings, M. C., and Krentz, S. E. (1985). Financing care for the elderly: Federal government programs. In J. Tedesco (Ed.), *Financing quality care for the elderly* (pp. 64–93). Chicago: American Hospital Assoc.; and U.S. Senate Special Committee on Aging. (1983). *Developments in aging: 1983* (98th Cong., Rep. 98-360, vol. 1, p. 432). Washington, DC: U.S. Government Printing Office.

49. O'Shaughnessy, Price, and Griffith, *Financing and delivery of long-term care services for the elderly;* and American Public Welfare Association. Voluntary Cooperative Information System, 1983 Figures.

50. O'Shaughnessy, Price, and Griffith, *Financing and delivery of long-term care services for the elderly,* p. 27.

51. Mather, J. H. (1984). An overview of the Veterans Administration and its services for older veterans. In T. Wetle and J. Rowe (Eds.), *Older veterans: Linking VA and community resources* (pp. 35–48). Cambridge, MA: Harvard Univ. Press.

52. Special Medical Advisory Group. (1983, May 11). *Task force of the VA geriatric plan. Caring for the older veteran.* Washington, DC: Veterans Administration.

53. Besdine, R. W., Levkoff, S. E., and Wetle, T. (1984). Health and illness behaviors in elder veterans. In Wetle and Rowe, (Eds.), *Older veterans,* pp. 1–33.

54. MacAdam, M. A., and Piktialis, D. S. (1984). Mechanisms of access and coordination. In Wetle and Rowe (Eds.), *Older veterans,* pp. 159–203; and Georgeson, G. (1987). The Veterans Administration nurse-administered unit. In Vladeck and Alfano (Eds.), *Medicare and extended care,* pp. 79–83.

55. Davis and Rowland, *Medicare policy.*

56. Bang, A., Morse, J. H., and Campion, E. W. (1984). Transition of VA acute care hospitals into acute and long term care. In Wetle and Rowe (Eds.), *Older veterans,* pp. 69–91.

57. O'Shaughnessy, Price, and Griffith, *Financing and delivery of long-term services for the elderly;* Jennings and Krentz, Financing care for the elderly; and Wallack, S. (1983). Where are the new resources for financing long term care? *PRIDE Inst J, 2*(2):21–28.

58. Wallack, Where are the new resources for financing long term care? p. 22.

59. U.S. Bureau of the Census, 1980 census of population and housing.

60. U.S. Bureau of the Census. (1985). After-tax money income estimates of households: 1983 *Current population reports* (ser. P-23, no. 143). Washington, DC: U.S. Government Printing Office.

61. McNerney, W. J. (1985). Critical underlying issues affecting the financing and delivery of care for the elderly. In Tedesco, (Ed.), *Financing quality care for the elderly,* pp. 6–24.

62. Kosterlitz, J. (1985, July). "Disaster" stories may spur Congress to protect health benefits for retirees. *Natl Journal,* 1743–1746.

63. U.S. Bureau of the Census, *1980 census of population and housing.*

64. Davis and Rowland, *Medicare policy;* and Estes, C. L., and Lee, P. R. (1986). Health problems and policy issues of old age. In L. H. Aiken and D. Mechanic (Eds.), *Applications of social science to clinical medicine and health policy* (pp. 335–355). New Brunswick, NJ: Rutgers Univ. Press.

65. Waldo, D., and Lazenby, H. (1984, Sept.). Demographic characteristics and health care use and expenditures by the aged in the United States: 1977–1984. Office of Research and Demonstrations, HCFA. Washington, DC: HCFA Pub. no. 03176.

66. National Center for Health Statistics, HCFA, 1980.

67. O'Shaughnessy, Price, and Griffith, *Financing and delivery of long-term services for the elderly.*

68. Wallack, Where are the new resources for financing long term care?; Home equity. (1987, Spring). Manufacturers Hanover (NY) Financial Resource, pp. 6–9; and Scholen, K. (1983.) Financing home care with home equity. *PRIDE Inst J, 2*(2):43–45.

69. Beirne, K. (1985, Jan. 28). Testimony before House Select Committee on Aging. Hearings on Home Equity Conversion: Issues and Options for the Elderly Homeowner (House Pub. no. 99-513). Washington, DC.

70. Scholen, Financing home care with home equity, p. 43.

71. Jacobs, B., and Weissert, W. (1985). Home equity financing of long-term care for the elderly. In P. Feinstein, M. Gornick, and J. Greenberg (Eds.), *Long-term care financing and delivery systems: Exploring some alternatives* (pp. 82–94). Washington, DC: U.S. Government Printing Office.

72. U.S. Senate Special Committee on Aging. (1984, July). *Turning home equity into income for older homeowners: An information paper* (S. Rep. 98-216). Washington, DC.

73. Firman, J. (1983). Reforming community care for the elderly and disabled. *Health Affairs, 2:*66–82.

74. Scholen, Financing home care with home equity.

75. O'Shaughnessy, Price, and Griffith, *Financing and delivery of long-term services for the elderly.*

76. Wessel, P. (1985). IRMA: A long term home equity conversion program. *PRIDE Inst J, 4*(2):29–31.

77. Scholen, K. (1984, Sept.). *A financial guide to the Century plan* (3rd ed.). Madison, WI: National Center for Home Equity Conversion.

78. Ibid.

79. Wessel, IRMA, p. 31.

80. Lane, L. F. (1985). Private long-term care insurance. *Long-Term Care Currents, 8:*9–12. Quote from p. 9.

81. Lane, L. F. (1985). The potential of private long term care insurance. *PRIDE Inst J, 4*(3):15–24; Washington report: Roybal introduces bill for broad health insurance coverage.

Chicago, IL: American Hospital Association: Aging and Long-Term Care [newsletter] *2*(5):6; and Freudenheim, M. (1987, Mar. 1). Insurance policies offered to help elderly infirm to remain at home. *New York Times,* p. 1

82. Meiners, M. (1986.) Long-term care insurance explored. *Aging and Long-Term Care, 2:* 2–3 Budnick, L. D., and Pickett, N. A., Jr. (1987). Home health care [letter to the editor]. *NEJM, 106:* 168; and Somers, A.R. (1987). Insurance for long-term care. *NEJM,* 317:23–29.

83. ICF Inc. (1984, Jan.). *Private financing of long term care: Current methods and resources.* Report to the Office of the Assistant Secretary for Planning and Evaluation, Dept. of Health and Human Services, Phase I.

84. Lane, Private long-term care insurance.

85. Ibid.; and Meiners, Long-term care insurance explored.

86. Lane, Private long-term care insurance.

87. Brickfield, C. F. (1985). Long term care financing solutions are needed now. *Am Health Care Assoc J, 11:* 11–15.

88. Matusz, W. (1985, Nov. 21–22). *Opportunities in the group market.* Summary of seminar on the emerging market in private long-term care insurance. San Francisco.

89. Kodner, D. (1986.) Long-term care insurance explored. *Aging and Long-Term Care, 2:* 2.

90. Gibson, R. M., Waldo, D. R., and Levit, K. R. (1983.) National health expenditures 1982. *Health Care Financing Rev, 5:* 1–31.

91. Lifson, A. (1983). Quoted in New dollars for long term care: Report of PRIDE Institute Conference. *PRIDE Inst J, 2*(2):33–36.

92. Haddow, C. M. (1985, Nov. 21–22). Report of the symposium on the emerging market in private long-term care insurance. San Francisco.

93. HR2293—Congressman Ron Wyden; S.1378—Senator Dave Durenberger.

94. Davis and Roland, *Medicare policy,* p. 86.

95. Ibid.

96. McNerney, Critical underlying issues affecting the financing and delivery of care for the elderly.

97. Michal, M. H. (1986). Commercial insurance for home care and nursing home care. In T. Fox, *Long term care and the law,* pp. 141–152. Owings Mills, MD: National Health Publishing.

98. Wallack, Where are the new resources for financing long term care?

99. Fullerton, W. (1982). Finding the money and paying for long-term-care services. In J. Meltzer, F. Farrow, and H. Richman (Eds.), *Policy options in long-term care,* pp. 182–208. Chicago: Univ. of Chicago Press.

100. Wallack, Where are the new resources for financing long term care?

101. Vladeck, B. C. (1985). Meeting the needs of the elderly: A client-based approach. In *Hospital research and educational trust. Financing quality care of the elderly,* p. 38. Chicago: American Hospital Assoc.

CHAPTER 3

1. Becker, P. M., and Cohen, H. J. (1984). The functional approach to the care of the elderly: A conceptual framework. *J Am Geriatric Soc, 32:* 923–928; and Engle, G. L. (1982). The biopsychosocial model and medical education. *NEJM, 306:* 802.

2. Goldstein, S., Moerman, E. J., Soeldner, J. S., et al. (1978). Chronologic and physiologic age affect replicative lifespan of fibroblasts from diabetic, prodiabetic, and normal donors. *Science, 199:* 781–782.

3. Rowe, J., and Besdine, R. W. (1982). *Health and disease in old age.* Boston: Little, Brown.

4. World Health Organization. (1984). *The use of epidemiology in the study of the elderly* (Technical Report Series 706). Geneva: WHO.

5. Manton, K. G. (1985, Nov.). Future patterns of chronic diseases incidence, disability and mortality among the elderly. *NY State J Med,* pp. 623–633.

6. Schneider, E., Vining, E. M., Hadley, E. C., et al. (1986). Recommended dietary allowances and the health of the elderly. *NEJM, 314:*157–160.

7. Eaton, S. B., and Konner, M. (1985). Paleolithic nutrition: A consideration of its nature and current implications. *NEJM, 312:*283–289.

8. Garry, P. J., Goodwin, J. S., Hunt, W. C., et al. (1982). Nutritional status in a healthy elderly population: Dietary and supplemental intakes. *Am J Clin Nutrition, 36:*319–331; Food and Nutrition Board, National Research Council. (1980). *Recommended dietary allowances,* 9th review ed. Washington, DC: National Academy of Sciences; and Sherman, M. N., Lechich, A., Brickner, P. W., et al. (1983). Nutritional parameters in homebound persons of greatly advanced age. *J Parenteral and Enteral Nutrition, 7:*378–380.

9. Chumlea, W. C., Roche, A. F., and Mukherjee, D. (1986). Some anthropometric indices of body composition for elderly adults. *J Gerontology, 41:*36–39.

10. Schorah, C. J., and Hay, A. W. M. (1986). Recommended dietary allowances for the elderly [Letter to the editor]. *NEJM, 314:*1707.

11. Ray, W. A., Griffin, M. R., Schaffner, W., et al. (1987). Psychotropic drug use and the risk of hip fracture. *NEJM, 316:*363–369; and Kelsey, J. L., and Hoffman, S. (1987). Risk factors for hip fracture. *NEJM, 316:*404–406.

12. Serfass, R. C., Agre, J. C., and Smith, E. (1985). Exercise testing for the elderly. *Topics for Geriatric Rehab, 1:*58–67; and Cress, E. M., and Schultz, E. (1985). Aging muscle: Functional, morphologic, biochemical, and regenerative capacity. *Topics for Geriatric Rehab, 1:*11–18.

13. Lieberman, M. A., and Tobin, S. S. (1983). *The experience of old age, stress, coping and survival.* New York: Basic Books.

14. Brickner, P. W. (1978). *Home health care for the aged.* New York: Appleton-Century-Crofts.

15. Segerberg, O. (1981). *Living to be 100.* New York: Charles Scribner's Sons.

16. Barter, C. E., and Campbell, A. H. (1976). Relationship of constitutional factors and cigarette smoking to decrease in 1-second forced expiratory volume. *Am Rev Respir Dis, 113:*305.

17. Rowe and Besdine, *Health and disease in old age.*

18. Nickens, H. (1985). Intrinsic factors in falling among the elderly. *Arch Int Med, 145:*1089–1093.

19. Brody, J. E. (1984, Oct. 2). Hope grows for a vigorous old age. *New York Times.*

20. Phillip, P. A., Rolls, B. J., Ledingham, J. G. G., et al. (1984). Reduced thirst after water deprivation in healthy elderly men. *NEJM, 311:*753–759; and Leaf, A. (1984). Dehydration in the elderly. *NEJM, 311:*791–792.

21. PRIDE Institute Journal Staff, in cooperation with Upjohn Healthcare Services, and the East Kentucky Health Services Center. (1982). Home health care for the rural elderly: Experiences in Florida and Kentucky. *PRIDE Inst J, 1*(2):12–19.

22. Long Term Case Mix Reimbursement Project. (1985, April). *PRI reference manual: RUG II training program.* Albany: N.Y. State Dept. of Health; and Rudder, C. (1987). Case-mix re-imbursement and resource utilization groups (RUGS). Nursing Home Community Coalition of NY State.

23. Rubenstein, L. Z., Josephson, K. R., and Wieland, G. D. (1984). Effectiveness of a geriatric evaluation unit. *NEJM, 311:*1664; Campion, E. W., Jette, A., and Beckman, B. (1983). An interdisciplinary geriatric consultation service. *J Am Geriatric Soc, 31:*792–796; Gupta, K. L., Gambert, S. R., and Powell, F. (1987). The importance of a specialized assessment unit within the nursing home. *NY Med Quart, 7*(1):32–36; George, L. K., and Fillenbaum, G. G. (1985). OARS methodology: A decade of experience in geriatric assessment. *J Am Geriatric Soc, 33:*611–615; Kane, R. A., and Kane, R. S. (1981). *Assessing the elderly: A practical guide to measurement.* Lexington, MA: Lexington Books; Martin, D. C., Morycz, R. K., McDowell, J. B., et al. (1985). Community-based geriatric assessment. *J Am Geriatric Soc, 33:*602–606; Williams, M. E., and Williams, T. T. (1986). Evaluation of older persons in the ambulatory setting. *J Am Geriatric Soc, 34:*37–43; and Williams, M. E. (1986). Geriatric assessment. *Ann Intern Med, 104:*720–721.

24. Bonanno, J. B. (1984). Legislation regarding health care for the older veteran. In T. Wetle and J. Rowe (Eds.), *Older veterans: Linking VA and community resources,* pp. 49–68. Cam-

bridge, MA: Harvard Univ. Press; Bang, A., Morse, J. H., and Campion, E. W. (1984). Transition of VA acute care hospitals into acute and long term care. In Wetle and Rowe (Eds.), *Older veterans*, pp. 69–91; and MacAdam, M. A., and Piktialis, D. S. (1984). Mechanisms of access and coordination. In Wetle and Rowe (Eds.), *Older veterans*, pp. 159–203.

25. Health and Public Policy Committee, American College of Physicians. (1984). Position paper, long-term care of the elderly. *Ann Int Med, 100:*760–763.

26. Coolidge, C. P. (1986). Clinical decisions in geriatric patients [Letter to the editor]. *NEJM, 314:*1519.

27. Rubenstein, Josephson, and Wieland, Effectiveness of a geriatric evaluation unit.

28. The 1981 White House Conference on Aging. (1981, Nov. 30–Dec. 3). Final Report, vol. 1, p. 114.

29. Resnick, N. M., and Yalla, S. V. (1985). Current concepts in management of urinary incontinence in the elderly. *NEJM, 313:*800–805; Ouslander, J. G., Kane, R. L., and Abrass, I. B. (1982). Urinary incontinence in elderly nursing home patients. *JAMA, 248:*1194–1198; and Mitteness, L. S. (1987). The management of urinary incontinence by community-living elderly. *Gerontologist, 27:*185–193.

30. Burgio, K. L., Whitehead, W. E., and Engel, B. T. (1985). Urinary incontinence in the elderly. *Ann Int Med, 104:*507–515.

31. Riley, M. W. (1985). Introductory statement. *Nature and extent of alcohol problems among the elderly.* New York: Springer.

32. Barnett, R. N. (1984). Laboratory reference ranges for elderly persons. *JAMA, 252:*826; and Tietz, M. W. (1983). Clinical guide to laboratory tests. Philadelphia: W. B. Saunders.

33. Brewer, V., Meyer, B. M., Keele, M. S., et al. (1983). Role of exercise in prevention of involutional bone loss. *Med Sci Sports Exercise, 15:*445–449; and Aloia, J. F., Cohn, S. H., Ostuni, J. A., et al. (1978). Prevention of involutional bone loss by exercise. *Ann Int Med, 89:* 356–358.

34. Mold, J. W., and Stein, H. F. (1986). The cascade effect in the clinical care of patients. *NEJM, 314:*512–514; and Scialli, A. R. (1986). The cascade effect in the clinical care of patients [Letter to the editor]. *NEJM, 315:*320.

35. Mold and Stein, The cascade effect in the clinical care of patients.

36. Applegate, W. B., Graves, S., Collins, T., et al. (1984). Acute myocardial infarction in elderly patients. *Southern Med, 77:*1127–1129.

37. Williams, B. O., Begg, T. B., Semple, T., et al. (1976). The elderly in a coronary unit. *Brit Med J, 2:*451.

38. Public Health Service, National Institutes of Health. (1985, June). *Cholesterol counts: Principles from the coronary primary prevention trial* (NIH Pub No. 85-2699). Bethesda, MD: U.S. Dept. of Health and Human Services; Atherosclerosis Study Group. (1984). Optimal resources for primary prevention of atherosclerotic diseases. *Circulation, 70:*157A–205A; and Rifkind, B., and Segal, P. (1983). Lipid research clinics program reference values for hyperlipidemia and hypolipidemia. *JAMA, 250:*1869–1872.

39. Gentry, D., Foster, S., and Haney, T. (1972). Denial as a determinant of anxiety and perceived health in the coronary care unit. *Psychosomatic Med, 34–39.*

40. Baum, A., Taylor, S. E., and Singer, J. E. (1984). *Handbook of psychology and health.* Hillsdale, NJ: Lawrence Earlbaum Associates; Lefton, E., Bonstelle, S., and Frengley, J. D. (1983). Success with an inpatient geriatric unit: A controlled study of outcome and follow-up. *J Am Geriatric Soc, 31:*149–155; and Teasdale, T. A., Shuman, L., and Luchi, R. J. (1983). A comparison of placement outcomes in geriatric cohorts receiving care in a geriatric assessment unit and on general medicine floors. *J Am Geriatric Soc, 31:*529–534.

41. Rubenstein, Josephson, and Wieland, Effectiveness of a geriatric evaluation unit; George and Fillenbaum, OARS methodology; Williams and Williams, Evaluation of older persons in the ambulatory setting; Teasdale, Shuman, and Luchi, A comparison of placement outcomes; and Lefton, Bonstelle, and Frengley, Success with an inpatient geriatric unit.

42. *PRI reference manual: RUG II training program;* and Rubenstein, Josephson, and Wieland, Effectiveness of a geriatric evaluation unit.

43. Steinberg, A., Fitten, L., and Kachuck, N. (1986). Patient participation in treatment decision-making in the nursing home: The issue of competence. *Gerontologist, 26:*362–366; Libow, L. S., and Waife, M. M. (1985, Oct.). Geriatric medicine: A mechanism for quality care. *Business and Health,* pp. 38–40; and Meier, D. E., and Cassel, C. K. (1986). Nursing home placement and the demented patient. *Ann Intern Med, 104:*98–105.

44. Rantakokko, V., Havia, T., Inberg, M. V., et al. (1983). Abdominal/aortic aneurysms: A clinical and autopsy study of 408 patients. *Acta Chir Scand, 149:*151–155.

45. Baranovsky, A., and Myers, M. H. (1986). Cancer incidence and survival in patients 65 years of age and older. *CA-A Cancer J for Clinicians, 36*(1):26–41; and Adami, H., Malken, B., Holmberg, L., et al. (1986). The relation between survival and age at diagnosis in breast cancer. *NEJM, 315:*359–363.

46. Eaton and Konner, Paleolithic nutrition; Baker, H., Jaslow, S. P., and Frank, O. (1978). Severe impairment of dietary folate utilization in the elderly. *J Am Geriatric Soc, 26:*218–221; Stiedmann, M., Jansen, C., and Harrill, I. (1978). Nutritional status of elderly men and women. *J Am Diet Assoc, 73:*132–139; and Vir, S. C., and Love, A.H.G. (1978). Nutritional evaluation of B groups of vitamins in institutionalised aged. *Int J. Vitam Nut Res, 48:*274–280.

47. Stead, W. W. (1981). Tuberculosis among elderly persons: An outbreak in a nursing home. *Ann Int Med, 94:*606.

48. Waxman, H. M., Klein, M., Kennedy, R., et al. (1985). Institutional drug abuse: The overprescribing of psychoactive medications in nursing homes. In E. Gottheil, K. A. Druley, T. E. Skoloda, and H. M. Waxman (Eds.), *The combined problems of alcoholism, drug addiction and aging,* pp. 173–190. Springfield, IL: Charles C Thomas.

49. Schwartz, T. B. (1982). For fun and profit: How to install a first-rate doctor in a third-rate nursing home. *NEJM, 306:*743–744.

50. Living Will Declaration. Society for the Right to Die, 250 West 57th Street, New York, NY 10107; and Gatza, G. A. (1986, Summer). Living wills. *New York Medicine,* p. 15.

51. Swick, T. (1986, June). Interpreting the Quinlan decision 10 years after. *ACP Observer,* pp. 18–22; Cassel, C. K., and Harrison, R. L. (1986). Views on use of life support methods. *Provider, American Health Care Assn., 12:*24–28; Cohen, E. S. (1986). Sound ethics must balance programs. *Provider, American Health Care Assn., 12:*4–7; Dubler, N. N. (1986). Honoring preference for the right to die. *Provider, American Health Care Assn, 12:*20–23; Falek, J. I. (1986). Ensuring delivery of care as chosen. *Provider, American Health Care Assn., 12:*8–11; Greenlaw, J. (1986). Nursing: Matching solution with need. *Provider, American Health Care Assn, 12:*11–14; Haddad, A. M. (1986). Ethical considerations in long term home care for ventilator-dependent clients. *PRIDE Inst J, 5*(2):3–7; and Lo, B., and Dornbrand, L. (1986). The case of Claire Conroy: Will administrative review safeguard incompetent patients? *Ann Int Med, 104:*869–873.

52. Annas, G. J. (1986). Do feeding tubes have more rights than patients? *Hastings Center Report, 16:*26–32.

53. Libow and Waife, Geriatric medicine; and Wetle, T. (1987). Age as a risk factor for inadequate treatment. Editorial. *JAMA, 258:*516.

CHAPTER 4

1. American Psychiatric Association. (1980). *Diagnostic and Statistical Manual of Mental Disorders,* 3rd ed. Washington, DC: APA.

2. Lander, R. (1983). *The diagnosis and evaluation of dementia in a homebound population.* (Available from Dept. of Community Medicine, St. Vincent's Hospital, New York.)

3. Bergmann, K. (1975). The epidemiology of senile dementia. *Brit J Psychiat, 9:*100–109; Council on Scientific Affairs, American Medical Association (1986). Dementia (Council Report). *JAMA, 256:*2234–2238; Gilmore, A. J. J. (1974). Community surveys and mental health. In W. F. Anderson and T. G. Judge (Eds.), *Geriatric medicine,* pp. 77–93. New York: Academic Press; Gruenberg, E. M. (1978). Epidemiology of senile dementia. In B. S. Schoenberg (Ed.), *Advances in neurology,* pp. 437–457. New York: Raven Press; Kay, D. W. K. (1977). The epidemiology of brain deficit in the aged: Problems in patient identification. In C. Eisdorfer and R.

O. Freidel (Eds.), *The cognitively and emotionally impaired elderly,* pp. 11–26. Chicago: Yearbook Medical Publishers; Preston, G. A. N. (1986). Dementia in elderly adults: Prevalence and institutionalization. *J of Gerontology, 41:*261–267; and Roth, M. (1978). Diagnosis of senile and related forms of dementia. In R. Katzman, R. D. Terry, and K. L. Bick, (Eds.), *Alzheimer's disease: Senile dementia and related disorders,* pp. 71–85. New York: Raven Press.

4. Katzman, R. (1981, June). Early detection of senile dementia. *Hosp Practice,* pp. 66–71; Stone, J. (1984). Cited in Medical News: Attempts to vanquish Alzheimer's disease intensify, take new paths. *JAMA, 251:*1805–1840; and Task Force sponsored by the National Institute on Aging. (1980). Senility reconsidered. *JAMA, 244:*259–263.

5. Strong, J. (1985, May 21). *Caring for America's Alzheimer's victims.* Hearing before the Select Committee on Aging, House of Representatives, 99th Congress, Washington, DC: U.S. Government Printing Office.

6. Wells, C. E. (1983). Differential diagnosis of Alzheimer's dementia: Affective disorder. In B. Reisberg (Ed.), *Alzheimer's disease: The standard reference,* pp. 193–197. New York: Free Press.

7. Ibid.; and Kling, A. (1981). Mental illness in the elderly. In A. R. Somers and D. R. Fabian (Eds.), *The geriatric imperative,* pp. 221–235. New York: Appleton-Century-Crofts.

8. Benson, D. F. (1982). Clinical aspects of dementia. In J. C. Beck (moderator), Dementia in the elderly: The silent epidemic. *Ann Intern Med, 97:*231–241. Quote from p. 232.

9. Torack, R. M. (1983). The early history of senile dementia. In Reisberg (Ed.), *Alzheimer's disease,* p. 24.

10. Ibid.

11. White, J. S. (Ed.). (1883). *Plutarch's "Lives."* New York: G. P. Putman Sons, p. 73.

12. Esquirol, J. E. D. (1976). *Des maladies mentales,* vol. 2. New York: Arno Press.

13. Cohen, G. D. (1983). Historical views and evolution of concepts. In Reisberg (Ed.), *Alzheimer's disease,* pp. 29–33.

14. Torack, the early history of senile dementia; and Alzheimer, A. (1907). Uber eine eigenartige erkrankung der hirnrinde. *Allg A Psychisch-Gerintlich Med, 64:*146–148.

15. Reisberg, B. (1983). Preface. In Reisberg (Ed.), *Alzheimer's disease,* pp. xvii–xix.

16. Thomas, L. Cited by J. P. Hammerschmidt, in *Caring for America's Alzheimer's victims.*

17. Mohs, R. C., Davis, K. L., and Dunn, D. D. (1984). A medical overview of Alzheimer's disease. *PRIDE Inst J, 3*(4):11–22; Campbell, A. J., McCosh, L. M., Reinken, J., et al. (1983). Dementia in old age and the need for services. *Age and Aging, 12:*11–16; and Gurland, B. J., and Cross, P. S. (1982). Epidemiology of psychopathology in old age. *Psychiat Clin N Am, 5:*11–26.

18. Mohs, Davis, and Dunn, A medical overview of Alzheimer's disease.

19. Stone, cited in Attempts to vanquish Alzheimer's disease intensify; Mohs, Davis, and Dunn, A medical overview of Alzheimer's disease; and Mortimer, J. A. (1983). Alzheimer's disease and senile dementia: Prevalence and incidence. In Reisberg (Ed.), *Alzheimer's disease,* pp. 141–48.

20. Mortimer, Alzheimer's disease and senile dementia; and Go, R. C. P., Todorov, A. B., Elston, R. C., et al. (1978). The malignancy of dementias. *Ann Neurol, 6:*559–561; Jarvik, L. F., Ruth, V., and Matsuyama, S. S. (1980). Organic brain syndrome and aging: A six-year follow-up of surviving twins. *Arch Gen Psychiat, 37:*280–286; and Kay, D. W. K. (1972). Epidemiological aspects of organic brain disease in the aged. In C. M. Gaitz (Ed.), *Aging and the brain.* New York: Plenum.

21. Reisberg, Preface.

22. Gruenberg, E. M. (1978). Epidemiology. Katzman, Terry, and Bick (Eds.), *Alzheimer's disease.*

23. Reisberg, Preface; Campbell, McCosh, Reinken, et al., Dementia in old age and the need for services; and Breckenridge, M. B. The senile dementias: A dual perspective on their epidemiology. In Somers and Fabian (Eds.), *The geriatric imperative,* pp. 153–170.

24. Sister Teresita Duque, R. N. Chelsea-Village Program, St. Vincent's Hospital, New York, personal communication, April 1987.

25. Campbell, McCosh, and Reinken, Dementia in old age and the need for services.

26. Breckenridge, The senile dementias.

27. Csank, J. Z., and Zweig, J. P. (1980). Relative mortality of chronically ill geriatric patients with organic brain damage, before and after relocation. *J Amer Geriat Soc, 28:*76–83.

28. Morscheck, P. (1984). Introduction: An overview of Alzheimer's disease and long term care. *PRIDE Inst J, 3*(4):4–10.

29. Rango, N. (1985). The nursing home resident with dementia. *Ann Intern Med, 102:*835–841.

30. Sulkava, R., Haltia, M., Paetau, A., et al. (1983). Accuracy of clinical diagnosis in primary degenerative dementia: Correlation with neuropathological findings. *J Neurol Neurosurg Psychiat, 46:*9; and Fox, J. H., Penn, R., Claasen, R., et al. (1985). Pathological diagnosis in clincially typical Alzheimer's disease. [Letter to the editor]. *NEJM, 313:*1419–1420.

31. Stone, cited in Attempts to vanquish Alzheimer's disease intensify.

32. Reisberg, B. (1983). An overview of current concepts of Alzheimer's disease, senile dementia, and age-associated cognitive decline. In Reisberg (Ed.), *Alzheimer's disease*, pp. 3–20.

33. Ibid., p. 8.

34. Kral, V. A. (1978). Benign senescent forgetfulness. *Aging NY, 7:*47–51; and Kral, V. A. (1962). Senescent forgetfulness: Benign and malignant. *Can Med Assoc J, 86:*257–260.

35. Lander, The diagnosis and evaluation of dementia; Roth, Diagnosis of senile and related forms of dementia; and Council on Scientific Affairs, Dementia.

36. Reisberg, An overview of current concepts, p. 7.

37. Katzman, R. (1976). The prevalence and malignancy of Alzheimer's disease. *Arch Neurol, 33:*217–218.

38. Terry, R. D. (1976). Dementia: A brief and selective review. *Arch Neurol, 33:*1–4.

39. Reisberg, An overview of current concepts.

40. Shuttleworth, E. C. (1984). Atypical presentations of dementia of the Alzheimer type. *J Amer Geriat Soc, 32:*485–490.

41. Ibid.

42. Soininen, H., Partanen, J. V., Puranen, M., et al. (1982). EEG and computed tomography in the investigation of patients with senile dementia. *J Neurol Neurosurg Psychiat, 45:*711–714; and Creasey, H., and Rapoport, S. I. (1985). The aging human brain. *Annals of Neurology, 17:*2–10.

43. Takeda, S., and Matsuzawa, T. (1984). Brain atrophy during aging: A quantitative study using computed tomography. *J Amer Geriat Soc, 32:*520–524.

44. Brun, A. (1983). An overview of light and electron microscopic changes. In Reisberg (Ed.), *Alzheimer's disease*, pp. 37–47.

45. Wilcock, G. K., and Esiri, M. M. (1982). Plaques, tangles and dementia. *J Neurol Sciences, 56:*343–356; and Katzman, R. (1986). Alzheimer's disease. *NEJM, 314:*964–973.

46. Brun, An overview of light and electron microscopic changes, pp. 37–47.

47. Cummings, J. L., and Benson, D. F. (1983). *Dementia. A clinical approach.* Boston: Butterworths; and Mori H., Kondo, J., and Ihara, Y. (1987). Ubiquitin is a component of paired helical filaments in Alzheimer's Disease. *Science, 235:*1641–1644.

48. Scheibel, A. B. (1982). Structural changes in the brain with aging and dementia. In Beck (moderator), Dementia in the elderly, p. 233.

49. Gajdusek, D. C. (1985). Hypothesis: Interference with axonal transport of neurofilament as a common pathogenetic mechanism in certain diseases of the central nervous system. *NEJM, 312:*714–719.

50. Wurtman, R. J. (1985). Alzheimer's disease. *Scientific American, 252:*62–74.

51. Igbal, K., and Wisniewski, H. M. (1983). Neurofibrillary tangles. In Reisberg (Ed.), *Alzheimer's disease,* pp. 48–56; and Wisniewski, H. M. (1983). Neuritic (senile) and amyloid plaques. In Reisberg (Ed.), *Alzheimer's disease,* pp. 57–61.

52. Khadraturan, Z. S. (1985). Diagnosis of Alzheimer's disease. *Arch Neurol, 42:* 1097–1105.

53. Brody, H. (1955). Organization of the cerebral cortex: III: A study of aging in the human cerebral cortex. *J Comp Neurol, 102:* 511–556; and Henderson, G., Tomlinson, B. E., and Gibson, P. H. (1980). Cell counts in human cerebral cortex in normal adults throughout life using an image analyzing computer. *J Neurol Sci, 46:* 113–136.

54. Ball, M. J., Fisman, M., Hachinski, V., et al. (1985). A new definition of Alzheimer's disease: A hippocampal dementia. *Lancet, 1:* 14–16; and Bahmanyar, S., Higgins, A., Goldgaber, D., et al. (1987). Localization of amyloid β protein messenger RNA in brains from patients with Alzheimer's disease. *Science, 237:* 77–80.

55. Wurtman, Alzheimer's disease, p. 74.

56. Bondareff, W. (1984). Cited in Medical News: Attempts to vanquish Alzheimer's disease intensify, take new paths. *JAMA, 251:* 1805–1840.

57. Hyman, B. T., Van Hoesen, G. W., Damasio, A. R., et al. (1984). Alzheimer's disease: Cell specific pathology isolates the hippocampal formation. *Science, 225:* 1168–1170.

58. Ibid., p. 1170.

59. Bowen, D. M., and Davison, A. N. (1983). The failing brain. *J Chronic Dis, 36:* 3–13.

60. Holman, B. L., Gibson, R. E., Hill, T. C., et al. (1985). Muscarinic acetylcholine receptors in Alzheimer's disease. *JAMA, 254:* 3063–3066; and Francis, P. T., Palmer, A. M., Sims, N. R., et al. (1985). Neurochemical studies of early-onset Alzheimer's disease. *NEJM, 313:* 7–11.

61. Katzman, Alzheimer's disease; Scheibel, Structural changes in the brain with aging and dementia; and Perry, E., and Perry, R. H. (1983). Acetylcholinesterase in Alzheimer's disease. In Reisberg (Ed.), *Alzheimer's disease,* pp. 93–99.

62. Gajdusek, Hypothesis; and Mozar, H. N., Bal, D. G., and Howard, J. T. (1987). Perspectives on the etiology of Alzheimer's disease. *JAMA, 257:* 1503–1507.

63. Francis, Palmer, Sims, et al., Neurochemical studies of early-onset Alzheimer's disease.

64. Summers, W. K., Majovski, L. V., Marsh, G. M., et al. (1986). Oral tetrahydroaminoacridine in long term treatment of senile dementia, Alzheimer type. *NEJM, 315:* 1241–1245.

65. Brown, P. (1985). Synopsis of a 16-year experience in the primary transmission of Creutzfeldt-Jakob disease. In J. Tateishi (Ed.), *Proceedings of workshop on slow transmissible diseases,* pp. 27–31. Tokyo: Japanese Ministry of Health and Welfare; Brown, P., Coker-Vann, M., Pomeroy, K., et al. (1986). Diagnosis of Creutzfeldt-Jakob disease by Western blot identification of marker protein in human brain tissue. *NEJM, 314:* 547–551; Manuelidis, L. (1985). Creutzfeldt-Jakob disease prion proteins in human brains [Letter to the editor]. *NEJM, 312:* 1643–1644; Roberts, G. W., Lofthouse, R., Brown, R., et al. (1986). Prion-protein immunoreactivity in human transmissible dementias [Letter to the editor]. *NEJM, 315:* 1231–1233; and Southern, P., and Oldstone, M.B.A. (1986). Medical consequences of persistent viral infection. *NEJM, 314:* 359–367.

66. Salazar, A. M., Brown, P., Gajdusek, D. C., et al. (1983). Relation to Creutzfeldt-Jakob disease and other unconventional virus diseases. In Reisberg (Ed.), *Alzheimer's disease,* pp. 311–318.

67. Ibid.

68. Ibid., p. 313.

69. Gajdusek, D. C. (1977). Unconventional viruses and the origin and disappearance of kuru. *Science, 197:* 943–960.

70. Brown, Coker-Vann, Pomeroy, et al., Diagnosis of Creutzfeldt-Jakob disease; and Southern and Oldstone, Medical consequences of persistent viral infection.

71. Wisniewski, H. M., Moretz, R. C., and Lossinsky, A. S. (1981). Evidence for induction of localized amyloid deposits and neuritic plaques by an infectious agent. *Ann Neurol, 10:* 517–522.

72. Prusiner, S. B. (1982). Novel proteinaceous infectious particles cause scrapie. *Science, 216:*136–144; and Bockman, J. M., Kingsbury, D. T., McKinley, M. P., et al. (1985). Creutz-feldt-Jakob disease prion proteins in human brains. *NEJM, 312:*73–78.

73. Wurtman, Alzheimer's disease; and Prusiner, S. B. (1984). Some speculations about prions, amyloid, and Alzheimer's disease. *NEJM, 310:*661–663.

74. Prusiner, Some speculations about prions, amyloid, and Alzheimer's disease.

75. Ibid., p. 662.

76. Manuelidis, Creutzfeldt-Jakob disease prion proteins in human brains; and Roberts, Lofthouse, Brown, et al., Prion-protein immunoreactivity in human transmissible dementias.

77. Prusiner, Some speculations about prions, amyloid, and Alzheimer's disease, p. 662.

78. Goudsmit, J., Morrow, C. H., Asher, D. M., et al. (1980). Evidence for and against the transmissibility of Alzheimer's disease. *Neurology (NY), 30:*945–950.

79. Prusiner, Some speculation about prions, amyloid, and Alzheimer's disease, p. 663.

80. Katzman, Alzheimer's disease.

81. Prusiner, Some speculations about prions, amyloid, and Alzheimer's disease; Bowen, D. M., White, P., Spillane, J. A., et al. (1979). Accelerated aging or selective neuronal loss as an important cause of dementia? *Lancet, 1:*11–14; Growdon, J. H., Cohen, E. L., and Wurtman, R. J. (1977). Treatment of brain disease with dietary precursors of neurotransmitters. *Ann Intern Med, 86:*337–339; Perry, E., Perry, R. H., Blessed, G., et al. (1977). Necropsy evidence of central cholinergic deficits in senile dementia [Letter to the editor]. *Lancet, 1:*189; and Sims, N. R., and Bowen, D. M. (1983). Changes in choline acetyltransferase and in acetylcholine synthesis. In Reisberg (Ed.), *Alzheimer's disease,* pp 88–92.

82. Coyle, J. T., Price, D. L., and De Long, M. R. (1983). Alzheimer's disease: A disorder of cortical cholinergic innervations. *Science, 219:*1184–1190; Davies, P. (1979). Neurotrans-mitter-related enzymes in senile dementia of the Alzheimer type. *Brain Res, 138:*385–392; and Sims and Bowen, Changes in choline acetyltransferase and in acetylcholine synthesis.

83. Davies, Neurotransmitter-related enzymes in senile dementia of the Alzheimer type.

84. Ibid.

85. Chase, G. A., Folstein, M. F., Breitner, J.C.S., et al. (1983). The use of life tables and survival analysis in testing genetic hypotheses, with an application to Alzheimer's disease. *Am J Epidemiology, 117:*590–597.

86. Davies, P. (1984). Cited in Attempts to vanquish Alzheimer's disease intensify, pp. 1805–1840.

87. Larsson, T., Sjogren, T., and Jacobson, G. (1963). Senile dementia: A clinical, sociomedi-cal and genetic study. *Acta Psych Scand, 39* (suppl. 167):1–259.

88. Kallmann, F. J. (1953). *Heredity in health and mental disorder.* New York: Norton; and Kallman, F. J. (1956). *Genetic aspects of mental disorders in later life,* 2nd ed. Stanford, CA: Stanford Univ. Press.

89. Jarvik, Ruth, and Matsuyama, Organic brain syndrome and aging.

90. Heston, L. L., and White, J. (1983). *Dementia: A practical guide to Alzheimer's disease and related illnesses.* New York: W. H. Freeman.

91. Goldsmith, M. F. (1984). Cited in Attempts to vanquish Alzheimer's disease intensify, pp. 1805–1840.

92. Wurtman, Alzheimer's disease, p. 63.

93. Folstein, M. F. (1982). Inheritability of Alzheimer's disease. *AFP, 26:*57; and Folstein, M. F., and Breitner, J. (1982). Language disorder predicts familial Alzheimer disease. *Johns Hopkins Med J, 149:*145–147.

94. Katzman, Alzheimer's disease.

95. Cutler, N. R. (1985). Alzheimer's disease and Down's syndrome: New insights. *Ann Intern Med, 103:*560–578.

96. Cohen, D., Eisdorfer, and Leverenz, J. (1982). Alzheimer's disease and maternal age. *J Am Geriat Soc, 30:*656–659.

97. Heston, L. L. (1977). Alzheimer's disease, trisomy 21 and myeloproliferative disorders: Associations suggesting a genetic diathesis. *Science, 196:*332; and Heston, L. L., and White, J. (1978). Pedigrees of 30 families with Alzheimer's disease: Associations with defective organization of microfilaments and microtubules. *Behav Genet, 8:*315.

98. Cohen, Eisdorfer, and Leverenz, Alzheimer's disease and maternal age.

99. Klatzo, I., Wisniewski, H., and Streicher, E. (1965). Experimental production of neurofibrillary degeneration: I. Light microscopic observations. *J Neuropathol Exp Neurol, 24:* 187–199.

100. Crapper, D. R., Krishnan, S. S., and Quittkat, S. (1976). Aluminum, neurofibrillary degeneration and Alzheimer's disease. *Brain, 99:*67–80; and Perl, D. R. (1983). Pathologic association of aluminum in Alzheimer's disease. In Reisberg (Ed.), *Alzheimer's disease,* pp. 116–121.

101. Alfrey, A. C., LeGendre, F. R., and Kaehny, W. D. (1977). The dialysis encephalopathy syndrome: Possible aluminum intoxication. *NEJM, 296:*184–188.

102. Katzman, Alzheimer's disease.

103. Spar, J. E. (1982). Pathophysiologic mechanism of dementia. In Beck, Dementia in the elderly, pp. 237–238; and Mann, D.M.A. (1983). Changes in protein synthesis. In Reisberg (Ed.), *Alzheimer's disease,* pp. 107–115.

104. Spar, Pathophysiologic mechanism of dementia.

105. Mann, Changes in protein synthesis.

106. Wurtman, Alzheimer's disease, p. 71.

107. Spar, Pathophysiologic mechanism of dementia.

108. Loeb, C. (1980). Clinical diagnosis of multi-infarct dementia. In L. Amaducci, A. N. Davison, and P. Antuono (Eds.), *Aging,* vol. 13: *Aging of the Brain and Dementia,* pp. 251–260. New York: Raven Press.

109. Corsellin, J.A.N. (1962). *Mental illness and the aging brain.* London: Oxford Univ. Press; Hachinski, V. C., Lassen, N. A., and Marshall, J. (1974). Multi-infarct dementia: A cause of mental deterioration in the elderly. *Lancet, 2:*207–209; and Worm-Peterson, J., and Pakkenberg, H. (1968). Atherosclerosis of cerebral arteries, pathological and clinical correlations. *J Geront, 23:*445.

110. Loeb, Clinical diagnosis of multi-infarct dementia; Judd, B. W., Meyer, J. S., Rogers, R. L., et al. (1986). Cognitive performance correlates with cerebro vascular impairments in multi-infarct dementia. *J Amer Geriatric Soc, 34:*355–360; and Meyer, J. S., Judd, B. W., Tawaklna, T., et al. (1986). Improved cognition after control of risk factors for multi-infarct dementia. *JAMA, 250:*2203–2209.

111. Kistler, J. P., Ropper, A. H., and Heros, R. C. (1984). Therapy of ischemic cerebral vascular disease due to atherothrombosis. *NEJM, 311:*29–34.

112. Hachinski, Lassen, and Marshall, Multi-infarct dementia.

113. Rubenstein, L. Z. (1982). Reversible dementia. In Beck (moderator), *Dementia in the elderly,* pp. 235–237.

114. Mesulam, M. (1985). Dementia: Its definition, differential diagnosis, and subtypes. *JAMA, 253:*2559–2561.

115. Meyer, Judd, Tawaklna, et al. Improved cognition after control of risk factors for multi-infarct dementia.

116. Hachinski, V. C. (1983). Differential diagnosis of Alzheimer's dementia: Multiinfarct dementia. In Reisberg (Ed.), *Alzheimer's disease,* pp. 188–192.

117. Ibid., p. 189.

118. Lieberman, A. N. (1983). Parkinsonian dementia and Alzheimer's dementia: Clinical and epidemiological associations. In Reisberg (Ed.), *Alzheimer's disease,* pp. 303–310.

119. Fuld, P. A. (1983). Psychometric differentiation of the dementias: An overview. In Reisberg (Ed.), *Alzheimer's disease,* pp. 201–210.

120. Albert, M. L. (1978). Subcortical dementia. In Katzman and Terry (Eds.), *Alzheimer's disease.*

121. Teravainen, H., and Calne, D. B. (1983). Motor system in normal aging and Parkinson's disease. In Katzman and Terry (Eds.), *The neurology of aging,* pp. 85–109.

122. Ibid.; and Boller, F. (1983). Alzheimer's disease and Parkinson's disease: Clinical and pathological associations. In Reisberg (Ed.), *Alzheimer's disease,* pp. 295–302.

123. Parkinson, J. (1817). *An essay on the shaking palsy.* London: Sherwood, Nelly and Jones. Cited in Sroka, H., Elizan, T. S., Yahr, M. D., et al. (1981). Organic mental syndrome and confusional states in Parkinson's disease. *Arch Neurol, 38:* 339–342.

124. Albert, Subcortical dementia; and Bowen, F. P. (1976). Behavioral alterations in patients with basal ganglia lesions. In M. Yahr (Ed.), *The basal ganglia,* pp. 169–180. New York: Raven Press.

125. Boller, Alzheimer's disease and Parkinson's disease; Larson, E. B., Reifler, B. V., and Featherstone, H. J. (1984). Dementia in elderly outpatients. *Ann Intern Med, 100:* 417–423; and Sroka, Elizan, Yahr, et al. Organic mental syndrome and confusional states in Parkinson's disease.

126. Lieberman, Parkinsonian dementia and Alzheimer's dementia.

127. Ibid., p. 305.

128. Boller, Alzheimer's disease and Parkinson's disease.

129. Lieberman, Parkinsonian dementia and Alzheimer's dementia, p. 308.

130. Fahn, S. (1984). Huntington's disease and other forms of chorea. In L. P. Roland (Ed.), *Merritt's textbook of neurology,* 7th ed., pp. 517–521. Philadelphia: Lea and Febiger; Martin, J. B., and Gusella, J. F. (1986). Huntington's disease. Pathogenesis and management. *NEJM, 315:* 1267–1276; and Mazziotta, J. C., Phelps, M. E., Pahl, J. J., et al. (1987). Reduced cerebral glucose metabolism in asymptomatic subjects at risk for Huntington's disease. *NEJM, 316:* 357–362.

131. Meyer, Judd, Tawaklna et al., Improved cognition after control of risk factors for multi-infarct dementia; Rubenstein, Reversible dementia; and Mesulam, Dementia.

132. Rubenstein, Reversible dementia.

133. Task Force, Senility reconsidered; Smith, J. S., and Kiloh, L. G. (1981). The investigation of dementia: Results in 200 consecutive admissions. *Lancet, 1:* 824–827; and Wells, C. E. (1978). Chronic brain disease: An overview. *Am J Psych, 135:* 1–12.

134. Meyer, J. S., Largen, J. W., Shaw, T., et al. (1984). Interactions of normal aging, senile dementia, multi-infarct dementia, and alcoholism in the elderly. In J. T. Hartford and T. Samorajski (Eds.), *Alcoholism in the elderly,* pp. 227–251; New York: Raven Press; and King, M. B. (1986). Alcohol abuse and dementia. *International J. Geriatric Psychiatry, 1:* 31–36.

135. Eckardt, M. J., Harford, T. C., Kaebler, C. T., et al. (1981). Health hazards associated with alcohol consumption. *JAMA, 246:* 648–666.

136. Ibid.; and Meyer, Largen, Shaw, et al., Interactions of normal aging.

137. Eckardt, Harford, Kaebler et al., Health hazards associated with alcohol consumption, p. 652.

138. Garraway, M., Dickson, R., Whisnant, J., et al. (1985). Impact of computed tomography on sub-dural hematoma. *JAMA, 253:* 2378–2381.

139. Brickner, P. W. (1978). *Home health care for the aged.* New York: Appleton-Century-Crofts, p. 98.

140. Adams, R. D., Fischer, C. M., Hakim, S., et al. (1965). Symptomatic occult hydrocephalus with "normal" cerebrospinal-fluid pressure: A treatable syndrome. *NEJM, 273:* 117–126.

141. Lieberman, Parkinsonian dementia and Alzheimer's dementia.

142. Jellinger, K. (1976). Neuropathological aspects of dementias resulting from abnormal blood and cerebrospinal fluid dynamics. *Acta Neuro Belg, 76:* 83.

143. Meyer, J. S., Kitagawa, Y., Tanahashi, N., et al. (1985). Evaluation of treatment of normal pressure hydrocephalus. *J Neurosurg, 65:* 513–521.

144. Wells, Chronic brain disease.

145. Wolfson, L. I., and Katzman, R. (1983). The neurologic consultation at age 80. In R. Katzman and R. D. Terry (Eds.), *The Neurology of Aging.* Philadelphia: F. A. Davis.

146. Council on Scientific Affairs, AMA, Dementia; and Katzman, Alzheimer's disease.

147. Small, G. W., and Jarvik, L. F. (1982). The dementia syndrome. *Lancet, 2:*1443–1446.

148. Ibid.; Spar, Pathophysiologic mechanism of dementia; Marsden, C. E., and Harrison, M.J.G. (1972). Outcome of investigation of patients with presenile dementia. *Br Med J, 2:*249–252; Wells, C. E. (Ed.). (1977). *Dementia,* 2nd ed. Philadelphia: F. A. Davis; and Wells, C. E. (1979). Diagnosis of dementia. *Psychosomatics, 20:*517–522.

149. Small and Jarvik, The dementia syndrome; and Charatan, F. B., Sherman, F. T., and Libow, L. S. (1981). Geriatric psychiatry. In L. S. Libow and F. T. Sherman (Eds.), *The core of geriatric medicine,* pp. 92–126. St. Louis: C. V. Mosby.

150. Wells, C. E. (1979). Pseudodementia. *Am J Psych, 136:*895–900.

151. Wells, Diagnosis of dementia.

152. Marsden and Harrison, Outcome of investigation of patients with presenile dementia.

153. Wells, C. E. (1979). Management of dementias. In R. Katzman (Ed.), *Congenital and acquired cognitive disorders.* New York: Raven Press.

154. Dahl, D. S. (1983). Diagnosis of Alzheimer's disease. *Postgraduate Medicine, 73:*217–221.

155. Ibid.

156. Rubenstein, Reversible dementia.

157. Friesen, A.D.J. (1983). Adverse drug reactions in the geriatric client. In L. A. Pagliaro and A. M. Pagliaro (Eds.), *Pharmacologic aspects of aging,* pp. 257–293. St. Louis: C. V. Mosby.

158. Lynch, H. T., Droszcz, C. P., Albano, W. A., et al. (1981). Organic brain syndrome secondary to 5-Fluorouracil toxicity. *Dis Colon Rectum, 24:*130–131.

159. Cummings, J., Benson, D. F., and LoVerne, S. (1980). Reversible dementia. *JAMA, 243:*2434–2439; and Gershon, S., and Herman, S. P. (1982). The differential diagnosis of dementia. *J Am Geriat Soc, 30* (supplement):58–66.

160. Block, L. H. (1983). Drug interactions in the geriatric client. In Pagliaro and Pagliaro (Eds.), *Pharmacologic aspects of aging,* pp. 140–191.

161. Peto, J. J., and Skelton, D. (1983). Drug selection and dosage in the elderly. In Pagliaro and Pagliaro (Eds.), *Pharmacologic aspects of aging,* pp. 294–336.

162. Task Force, Senility reconsidered, p. 260.

163. Ibid.

164. Damasio, A. R., and Demeter, S. (1981). Dementia due to systemic illness. *Res & Staff Physician, 7:*36–41.

165. Blass, J. P. Metabolic dementias. In Amaducci, Davison, and Antuono (Eds.), *Aging,* vol. 13, pp. 261–270.

166. Zarit, S. H., Horr, N. K., and Zarit, J. M. (1985). The hidden victims of Alzheimer's disease. Families under stress. New York: New York Univ. Press; Cohn, D. (1986). Guest editor's perspective. *PRIDE Inst J, 5*(3):2–3; and Mace, N. L. (1986). Families: The other side of Alzheimer's. *Provider, 12*(5):22–25.

167. Melnic, V. L., Dubler, N., Weisbard, A., et al. (1984). Clinical research in senile dementia of the Alzheimer type. *J Am Geriat Soc, 32:*531–536. Quote from p. 531.

168. Hemsi, L. (1982). Living with dementia. *Postgraduate Med J, 58:*610–617. Quotes from pp. 610, 611.

169. Ibid.

170. Ibid., p. 613.

171. Cohen, D., Coppel, D., and Eisdorfer, C. (1983). Management of the family. In Reisberg (Ed.), *Alzheimer's disease,* pp. 445–448; and Caserta, M. S., Lund, D. A., Wright, S. D., et al. (1987). Caregivers to dementia patients. *Gerontologist, 27:*209–214.

172. Sheldon, F. (1982). Supporting the supporters: Working with the relatives of patients with dementia. *Age and Aging, 11:*184–188.

173. Wasow, M. (1986). Support groups for family care givers of patients with Alzheimer's disease. *Social Work, 31:*93–97.

174. Powell, L. S., and Courtice, K. (1983). *Alzheimer's disease: A guide for families.* Reading, MA: Addison-Wesley; Barnes, R. F., Raskind, M. A., Scott, M., et al. (1981). Problems of families caring for Alzheimer patients: Use of a support group. *J Amer Geriat Soc, 29:* 80–85; Haycox, J. A. (1983). Social management. In Reisberg (Ed.), *Alzheimer's disease,* pp. 439–444; and Steinberg, G. (1983). Long term continuous support for family members of Alzheimer patients. In Reisberg (Ed.), *Alzheimer's disease,* pp. 455–458.

175. Hemsi, Living with dementia.

176. Aronson, M. K., and Lipkowitz, R. (1981). Senile dementia, Alzheimer type: The family and the health care delivery system. *J Amer Geriat Soc, 29:* 568–571; and Rosin, A. J., Abramowitz, L., Diamond, J., et al. (1986). Environmental management of senile dementia. *Social Work in Health Care, 11:* 33–43.

177. Dobrof, R. (1985/86). Editorial. Social work and Alzheimer's disease. *J of Gerontological Social Work, 9:* 1–4; Greenlaw, J. (1986). Nursing: Matching solution with need. *Provider, 12* (10):11–14; and Jahnigen, D. W. (1986). The doctor-patient relationship is key. *Provider, 12* (10):14–16.

178. Hemsi, Living with dementia, p. 616.

179. Hinchman, A. (1986). The role of the paraprofessional in mental health home care. *Caring, 5* (7):49–54.

180. DiCicco-Bloom, B., and Coven, C. R. (1982). *Innovative approaches: Group work with personal care workers of the homebound elderly.* (Available from Dept. of Community Medicine, St. Vincent's Hospital, New York.)

181. Waxman, H. M., Klein, M., Kennedy, R., et al. (1985). Institutional drug abuse: The overprescribing of psychoactive medications in nursing homes. In E. Gottheil, K. A. Druley, T. E. Skolada, and H. M. Waxman (Eds.), *The combined problems of alcoholism, drug addiction and aging,* pp. 179–190. Springfield, IL: Charles C Thomas.

182. Hemsi, Living with dementia.

183. Folsom, J. C. (1983). Reality orientation. In Reisberg (Ed.), *Alzheimer's disease,* pp. 449–454. Quote from p. 449.

184. Greene, J. G., Timbury, J. C., Smith, R., et al. (1983). Reality orientation with elderly patients in the community: An empirical evaluation. *Age and Aging, 12:* 38–43.

185. Folsom, J. C. (1968). Reality orientation for the elderly mental patient. *J Geriat Psychiat, 1:* 291–307; Folsom, J. C. (1981). *Help begins at home.* New York: International Center for the Disabled.

186. Dunn, L. (1986). Senior respite care programs. *PRIDE Inst J, 5* (3):7–12; French, C. J. (1986). The development of special services for victims and families burdened by Alzheimer's disease. *PRIDE Inst J, 5* (3):19–27; and Sanborn, B. (1986). San Diego's Alzheimer's family center. *PRIDE Inst J, 5* (3):13–18.

187. D. Cohn, Guest editor's perspective.

CHAPTER 5

1. Goldstein, D. B. (1983). *Pharmacology of alcohol.* New York: Oxford Univ. Press, p. 1.

2. Blose, I. L. (1978). The relationship of alcohol to aging and the elderly. *Alcoholism: Clinical and Experimental Research, 2:* 17–21. Quote from p. 17.

3. Schuckit, M. A. (1982). A clinical review of alcohol, alcoholism, and the elderly patient. *J Clin Psych, 43:* 396–399.

4. Garver, D. L. (1984). Age effects on alcohol metabolism. In J. T. Hartford and T. Samorajski (Eds.), *Alcoholism in the elderly: Social and biomedical Issues,* pp. 153–159. New York: Raven Press.

5. Seixas, F. A. (1978). Alcoholism in the elderly: Introduction. *Alcoholism: Clin & Exper Res, 2* (1):15.

6. Kafetz, K., and Cox, M. (1978). Alcohol excess and the senile squalor syndrome. *J Am Geriat Soc, 30:* 706.

7. Glatt, M. M. (1978). Experiences with elderly alcoholics in England. *Alcoholism: Clin & Exper Res, 2:*23–26.

8. Mishara, B. L., and Kastenbaum, R. (1980). *Alcohol and Old Age.* New York: Grune & Stratton.

9. Ibid., pp. 90–91.

10. Butler, R. A. (1975). *Why survive?* New York: Harper & Row.

11. Chelsea-Village Program. (1987). Department of Community Medicine, St. Vincent's Hospital and Medical Center of New York.

12. Blose, The relationship of alcohol to aging and the elderly.

13. Riley, M. W. (1986). Cited in G. Maddox, L. N. Robins, and N. Rosenberg (Eds.), *Nature and extent of alcohol problems among the elderly,* pp. 1–3. New York: Springer.

14. Glenn, N. D. (1981). Age, birth cohorts, and drinking: An illustration of the hazards of inferring effect from cohort data. *J of Gerontology, 36:*362–269.

15. Proust, M. (1920). *The Guermantes Way,* p. 191. T. Kilmartin, trans. New York, Random House.

16. Public Health Service. (1986). *Women's Health: Report of the Public Health Services Task Force on women's issues.* Chapter 4: Alcohol, drug use and abuse, and the mental health of women. Washington, DC: U.S. Dept. of Health and Human Services; and Rabinowitz, E. (1984). Women and alcoholism. *Directions in Psychiatry, 4:*1–7.

17. Blose, The relationship of alcohol to aging and the elderly, p. 19.

18. Schuckit, M. A. (1985). Genetics and the risk for alcoholism. *JAMA, 254:*2614–2617; and Rutstein, D. D., and Veech, R. L. (1978). Genetics and addiction to alcohol. *NEJM, 298:*1140–1141.

19. Goldstein, *Pharmacology of alcohol.*

20. Mishara and Kastenbaum, *Alcohol and old age,* p. 99.

21. Brown, B. B. (1982). Professional's perceptions of drug and alcohol abuse among the elderly. *Gerontologist, 22:*519–525.

22. Public Health Service, Alcohol, Drug Abuse, and Mental Health Administration. (1981). *Fourth Special Report to the U.S. Congress on Alcohol and Health.* Rockville, MD: U.S. Dept. of Health and Human Services.

23. Goldstein, Pharmacology of alcohol.

24. Williams, E. P. (1973). Alcoholism and problem drinking among older persons: Community agency study. In E. P. Williams (Ed.), *Alcohol and problem drinking among older persons.* Springfield, VA: National Technical Information Service.

25. Rosin, A. J., and Glatt, M. M. (1971). Alcohol excess in the elderly. *Q J Stud Alcohol, 32:*53–59.

26. Reuler, J. B., Girard D. E., and Conney, T. G. (1985). Wernicke's encephalopathy. *NEJM, 312:*1035–1039.

27. Hartford, J. T., and Thienhaus, O. J. (1984) Psychiatric aspects of alcoholism in geriatric patients. In Hartford and Samorajski (Eds.), *Alcoholism in the elderly,* pp. 253–262.

28. Peto, J., and Skelton, D. (1983). Drug selection and dosage in the elderly. In L. A. Pagliaro and A. M. Pagliaro (Eds.), *Pharmacologic aspects of aging,* pp. 294–336. St. Louis: C. V Mosby.

29. American Medical Association. (1977). *Manual on alcoholism,* 3rd ed. Chicago: AMA.

30. Miller, M. (1979). *Suicide after 60.* New York: Springer.

31. Schuckit, M. A. (1977). Geriatric alcoholism and drug abuse. *Gerontologist, 17:*168–174; and The 1981 White House Conference on Aging. (1981). Executive summary of technical committee on health maintenance and promotion. Washington, DC: U.S. Government Printing Office.

32. Schuckit, A clinical review of alcohol, alcoholism, and the elderly patient.

33. Blose, The relationship of alcohol to aging and the elderly.

34. Schuckit, A clinical review of alcohol, alcoholism, and the elderly patient.

35. Gomberg, E. L. (1980). Drinking and problem drinking among the elderly. Ann Arbor: Institute of Gerontology, University of Michigan.

36. Gomberg, E. L. (1975). Prevalence of alcohol among ward patients in a Veteran's Administration Hospital. *J Stud Alcohol, 36:*1458–1467.

37. Corrigan, E. M. (1974). *Problem drinkers seeking treatment.* Rutgers Center of Alcohol Studies, Publications Div., Monograph no. 8.

38. Williams, E. P., Carruth, B., and Hyman, M. M. (1973). Community care providers and the older problem drinker. In Williams (Ed.), *Alcoholism and problem drinking among older persons.*

39. Bailey, M. P., Haberman, P. W., and Alksne, H. (1965). The epidemiology of alcoholism in an urban residential area. *Q J Study on Alcohol, 26:*19–40.

40. Gomberg, Drinking and problem drinking among the elderly.

41. Lefkowitz, P., Isenberg, Y., and Brickner, P. W. (1986, June 30). *The prevalence of alcoholism among the homebound elderly.* (Available from Dept. of Community Medicine, St. Vincent's Hospital, New York.)

42. Mayfield, D., McLeod, G., and Hall, P. (1974). The CAGE questionnaire: Validation of a new alcoholism screening instrument. *Am J Psychiat, 131:*1121–1123.

43. Cahalan, D., Cisin, H., and Crossley, H. M. (1969). *American drinking practices.* New Brunswick, NJ: Rutgers Center of Alcohol Studies.

44. Mayer, J. (1979). Alcohol and the elderly: A review. *Health and Social Work, 4:*129–143.

45. Ibid.

46. Weiss, K. M. (1984). The evolutionary basis of alcoholism: A question of the neocortex. In Hartford and Samorajski (Eds.), *Alcoholism in the elderly,* p. 19.

47. Schuckit, M. A., and Pastor, P. A. (1978). The elderly as a unique population. *Alcoholism: Clin & Exp Research, 2*(1):31–38; and (1985). Surveillance and assessment of alcohol-related mortality—United States, 1980. *MMWR, 34:*161–163.

48. Bahr, H. M. (1969). Lifetime affiliation patterns of early and late-onset heavy drinkers on skid row. *Q J Study on Alcoholism, 30:*645–656.

49. Mishara and Kastenbaum, *Alcohol and old age;* and Lefkowitz, Eisenberg, and Brickner, The prevalence of alcoholism among the homebound elderly.

50. Gomberg, Drinking and problem drinking among the elderly.

51. Goldstein, *Pharmacology of alcohol.*

52. Bailey, Haberman, and Alksne, The epidemiology of alcoholism in an urban, residential area.

53. Public Health Service, *Women's Health: Report of the Public Health Services Task Force on Women's Issues;* and Rabinowitz, Women and alcoholism.

54. Rathbone-McCuan, E., and Roberds, L. A. (1980). Treatment of the older female alcoholic. *J Addiction and Health, 1:*104–128.

55. Keller, M., and Gurioli, C. (1976). Statistics on consumption of alcohol and on alcoholism. *J Study of Alcohol.* Rutgers Center of Alcohol Studies.

56. Cahalan, Cisin, and Crossley, *American drinking practices.*

57. Schuckit and Pastor, The elderly as a unique population, p. 36.

58. Ibid., p. 37.

59. Gomberg, Drinking and problem drinking among the elderly, p. 6.

60. Mayer, Alcohol and the elderly.

61. Zimberg, S. (1978). Treatment of the elderly alcoholic in the community and in the institutional setting. *Addict Dis, 3:*417–427; and Blazer, D. G., and Pennybacker, M. R. (1984). Epidemiology of Alcoholism in the elderly. In Hartford and Samorajski, (Eds.), *Alcoholism in the elderly,* pp. 25–33.

62. Mann, T. (1957). *Confessions of Felix Krull, confidence man.* New York: Signet.

63. Blazer and Pennybacker, Epidemiology of alcoholism in the elderly.

64. Gomberg, Drinking and problem drinking among the elderly.

65. National Council on Alcoholism. (1981, Feb.) *Preliminary report on aging and alcoholism.* Washington, DC: National Council on Alcoholism.

66. Criteria Committee, National Council on Alcoholism. (1972). *Criteria for the diagnosis of alcoholism. Am J Psych, 129:*127–135.

67. American Psychiatric Association. (1980). *Diagnostic and statistical manual of mental disorders,* 3rd ed. Washington, DC: APA; and Robin, L. N. (1981). The diagnosis of alcoholism after DSM-III. In R. E. Meyer, T. F. Babor, B. C. Blueck, et al. (Eds.), *Evaluation of the alcoholic: Implications for treatment.* Research Monograph no. 5. National Institute on Alcohol Abuse and Alcoholism, pp. 85–105.

68. Zimberg, S. (1978). Diagnosis and treatment of the elderly alcoholic. *Alcoholism: Clin & Exp Research, 2*(1):27–29. Table from p. 28.

69. Ibid., p. 27.

70. Blose, The relationship of alcohol to aging and the elderly; and Williams, Carruth, and Hyman, Community care providers and the older problem drinker.

71. Schuckit and Pastor, The elderly as a unique population.

72. Lambert, A. (1907). Alcohol. In *Osler's modern medicine,* vol. 1, pp. 157–202. Philadelphia: Lea Brothers.

73. Davis, J. S. (1957). The medicinal benefits of beverage alcohol. *Va Med, 84:*3–9.

74. Gomberg, Drinking and problem drinking among the elderly.

75. Hennekens, C. H., Willett, W., Rosner, B., et al. (1979). Effects of beer, wine, and liquor in coronary deaths. *JAMA, 242:*1973–74; Haskell, W. L., Camargo, C., Jr., Williams, P. T., et al. (1984). The effects of cessation and resumption of moderate alcohol intake on serum high-density-lipoprotein subfractions: A controlled study. *NEJM, 310:*805–810; and Mikhailidis, D. P., Jenkins, W. J., Jeremy, J., et al. (1984). Ethanol and arterial disease [Letter to the editor]. *NEJM, 311:*536–537.

76. Hennekens, Willett, Rosner et al., Effects of beer, wine, and liquor in coronary deaths.

77. Haskell, Camargo, Williams et al., The effects of cessation and resumption of moderate alcohol intake.

78. Mikhailidis, Jenkins, Jeremy et al., Ethanol and arterial disease.

79. Forbes, G. B., and Reina, J. C. (1970). Adult lean body mass declines with age: Some longitudinal observations. *Metabolism, 19:*653–663.

80. Long, C., Ham, R. J., and Smith, M. R. (1983). The management of elderly patients with multiple medical problems. In R. J. Ham (Ed.), *Primary care geriatrics,* pp. 215–233. Boston: PSG Inc.

81. Gambert, S. R., Newton, M., and Duthie, E. H., Jr. (1984). Medical issues in alcoholism in the elderly. In Hartford and Samorajski (Eds.), *Alcoholism in the elderly,* pp. 175–191.

82. Garver, D.L. Age effects on alcohol metabolism; and Vestal, R. E., McGuire, E. A., Tobin, J. D., et al. (1977). Aging and ethanol metabolism. *Clin Pharm Ther, 31:*343–354.

83. Gomberg, Drinking and problem drinking among the elderly; and Cahalan, Cisin, and Crossley, *American drinking practices.*

84. Thomas, J. (1986, Apr. 12). Living in a castle by royal favor. *New York Times.*

85. Samorajski, T., Persson, K., Bissell, C., et al. (1984). Biology of alcoholism and aging in rodents: Brain and liver. In Hartford and Samorajski (Eds.), *Alcoholism in the elderly,* pp. 43–63.

86. Lundin, D. V. (1983). Medication-taking behavior and compliance in the elderly. In Pagliaro and Pagliaro (Eds.), *Pharmacologic aspects of aging,* pp. 7–33.

87. Gomberg, Drinking and problem drinking among the elderly.

88. Mellinger, G. E., Balter, M. B., and Manheimer, D. I. (1971). Patterns of psychotherapeutic drug use among adults in San Francisco. *Arch Gen Psych, 25:*385–349; and Aoki, F. Y., Hildahl, V. K., Large, G. W., et al. (1983). Aging and heavy drug use: A prescription survey in Manitoba. *J Chron Dis, 36:*75–84.

89. Richmond, J. B. (1979). *Surgeon General's Advisory.* U.S. Dept. of Health, Education and Welfare [HEW], Public Health Service.

90. Bosman, H. B. (1984). Pharmacology of alcoholism and aging. In Hartford and Samorajski (Eds.), *Alcoholism in the elderly*, pp. 161–174.

91. Gill, J. S., Zezulka, A. V., Shipley, J. M., et al. (1986). Stroke and alcohol consumption. *NEJM, 315*:1041–1046; and Wolf, P. A. (1986). Cigarettes, alcohol, and stroke. *NEJM, 315*: 1087–1089.

92. Meyer, J. S., Largen, J. W., Jr., Shaw, T., et al. (1984). Interactions of normal aging, senile dementia, multi-infarct dementia and alcoholism in the elderly. In Hartford and Samorajski (Eds.); Rogers, R. L., Meyer, J. S., Shaw, T. G., et al. (1983). Reductions in regional cerebral blood flow associated with chronic consumption of alcohol. *J Amer Geriatric Soc, 31*:540–543. *Alcoholism in the elderly*, pp. 227–251; and King, M. B. (1986). Alcohol abuse and dementia. *International J. Geriatric Psychiatry, 1*:31–36.

93. Flinn, G. A., Reisberg, B., and Ferris, S. H. (1984). Neuropsychological models of cerebral dysfunction in chronic alcoholics. In Hartford and Samorajski (Eds.), *Alcoholism in the elderly*, pp. 193–200; and Wood, W. G., Armbrecht, H. J., and Wise, R. W. (1984). Aging and the effects of ethanol: The role of brain membranes. In Hartford and Samorajski (Eds.), *Alcoholism in the elderly*, pp. 139–151.

94. Freund, G. (1984). Neuro transmitter function in relation to aging and alcoholism. In Hartford and Samorajski (Eds.), *Alcoholism in the elderly*, p. 67.

95. Ibid.

96. Wilkins, J. N., and Gorelick, D. A. (1986). Clinical neuroendocrinology and neuropharmacology of alcohol withdrawal. In M. Galanter (Ed.), *Recent developments in alcoholism*, vol. 4, pp. 241–263. New York: Plenum Press.

97. Ryan, C., and Butters, N. (1980). Learning and memory impairments in young and old alcoholics: evidence for the premature aging hypothesis. *Alcohol: Clin & Exp Research, 4*:288–293; and Burger, M. C., Botwinick, J., and Storandt, M. (1987). Aging, alcoholism, and performance on the Luria-Nebraska neuropsychological battery. *J of Gerontology, 42*:69–72.

98. Jones, B., and Parsons, O. A. (1971). Impaired abstracting ability in chronic alcoholics. *Arch Gen Psych, 24*:71–75.

99. Sun, A. Y., and Samorajski, T. (1977). The effects of age and alcohol on $(NA^+$ and $K^+)$-ATPase activity of whole homogenate and synaptosomes prepared from correlates of chronic alcoholism and aging. *J Neur Ment Dis, 165*:348–355.

100. Ibid.

101. Blusewicz, M. J., Dustman, R. E., Schenkenberg, T., et al. (1975). Neuropsychological correlates of chronic alcoholism and aging. *J Neurochem, 24*:161–164; Blusewicz, M. J., Schenkenberg, T., Dustman, R. E., et al. (1977). Alcoholic and elderly normal groups: An evaluation of organicity and mental aging indices. *J Clin Psych, 33*:1149–1153; Cala, L. A., Jones, B., Mastaglia, F. L., et al. (1978). Brain atrophy and intellectual impairment in heavy drinkers. *Aust NZ J Med, 8*(2):147–153; and Migiolo, M., Buchtel, H. A., Campanini, T., et al. (1979). Cerebral hemispheric lateralization of cognitive deficits due to alcoholism. *J Nerv Ment Dis, 167*(4):212–217.

102. Ryan, C., and Butters, N. (1980). Further evidence of a continuum-of-impairment encompassing alcoholic Korsakoff patients and chronic alcoholics. *Alcoholism, 4*:190–198.

103. Cala, L. A., and Mastaglia, F. L. (1980). Computerized axial tomography in the detection of brain damage. *Med J Aust, 2*:193–198; and von Gall, M., Becker, H., Artmann, H., et al. (1978). Results of computer tomography on chronic alcoholics. *Neuroradiology, 16*:329–331.

104. Meese, W., Kluge, W., Grumme, T., et al. (1980). CT evaluation of the CSF spaces of healthy persons. *Neuroradiology, 19*(3):131–136.

105. Brickner, R. M. (1936). *The intellectual functions of the frontal lobes.* New York: Macmillan.

106. Cala and Mastaglia, Computerized axial tomography in the detection of brain damage.

107. Courville, C. B. (1966). *Effects of alcohol on the nervous system of man.* Los Angeles: San Lucas Press.

108. Flinn, Reisberg, and Ferris, Neuropsychological models of cerebral dysfunction in chronic alcoholics, p. 198.

109. Garver, Age effects on alcohol metabolism.

110. Ibid.

111. Kalant, H., Khanna, J. M., and Isreal, Y. (1980). The alcohols. In P. Seeman, E. M. Sellers, and W.H.E. Ropschlau, *Principles of medical pharmacology,* 3rd ed. Toronto: Univ. of Toronto Press.

112. Glatt, Experiences with elderly alcoholics in England.

113. Gambert, Newton, and Duthie, Medical issues in alcoholism in the elderly; and Barboriak, J. J., Rooney, C. B., Leitschuh, T. H., et al. (1978). Alcohol and nutrient intake of elderly men. *J Am Diet Assoc, 72:*493–495.

114. Bosman, Pharmacology of alcoholism and aging.

115. Gorelick, D. A. and Wilkins, J. N. (1986). Special aspects of human alcohol withdrawal. In Galanter (Ed.), *Recent developments in alcoholism,* pp. 283–305.

116. Finkle, B. S. (1969). Drugs in drinking drivers: A study of 2500 cases. *J Safety Res, 1:*179–183; Seixas, F. A. (1979). Drug/alcohol interactions: Avert potential dangers. *Geriatrics, 34:*89–102; and Seixas, F. A. (1975). Alcohol and its drug interactions. *Ann Intern Med, 83:*86–92.

117. Gomberg, Drinking and problem drinking among the elderly, p. 20.

118. Vaillant, G. (1983). Prospective study of alcoholism treatment. *Am J Med, 75:*455–463.

119. Mishara and Kastenbaum, *Alcohol and old age.*

120. DiClemente, C. C., Gordon, J. R. (1984). Aging, alcoholism, and addictive behavior change: Diagnostic treatment models. In Hartford and Samorajski (Eds.), *Alcoholism in the elderly,* p. 268.

121. DiCicco-Bloom, B., Space, S., and Zahourek, R. P. (1986). The homebound alcoholic. *Am J Nursing, 86:*167–169.

122. Gomberg, Drinking and problem drinking among the elderly, p. 15.

123. National Council on Alcoholism. (1981, Feb.). Preliminary report on aging and alcoholism by the blue ribbon study commission on aging and alcoholism. Washington, DC: NCA.

124. Gomberg, Drinking and problem drinking among the elderly; and Pascarelli, E. F., and Fischer, W. (1974). Drug dependence in the elderly. *International J of Aging and Human Devel, 5:*347–356.

125. Schuckit, M. A. (1976, June 7). An overview of alcohol and drug abuse problems in the elderly. Testimony before the Senate Subcommittee on Alcoholism and Narcotics, and the Subcommittee on Aging of the Senate Committee on Labor and Public Welfare.

126. Ciompi, L., and Eisert, M. (1971). Retrospective long term studies on the health status of alcoholics in old age. *Social Psych, 6:*129–151.

127. Ibid.; and Mishara and Kastenbaum, *Alcohol and old age.*

128. Chelsea-Village Program.

129. Sellers, E. M., Naranjo, C. A., and Peachey, J. E. (1981). Drugs to decrease alcohol consumption. *NEJM, 305:*1255–1262.

130. Goldstein, *Pharmacology of alcohol.*

131. Rathbone-McCuan, E., and Triegaardt, J. (1979, summer). The older alcoholic and the family. *Alcohol Health and Research World* (Dept. of HEW), pp. 7–12.

132. Hartford and Thienhaus, Psychiatric aspects of alcoholism in geriatric patients.

133. Blume, S. B. (1978). Group psychotherapy in the treatment of alcoholism. In S. Zimberg, J. Wallace, and S. B. Blume (Eds.), *Practical approaches to alcoholism psychotherapy.* New York: Plenum Press.

134. Hartford and Thienhaus, Psychiatric aspects of alcoholism in geriatric patients, p. 259.

135. *A.A., Alcoholics Anonymous.* New York: Works Publishing Co. 1939; Alibrandi, L. A. (1978) The folk psychotherapy of Alcoholics Anonymous. In Zimberg, Wallace, and Blume (Eds.), *Practical approaches to alcoholism psychotherapy;* and Leach, B. (1973). Does Alcoholics Anon-

ymous really work? In P. G. Bourn (Ed.), *Alcoholism: Progress in research and treatment,* pp. 245–284. New York: Academic Press.

136. Ciompi and Eisert, Retrospective long-term studies on the health status of alcoholics in old age.

137. Dept. of HEW. (1975, spring). Older problem drinkers: Their special needs and a nursing home geared to those needs. *Alcohol Health and Research World,* pp. 12–17.

138. Ibid., p. 15.

139. Nerviano, V. J., and Gross, H. W. (1983). Personality types of alcoholics on objective inventories. *J Stud Alcohol, 44:*837–851.

140. Horn, J. L., and Wanberg, K. W. (1969). Symptom patterns related to excessive use of alcohol. *QJ Stud Alcohol, 30:*35–58; Hesselbrock, M. N. (1986). Alcoholic typologies. A review of empirical evaluations of common classification schemes. In Galanter (Ed.), *Recent developments in alcoholism,* pp. 191–206; and Kivlahan, D. R., Donovan, D. M., and Walker, R. D. (1983). *Alcoholic subtypes: Validity of clusters based on multiple assessment domains.* Paper presented at the annual meeting of the American Psychological Association, Anaheim, California.

141. Parrish, J. (1883). *Alcoholic inebriety: From a medical standpoint.* Philadelphia: P. Blakiston; and LeGrain, P. M. (1889). *Heredite et alcoolisme.*

142. Jellinek, E. M. (1960). *The disease concept of alcoholism.* New Haven: College and University Press.

143. Babor, T. F., and Lauerman, R. J. (1986). Classification and forms of inebriety. Historical antecedents of alcoholic typologies. In Galanter (Ed.), *Recent developments in alcoholism,* pp. 113–144.

CHAPTER 6

1. General Accounting Office [GAO]. (1985). Summary of States Issues on Aging: An information paper to the Chairman of the Board of the Select Committee on Aging, House of Representatives, 98th Congress, Second Session, April 1985 (Comm. Pub. no. 99–491). Washington, DC: U.S. Government Printing Office; Brickner, P. W. (1978). *Home health care for the aged.* New York: Appleton-Century-Crofts; and GAO. (1979). *Entering a nursing home: Costly implications for Medicaid and the elderly* (Pub. no. PAD 80-12). Washington, DC: U.S. Government Printing Office.

2. Dickens, C. (1844). *Martin Chuzzlewit.* Boston: Dana Estes and Co., p. 286.

3. Stuart, M. R., and Snope, F. C. (1981). Family structure, family dynamics and the elderly. In A. R. Somers and D. R. Fabian (Eds.), *The geriatric imperative,* pp. 137–52. New York: Appleton-Century-Crofts; and Spiegel, A. D. (1983). *Home health care.* Owings Mills, MD: National Health Publishing.

4. Spiegel, *Home health care;* Borup, J. H., Gallego, D. T., and Heffernan, P. G. (1980). Relocation: Its effect on health, functioning and mortality. *Gerontologist, 20:*468–479; Bourestom, N., and Pastalan, L. (1981). The effects of relocation on the elderly. *Gerontologist, 21:*4–7;Damon, L. E. (1982). Effects of relocation on the elderly. *AFP, 26:*144–148; Ham, R. J., Marcy, M. L., and Pawlson, L. G. (1983). The health care system and the elderly. In R. J. Ham, J. M. Holtzman, M. L. Marcy and M. R. Smith (Eds.), *Primary care geriatrics,* pp. 73–87. Boston: John Wright-PSG Inc.; Linn, N. W., and Linn, B. S. (1980). Qualities of institutional care that affect outcome: A review of the literature. *Aged Care and Services Review, 2:*1–14; and Schulz, R., and Brenner, G. (1977). Relocation of the aged: A review and theoretical analysis. *J Gerontology, 32:*323–332.

5. Brickner, *Home health care for the aged,* p. 24.

6. Brody, E. M. (1979, Feb.). Long term care of the aged: Promises and prospects. *Health and Social Work,* pp. 29–59; Brody, E. M., Johnsen, P. T., Fulcomer, M. C., et al. (1983). Women's changing roles and help to elderly patients: Attitudes of three generations of women. *J. Gerontology, 38:*597–607; Cantor, M. H. (1983). Strain among caregivers: A study of experience in the United States. *Gerontologist, 23:*597–604; Caro, F. G. (1984, Sept. 6). *Structure and operation of New York City Human Resources Administration Home Care Program* [Draft]. New York:

Institute for Social Welfare Research, Community Service Society; Caro, F. G., and Blank, A. (1985, May). *Home care in New York City.* New York: Community Service Society; Eidus, R. (1981). The physician and the nursing home patient. In Somers and Fabian (Eds.), *The geriatric imperative,* pp. 269–280; Horowitz, A, and Dobrof, R. (1982). *The role of families in providing long term care to the frail and chronically-ill elderly living in the community. Final report.* New York: Brookdale Center of Aging of Hunter College; Johnson, C. L., and Catalano, D. J. (1981). Childless elderly and their family supports. *Gerontologist, 21:*610–618; Marks, R. (1987). The family dimension in long-term care. *PRIDE Inst J, 6*(1): in press; and Marshall, E. (1983, Nov. 20). *Post-hospital care arrangements for the functionally disabled elderly: A symposium.* New York: Community Service Society.

7. Stuart and Snope, Family structure, family dynamics and the elderly; Brody, E. M. (1978). The aging family. *Ann Amer Acad Pol and Soc Sci, 438:*13–27; Brody, E. M. (1981). Women in the middle and family help to older people. *Gerontologist, 21:*471–480; Chatters, L. M., Taylor, R. J., and Jackson, J. S. (1985). Size and composition of the informal helper networks of elderly blacks. *J Gerontology, 40:*605–614; Hartford, M. E., and Parsons, R. (1982). Groups with relatives of dependent older adults. *Gerontologist, 22:*394–398; Poulshock, S. W., and Deimling, G. T. (1984). Families caring for elders in residence: Issues in the measurement of burden. *J Gerontology, 39:*230–239; Quirke, E., and Stahl, I. (1978). The social worker. In Brickner, P. W. *Home health care for the aged,* pp. 109–140; Shanas, E. (1979). The family as a social support system in old age. *Gerontologist, 19:*169–174; Silverstone, B., and Burack-Weiss, A. (1982). The social work function in nursing homes and home care. *J Gerontological Soc Work, 5:*7–33; Soldo, B. (1983, July). The elderly home care population: National prevalence rates, select characteristics and alternative sources of assistance. In Dept. of Health and Human Services, *Project to analyze existing long-term care data, final report, vol. 3* (Contract No. 100-80-0158). Washington, DC: Dept. of Health and Human Services; Somers, A. R. (1982). Long term care for the elderly and disabled. *NEJM, 307:*221–226; Steuer, J. L., and Clark, E. O. (1982). Family support groups within a research project on dementia. *Clin Gerontologist, 1:*87–95; and Zarit, S. H., Reever, K. E., and Bach-Peterson, J. (1980). Relatives of the impaired elderly: Correlates of feelings of burden. *Gerontologist, 20:*649–655.

8. Vladeck, B. C. (1983). Two steps forward, one back: The changing agenda of long-term care reform. *PRIDE Inst J, 2*(3):3–9.

9. Feifel, H. (1971). The meaning of death in American society: Implications for education. In B. R. Green and D. P. Irish (Eds.), *Death education,* pp. 3–12. Cambridge, MA: Schenkman.

10. Brickner, P. W. (Ed). (1971). *Care of the nursing home patient.* New York: Macmillan, pp. 16–17.

11. *Taxonomy of long term care services.* St. Louis: Catholic Health Assn., 1983.

12. Eggert, G. M. (1985, March). *Monroe County Long Term Care Program* [abstract]. Miami: Alliance for Care, National Conference; ACCESS: A caring partnership for home care. *Caring,* Dec. 1984, pp. 29–37; Brown, T. E., and Learner, R. M. (1983). The South Carolina Community Long Term Care Project. In Zawadski, *Community-based systems of long term care,* pp. 73–89; Eggert, G. M., and Brodows, B. S. (1983). Five years of ACCESS: What have we learned. In R. T. Zawadski, *Community-based systems of long term care.* New York: Haworth Press, pp. 27–48; *Five-Hospital Program: Home Front.* Chicago, Five-Hospital Program, Fall 1985; Perkel, R. L., and Plumb, J. D. (1983). The urban community family medicine home visit program at Thomas Jefferson University Hospital. *PRIDE Inst J, 2*(3):10–17; Schreiber, M. S., and Hughes, S. (1982). The Chicago Five-Hospital Homebound Elderly Program: A long-term home care model. *PRIDE Inst J, 1*(1):12–20; Skellie, F. A. (1979). The impact of alternatives to nursing home care. *Am Health Care Assn, 3:*46–53; Weiss, L. J., and Sklar, B. W. (1983). Project OPEN: A hospital-based long-term care demonstration program for the chronically ill elderly. In Zawadski, *Community-based systems of long term care,* pp. 127–145; and Zimmer, J. G., Groth-Junker, A., and McCusker, J. (1985). A randomized controlled study of a home health care team. *Am J Public Health, 75:*134–141.

13. Spiegel, *Home health care;* and Skellie, The impact of alternatives to nursing home care.

14. Spiegel, *Home health care;* Feder, J. (1987). Background on financial perspectives: Medicare's skilled nursing benefit. In B. C. Vladeck and G. J. Alfano (Eds.), *Medicare and extended care,*

pp. 131–136. Owings Mills, MD: National Health Publ.; and Health Care Financing Administration [HCFA]. (N.D.). *Medicare Part A Intermediary Manual.* Washington, DC: Dept. of Health and Human Services.

15. Quirke and Stahl, The social worker; Moore, F. M., and Layzer, E. (1983). Supporting the homemaker-home health aide as a valuable player on the home care team. *PRIDE Inst J, 2*(3):19–23; and Turner, P. A. (1983). Homemaker-home health aides as members of the home care team. *PRIDE Inst J, 2*(3):26–27.

16. Smith, J. P. (1984). Oxygen therapy: Its uses and limitations. *PRIDE Inst J, 3*(2):8–13; Braun, N. (1984). Long-term mechanical ventilation. *PRIDE Inst J, 3*(2):13–19; Evashwick, C. (1987). Home health care: Current trends and future opportunities. In N. Goldfield and S. B. Goldsmith (Eds.). *Alternative delivery systems,* pp. 5–18. Rockville, MD: Aspen; Garvey, M. (1984). Evaluating patients for their applicability to home dialysis. *PRIDE Inst J, 3*(2):26–28; Goldman, P. (1982). Rate-controlled drug delivery. *NEJM, 307:*286–290; Goodspeed, N. B. H. (1984). CAPD: An evolving technology in home dialysis. *PRIDE Inst J, 3*(2):20–26; Javanovic, L. (1984). Insulin therapy. *PRIDE Inst J, 3*(2):38–44; Lokich, J. J. (1984). Chemotherapy. *PRIDE Inst J, 3*(2):33–38; Perry, S., Smith, J. P., Lokich, J. J., and Goodspeed, N. B. H. (1984). Current consequences of high technology. *PRIDE Inst J, 3*(2):45–49; Ruchlin, H. S., and Morris, J. N. (1981). Cost-benefit analysis of an emergency alarm and response system: A case study of a long-term care program. *Health Services Research, 16:*65–80; Timms, D., and Moser, K. (1981). An analysis of the practice of outpatient oxygen therapy. *Chest 80:*13; Turner, N. (1984). Home nutrition support: Parenteral and enteral nutrition. *PRIDE Inst J, 3*(2):29–33; and Weiss, S. M., Worthington, P. H., Prioleau, M., and Rosato, F. E. (1984). Home total parenteral nutrition in cancer patients. *Cancer, 50:*1210–1213.

17. U.S. Congress. House Select Committee on Aging. *Hearings on high technology and its benefits for an aging population.* 98th Cong., May 22, 1984. Comm. Pub. No. 98-459. Washington, DC: U.S. Government Printing Office; Laxton, C. (Ed.). (1986, Sept.). High tech, high touch. *Caring, 5;* and Symposium on high technology in home care. *Cleveland Clinic Quart, 52:*283–349, 1985.

18. Lechich, A. (1985). Applications of technology: Introduction. *PRIDE Inst J, 3*(2):6–7.

19. Kane, R. A., and Kane, R. L. (1985). The feasibility of universal long-term care benefits. *NEJM, 312:*1357–1364.

20. Ibid.; GAO, *Entering a nursing home;* HCFA. (1984). *Health Care Spending Bulletin* (no. 84-4); and Scanlon, W. J., and Feder, J. (1984, Jan.). The long-term care marketplace: An overview. *Healthcare Financial Management,* pp. 18–36.

21. Applebaum, R. A., Baxter, R. J., Callahan, J. J., Jr., et al. (1984). *Targeting services to chronically disabled elderly: The preliminary experiences of the National Long Term Care Channeling Demonstration.* Princeton, NJ: MPR; and Capitman, J. A. (1986). Community-based long-term care models, target groups, and impacts on service use. *Gerontologist, 26:*389–397.

22. Guterman, S., and Dobson, A. (1986). Impact of the Medicare prospective payment system for hospitals. *Health Care Financing Review, 7:*97–114; and Leader, S. (1986, Sept.). *Home health benefits under Medicare.* Washington, DC: AARP.

23. Scanlon and Feder, The long-term care marketplace; GAO. (1979, May 15). *Home health care services—Tighter fiscal controls needed* (HRD 79-17). Washington, DC: U.S. GAO; GAO. (1981, Oct. 26). *Improved knowledge base would be helpful in reaching policy decisions of providing long-term in-home services for the elderly* (HRD-82-4). Washington, DC: U.S. GAO; Hammond, J. (1979). Home health care cost effectiveness: An overview of the literature. *Public Health Reports, 94:*305–311; Skellie, F. A., Mobley, G. M., and Coan, R. E. (1979). Cost-effectiveness of community-based long-term care: Current findings of Georgia's alternative health services project. *Am J Public Health, 72:*353–358; Trager, B. (1980). Home health care and national health policy. *Home Health Care Q, 1:*1–103; U.S. Congress. Senate Committee on Labor and Human Resources. (1982, Dec. 7). *Report to the chairman: The elderly should benefit from expanded home health care but increasing these services will not insure cost reductions* (GAO/IPE-83-1). Washington, DC: U.S. GAO; Vladeck, B. C. (1987). History of the Medicare extended care benefit. In Vladeck and Alfano (Eds.), *Medicare and extended care,* pp. 5–13; Weissert, W. G. (1979). Long term care: An overview. In *Health United States, 1978.* Washington DC: USDEW, National Center for Health Statistics; Weissert, W. G., Wan, T.T.H., Livieratos, B. B. (1979, Aug.). Effects and cost of day care and homemaker service for the chronically ill: A randomized experiment (PHS 79-3250). Hyatts-

ville, MD: National Center for Health Services Research; and Weissert, W. G., Wan, T. T. H., Livieratos, B. B., et al. (1980). Cost effectiveness of homemaker services for the chronically ill. *Inquiry, 17*(3):230–243.

24. The cost-effectiveness of home care. (1986, Aug.). *Caring, 5:* 27–29.

25. Feller, B. A. (1983). Americans needing help to function at home. In *Advance data from vital and health statistics, 1983.* (DHHS Pub. No. [PHS] 83-1250). Hyattsville, MD: National Center for Health Statistics.

26. Eggert and Brodows, Five years of ACCESS; ACCESS: A caring partnership; Birnbaum, H., Gauner, G., Pratter, F., et al. (1984, Dec.). *Nursing Home Without Walls: Evaluation of the New York State Long Term Home Health Care Program.* Cambridge, MA: Abt Associates; Brown and Learner, The South Carolina Community Long Term Care Project; Dept. of Community Medicine. (1985). *Chelsea-Village Program 12 Year Report.* New York: St. Vincent's Hospital; Five-Hospital Program; O'Rourke, B., Raisz, H., and Segal, J. (1982). *Triage II: Coordinated delivery of services to the elderly. Final report.* Bristol, CT: N.P.; Perkel and Plumb, The urban community Family Medicine home visit program; Salzman, H., Langendorf, R., and Ravenna, P. (1987). Home health care [Letter to the editor]. *NEJM, 106:* 168; Schreiber and Hughes, The Chicago Five-Hospital Homebound Elderly Program; Skellie, The impact of alternatives to nursing home care; Weiss and Sklar, Project OPEN; and Zawadski, R. T., Shen, J., Yordi, C., et al. (1984, Dec.). *On Lok's community care organization for dependent adults.* San Francisco: On Lok Senior Health Services.

27. GAO, Home health care services; National Association of Home Health Agencies. (1980, Oct.). *Position statement on prospective reimbursement.* Washington, DC: National Assn. of Home Health Agencies; Upjohn Healthcare Services. (1979). *Home care under Medicare.* Kalamazoo, MI: Upjohn.

28. Diamond, L. M., and Berman, D. E. (1981). The social/health maintenance organization: A single-entry, prepaid, long-term care delivery system. In J. J. Callahan and S. Wallack (Eds.), *Reforming the long-term care system,* pp. 185–217. Lexington, MA: Lexington Books. Governor's Long Range Medicaid Planning Committee. (1982, March). *The feasibility of developing and operating social/health maintenance organizations in New York State.* Albany: New York State Health Planning Commission; Greenberg, J., and Lentz, W. N. (1983, Nov. 16). *The social/health maintenance organization: Its role in the long term care system.* Paper presented at the annual meeting of the American Public Health Association, Dallas, TX; Greenberg, J. N., Lentz, W. N., and Grahams, R. (1987). The national social health maintenance organization demonstration. In Goldfield and Goldsmith (Eds.), *Alternative delivery systems,* pp. 33–62; Harrington, C., Newcomer, R., and Newacheck, P. (1983, April). *Prepaid long term care plans: A policy option for California's Medi-Cal Program.* Berkeley: Institute of Governmental Studies, Univ. of California; Kodner, D. L. (1981). Who's a S/HMO: A look at Metropolitan Jewish Geriatric Center and its plans to develop a social/health maintenance operation. *Home Health Svcs Quart, 2*(4):57–68; Schneider, D. (1981). *Policy analysis of coordinative integrative services: The Social/HMO.* New York State Health Planning Commission, Albany; and S/HMOs: A new experiment in health care. *The Internist* (1986, Sept.), p. 20.

29. Kane and Kane, The feasibility of universal long-term care benefits; Thompson, R. H., Muller, E. M., and Seshagiri, V. (1985, May). *Studies of community-based long term care.* Health Systems Agency of New York City, New York; and U.S. Dept. of Health and Human Services. (1981). *Long term care: Background and future directions* (Pub. no. [HCFA] 81-20047). Washington, DC: U.S. Government Printing Office.

30. Lombardi, T. (1980, June 2). Long Term Home Health Care in New York State: The Experience of the Lombardi Program To Date: Report of the Symposium. New York: St. Vincent's Hospital, p. 69.

31. New York State Senate Health Committee. (1984, July 16). *Long term care—An issue facing us all.* (Health Bulletin No. 75). Albany, NY.

32. Birnbaum, Gauner, Pratter et al., *Nursing Home Without Walls.*

33. Bluestone, E. M. (1946). The place of the long term patient in the modern hospital: The use and misuse of hospital beds. *ACS Bull, 31:* 104; Cherkasky, M. (1947). Hospital service goes home. *Modern Hospital, 68:* 47–48; Cherkasky, M. (1981). Author's comment re hospital service

goes home. *Colloquium, 2:*7; and Jensen, F., Weiskottch, H. G., and Thomas, M. A. (1944). *Medical care of the discharged hospital patient.* New York: Commonwealth Fund.

34. Vladeck, B. C. (1980). *Unloving Care.* New York: Basic Books; and New York State Moreland Act Commission on Nursing Homes and Residential Facilities. (1976, Feb.). *Nursing home and domiciliary facility planning.*

35. Birnbaum, Gauner, Pratter et al., *Nursing Home Without Walls;* and Abt Associates, Inc. (1979, Aug. 27). *New York State's long term health care programs: Part 1: Technical Proposal* (RFP no. HCFA-79-ORDS-44/AG), Cambridge, MA: Abt Associates.

36. Chapter 895 of the Laws of 1977, New York State.

37. Birnbaum, Gauner, Pratter et al., *Nursing Home Without Walls;* and Abt Associates, *New York State's long term health care programs.*

38. New York State Senate Health Committee. (1985, Sept. 1). *Nursing Home Without Walls: An update.* (Health Bulletin No. 75-E). Albany, NY.

39. Barhydt, N. R. (1986, July 10). *LTHHCP status report.* Albany, NY: Office of Health Systems Management, Bureau of Home Health Care, NY State Dept. of Health.

40. Applebaum, Baxter, Callahan et al., *Targeting services for the chronically disabled elderly;* Capitman, Community-based long-term care models; Brown, R. S., Mossel, P. A., Schore, J., et al. (1986, Jan. 13). *Final report on the effects of sample attrition on estimates of channeling's impacts. Executive summary.* Princeton, NJ, Prepared for Dept. of Health and Human Services by Mathematica Policy Research Inc.; Brown, R. S. (1986, July). *Methodological issues in the evaluation of the National Long Term Care Demonstration. Executive Summary.* Princeton, NJ, prepared for the Dept. of Health and Human Services by Mathematica Policy Research Inc.; Clark, R. F. (1987). The costs and benefits of community care: A perspective from the Channeling demonstration. *PRIDE Inst J, 6*(2): in press; Horowitz, A., and Dono, J. E. (1984, May). *Delivery of medical and social services to the homebound elderly: A demonstration of interservice coordination.* New York: New York City Dept for the Aging; and Phillips, B. R., Stephens, S. A., and Cerf, J. J. (1986, May 7). *Survey data collection design and procedures: Overview of data collection in the National Long Term Care Demonstration. Executive Summary.* Princeton, NJ, prepared for the Dept of Health and Human Services by Mathematica Policy Research Inc.

41. Section 222, Public Law 93-403 [Authority for Medicare waivers]; Section 1115, 1974 Medicare Act; Section 1915, 1981 Omnibus Reconciliation Act [Authority for Medicaid waivers].

42. Capitman, J. A., Haskins, B., and Bernstein, J. (1986). Case management approaches in coordinated community-oriented long-term care demonstrations. *Gerontologist, 26:*398–404.

43. Zawadski, R. T. (1983). The long term care demonstration projects. In Zawadski, *Community-based systems of long term care,* pp. 5–19.

44. Quinn, J. (1978). Testimony before Select Committee on Aging, U.S. House of Representatives. Hearing on Home Care for the Elderly: *The need for a national policy* (Comm. Pub. no. 95-139). Washington, DC: U.S. Government Printing Office, p. 67.

45. Quinn, J. (1985, March). *Triage* [abstract]. Paper presented at the National Conference of the Alliance for Care, Miami; and Quinn, J., and Hodgson, J. H. (1983). Triage: A long term care study. In Zawadski, *Community-based systems of long term care,* pp. 171–191.

46. Shealy, M. J. (1979, Dec.). *Triage: Coordinated delivery of services to the elderly.* Hartford: Connecticut State Department on Aging.

47. Spiegel, *Home health care;* and Quinn, J. (1982, Feb. 28). *Triage II. Coordinated delivery of services to the elderly.* Final report, vol. 1. Wethersfield, CT: N. P.

48. Quinn, *Triage II,* p. 12.

49. Spiegel, *Home health care;* and Quinn and Hodgson, *Triage.*

50. Quinn, *Triage.*

51. Kodner, D. L. (1982, Jan.). *The integration of long term funding by channeling demonstration projects.* (Published for the National Long Term Care Channeling Demonstration Program by the Technical Assistance Contractor.) Philadelphia: Temple University, Institute on Aging.

52. National Long-Term Care Channeling Demonstration. (1986, July). *The planning and operational experience of the channeling projects,* vols. 1, 2. Plainsboro, NJ: Mathematica Policy Research, for the U.S. Dept. of Health and Human Services.

53. Quinn, *Triage.*

54. Ansak, M. L., and Zawadski, R. T. (1983). On Lok CCODA: A consolidated model. In Zawadski, *Community-based systems of long term care,* pp. 147–170; Ansak, M. L. (1983). On Lok Senior Health Services: A community care organization for dependent adults. *PRIDE Inst J* 2(1):7–12; Yordi, C. L., and Waldman J. (1982, Sept.). *A comparative study on the quality and cost of long term care for the frail elderly: The research design and sampling methodology* (On Lok Technical Report no. 306) San Francisco: On Lok; and Zawadski, R. T., and Ansak, M. L. (1983). Consolidating community-based long-term care: early returns from the On Lok demonstration. *Gerontologist, 23:*364–369;

55. Zawadski, R. T., Shen, J., Yordi, C., and Hansen, J. C. (1984, Dec.). *On Lok's CCODA: A research and development project: Final report, 1978–83.* San Francisco: On Lok. Quote from p. 2-1.

56. Ansak and Zawdski, On Lok CCODA.

57. Zawadski, Shen, Yordi, and Hansen, *On Lok's CCODA.*

58. Shen, J., and Zawadski, R. T. (1981, Dec.). Long term care costs in a consolidated model. (On Lok Technical Report no. 302). San Francisco: On Lok.

59. Ibid.

60. Zawadski, Shen, Yordi, and Hansen, *On Lok's CCODA.*

61. Ibid.

62. Ibid.

63. Ibid., pp. 4–15, 16.

64. Social Security Amendments of 1983, Section 603(c) of the Conference Report.

65. On Lok Senior Health Services (winter 1986). *On Lok News;* and On Lok announcement (Oct. 1986). On Lok Senior Health Services (spring 1986). *On Lok News;* and On Lok announcement, On Lok Senior Health Services risk-based long term care initiative, July 13, 1987.

66. Walsh, M. L. W., Sr. (1965). *With a great heart.* New York: St. Vincent's Hospital; and Ollstein, R., Haggerty, E. C., and Rosenthal, P. (1976). St. Vincent's Hospital and Medical Center of New York. *NY State J Med, 76:*306–309.

67. Brickner, P. W., Duque, T., Kaufman, A., et al. (1975). The homebound aged: A medically unreached group. *Ann Intern Med, 82:*1–6.

68. American College of Physicians. (1986). Home health care. Position paper. *Ann Intern Med, 105:*454–460; Koren, M. J. (1986). Home care—who cares? *NEJM, 314:*917–920; and Rovner, J. (1986, May 31). Long-term care: The true 'catastrophe.' *Congressional Quarterly,* pp. 1227–1231.

69. Brickner, *Home health care for the aged,* pp. 90–91.

70. Chelsea-Village Program Files. New York, St. Vincent's Hospital.

71. Department of Community Medicine. (1987). *Chelsea-Village Program 14-Year Report* New York: St. Vincent's Hospital.

72. Brickner, *Home health care for the aged,* p. 23.

CHAPTER 7

1. Winston, E. (1969). Homemaker service and social welfare. In *Readings for homemaker service.* New York: National Council for Homemaker Services.

2. Werner, A. A. (1965). Homemaker services. In *Encyclopedia of social work.* Washington, DC: National Association of Social Workers. Quote from p. 382; Aalberts, N. (1986). Overview. *Caring, 5:*5–6; Spiegel, A. D., and Domanowski, G. F. (1983). Beginnings of home health care: A brief history. *PRIDE Inst J, 2*(3):28–33; and U.S. Dept. of Health and Human Services. (1980). *A model curriculum and teaching guide for the instruction of the homemaker-home health aide.* Washington, DC: U.S. Dept. of Health and Human Services.

3. National HomeCaring Council. (1981). *History of homemaker-home health aide services.*

4. Spiegel and Domanowski, Beginnings of home health care, p. 32.

5. Ibid.; and Cherkasky, M. (1949). The Montefiore Hospital home care program. *Am J Pub Health, 39:*163–166.

6. Crystal, S. (1984). Preface. In *The management of publicly financed home care.* New York: New York City Human Resources Administration.

7. National HomeCaring Council, *History of homemaker–home health aide services.*

8. Moore, F. M., and Layzer, E. (1983). Supporting the homemaker-home health aide as a valuable player on the home care team. *PRIDE Inst J, 2*(3):19–23.

9. Ibid.

10. *Ford Foundation Letter 16:*1; 1985.

11. Robinson, N. (1986). Standard setting and accreditation. *Caring, 5:*34–39.

12. New York City Dept. for the Aging. (1983, Oct.). *Year 1 of a proposed four-year plan.* New York: New York City Dept. for the Aging; Hall, H. D. (1986). The definition and role of the paraprofessional in home care. *Caring, 5*(4):8–10; New York City Dept. for the Aging. (1986, October). Proposed home care plan for functionally impaired elderly under the New York State Expanded In-house Services for the Elderly Program [EISEP]. An addendum to the four-year plan for the Older Americans Act and New York State Community Services for the Elderly Program; and Spiegel, A. D. (1983). *Home health care.* Owings Mills, MD: National Health Publishing.

13. Jennings, M. C., and Krentz, S. E. (1985). Financing care for the elderly: Federal government programs. In *Financing quality care for the elderly: The hospital research and educational trust,* pp. 63–93. Chicago: American Hospital Association.

14. Hall, The definition and role of the paraprofessional in home care; and Hall, H. D. (1983). The National HomeCaring Council's standards for paraprofessional services: A critical guide. *PRIDE Inst J, 2*(3):24–25.

15. Hall, The National HomeCaring Council's standards for paraprofessional services, p. 24.

16. Hall, The definition and role of the paraprofessional in home care, p. 10.

17. Clark, A.N.G., Mankikar, G. D., and Grey, I. (1985). Diogenes syndrome: A clinical study of gross neglect in old age. *Lancet, 1:*366–368.

18. Hall, The definition and role of the paraprofessional in home care.

19. Fine, D. R. (1986). The home as the workplace. *Caring, 5:*(4)12–19.

20. State Education Department and the Bureau of Home Economics Department (1975). *Health occupations education: Home health assisting, program development guide no. 4.* Albany, NY: University of the State of New York.

21. Liu, K., Manton, K., and Liu, B. (1985, Apr. 23). *Home care expenses for non-institutional elderly with ADL and IADL limitations.* Unpublished manuscript.

22. Health Care Financing Administration. (1981, Jan.). *Long-term care: Background and future directions* (Pub. no. 81-20047). Washington, DC: Dept. of Health and Human Services.

23. Trager, B. (1968). *San Francisco Health Service: Position paper regarding health paraprofessionals.* Typescript, pp. 2–3.

24. Morlock, M. (1966). *Homemaker services: History and bibliography.* Washington, DC: U.S. Government Printing Office.

25. National HomeCaring Council, *History of homemaker–home health aide services,* p. 38.

26. Starr, J. E. (1985, Oct. 13). Testimony to forum on homemaker-home health aide issues. Las Vegas NV, Foundation for Hospice and Homecare. Cited in *Caring, 5*(4) (1986) :29.

27. Mootz, A. (1986). Do we support standards in the homemaker/home health aide field? *Caring, 5*(4):32–33.

28. Starr, J. E. (1986). Testimony to forum on homemaker-home health aide issues. Cited in *Caring, 5*(4):30.

29. Robinson, Standard setting and accreditation, p. 35.

30. Johnson-Pawlson, J., and Goodwin, M. (1986). Total approach to nurse aide training. *Provider, 12:*14–18.

31. Moore and Layzer, Supporting the homemaker-home health aide.

32. Ibid., p. 20.

33. *A model curriculum and teaching guide for the instruction of the homemaker-home health aide.* New York: National HomeCaring Council, 1982.

34. National HomeCaring Council, *History of homemaker–home health aide services.*

35. Robinson, Standard setting and accreditation.

36. Kanoti, G. A. (1985). Home care: A shifting of ethical responsibilities. *Cleveland Clin Q, 52:*351–354. Quote from p. 354.

37. Adapted from patient records of Chelsea-Village Program, St. Vincent's Hospital.

38. Lerea, L. E., and LiMauro, B. F. (1982). Grief among healthcare workers: A comparative study. *J Gerontology, 37:*604–608. Quote from p. 607.

39. Ibid., p. 607.

40. Adapted from patient records of Chelsea-Village Program, St. Vincent's Hospital.

41. Brickner, P. W. (1978). *Home health care of the aged.* New York: Appleton-Century Crofts, pp. 101–102.

42. Browdie, R., and Turwoski, A. (1986). The problems of providing services to the elderly in their own homes. In A. O. Pelham and W. F. Clark (Eds.), *Managing home care for the elderly.* New York: Springer. pp. 31–46.

43. Fine, The home as the workplace.

44. DiCicco-Bloom, B., and Coven, C. R. (1981). *Innovative approaches: Group work with personal care workers of the homebound elderly.* St. Vincent's Hospital Department of Community Medicine, New York, p. 1.

45. Ibid., p. 9.

46. Lonergan, E. C. (1982). *Group intervention.* New York: Jason Aronson.

47. DiCicco-Bloom and Coven, *Innovative approaches,* pp. 18–19.

48. St. George, J., and DiCicco-Bloom, B. (1985). Using dramatization to train caregivers for the elderly. *Nursing Outlook, 33:*302–304. Quote from p. 302.

49. Davis, K., and Rowland, D. (1986). *Medicare policy: New directions for health and long term care.* Baltimore, MD: Johns Hopkins Univ. Press; and Cohen, J. (1983, Jan.). *Public programs financing long term care* (Urban Institute Working Paper no. 1466-18). Washington, DC: Urban Institute.

50. Office of the Actuary, Health Care Financing Administration [HCFA]. (1985, Aug.). *Health care Financing Program statistics: Analysis of state Medicaid program characteristics, 1984.* Baltimore, MD: Dept. of Health and Human Services.

51. O'Shaughnessey, C., Price, R., and Griffith, J. (1985, Oct. 17). *Financing and delivery of long-term care services for the elderly* (Doc. 85-1033 EPW). Washington, DC: Congressional Research Service, Library of Congress; and Raphael, C. (1986, Feb. 14). Deputy Administrator, Medical Assistance Program, New York City Human Resources Administration. Testimony before the City Council Committee on Aging.

52. Caro, F. G., and Blank, A. (1985, May). *Home care in New York City.* New York: Community Service Society.

53. Caro, F. G. (1984, Sept. 6). *Structure and operation of New York City Human Resources Administration home care programs* [draft]. New York: Community Service Society.

54. Haslanger, K. (1984, Nov.). Two-tiered contracting in New York City. In *The management of publicly financed home care.* New York: New York City Human Resources Administration, pp. 65–72.

55. Caro, *Structure and operation of NYC Human Resources Administration home care programs.*

56. Ibid.

57. Ibid.

58. Ibid.

59. O'Shaughnessy, Price, and Griffith, *Financing and delivery of long-term care services for the elderly.*

60. Office of the Actuary, HCFA, *Health Care Financing Program Statistics.*

61. Gornick, M., Greenberg, J. N., Eggers, P. W., et al. (1985, Dec.). Twenty years of Medicare and Medicaid: Covered populations, use of benefits, and program expenditures. In Office of Research and Demonstrations, Health Care Financing Administration. *Health Care Financing Review, 1985 Annual Supplement: 20 Years of Medicare and Medicaid.* Baltimore, MD: U.S. Dept. of Health and Human Services.

62. Spiegel, *Home health care.*

63. O'Shaughnessy, Price, and Griffith, *Financing and delivery of long-term care services for the elderly.*

64. Spiegel, *Home health care.*

65. O'Shaughnessy, Price, and Griffith, *Financing and delivery of long-term care services for the elderly.*

66. Ibid., p. 30.

67. Ibid.

68. Ibid.

69. Davis and Rowland, *Medicare policy.*

70. Spiegel, *Home health care.*

71. U.S. Dept. of Health and Human Services. (1982, May 6). Press release.

72. Bonanno, J. B. (1984). Legislation regarding health care for the older veteran. In T. Wetle and J. Rowe (Eds.), *Older veterans: Linking VA and community resources,* pp. 49–68. Cambridge, MA: Harvard Univ. Press.

73. MacAdam, M. A., and Piktialis, D. S. (1984). Mechanisms of access and coordination. In Wetle and Rowe (Eds.), *Older veterans,* pp. 159–203; and Bang, A., Morse, J. H., and Campion, E. W. (1984). Transition of VA acute care hospitals into acute and long term care. In Wetle and Rowe (Eds.), *Older veterans,* pp. 69–91.

74. Davis and Rowland, *Medicare policy.*

CHAPTER 8

1. Browdie, R., and Turwoski, A. (1986). The problems of providing services to the elderly in their own homes. In A.O. Pelham and W. F. Clark (Eds.), *Managing home care for the elderly.* New York: Springer, pp. 31–46; Cantor, M. (1979). Neighbors and friends. *Research on Aging, 1:*434–436; and Pelham, A. L., and Clark, W. F. Introduction. In Pelham and Clark (Eds.), *Managing home care for the elderly,* pp. 1–11.

2. Liu, K., Manton, K., and Liu, B.. (1985, Apr. 23). *Home care expenses for non-institutionalized elderly with ADL and IADL limitations.* Unpublished ms. Cited in C. O'Shaughnessy, R. Price, and J. Griffith, (1985, Oct. 17). *Financing and delivery of long-term care services for the elderly* (Doc. 85-1033 EPW). Washington, DC: Congressional Research Service, Library of Congress, Government Division, p. 12; and Health Care Financing Administration. (1981, Jan.). *Long-term care: Background and future directions* (HCFA 81-20047). Washington, DC: Dept. of Health and Human Services.

3. Davis, K., and Rowland, D. (1986). *Medicare policy: New directions for health and long-term care.* Baltimore, MD: Johns Hopkins Univ. Press.

4. U.S. General Accounting Office. (1981, Oct. 26). *Improved knowledge base would be helpful in reaching policy decisions on providing long-term, in-home services for the elderly* (HRD-82-4). Washington, DC: U.S. GAO.

5. Brickner, P. W. (1978). *Home health care for the aged.* New York: Appleton-Century-Crofts, pp 27–28.

6. Ibid., pp. 29–30.

7. Stuart, M. R., and Snope, F. C. (1981). Family structure, family dynamics, and the elderly. In A. R. Somers and D. R. Fabian (Eds.), *The geriatric imperative.* New York: Appleton-Century-Crofts, pp. 137–152; Brody, E. M., Johnsen, P. T., Fulcomer, M. C., et al. (1983). Women's changing roles and help for elderly parents: Attitudes of three generations of women. *J Gerontology, 38*(5):597–607; Brody, E. M., and Schoonover, C. B. (1986). Patterns of parent-care when adult daughters work and when they do not. *Gerontologist, 26*(4):372–381;

Brody, E. M., Kleban, M. H., Johnsen, P. T., et al. (1987). Work status and parent care: A comparison of four groups of women. *Gerontologist, 27:*201–208; and Poulshock, S. W., and Deimling, G. T. (1984). Families caring for elders in residence: issues in the measurement of burden. *J Gerontology, 39*(2):230–239.

8. Stuart, and Snope, Family structure, family dynamics, and the elderly, p. 144.

9. Brody, E. M., and Brody, S. J. (1981). New directions in health and social supports for the aging. In M. A. Lewis (Ed.), *The aging: Medical and social supports in the decade of the 80's,* pp. 35–48. New York: Third Age Center, Fordham University.

10. Davis and Rowland, *Medicare policy.*

11. Brody, Johnsen, Fulcomer et al., Women's changing roles and help for elderly parents.

12. Lipman, A. (1979). *Impact of demographic changes of family: Recent advances in gerontology.* Amsterdam: Excerpta Medica.

13. Glasse, L. (1983, March). *Family caregiving and the elderly: Policy recommendations and research findings.* Albany, NY: New York State Office for the Aging.

14. Cantor, M., and Johnson, J. (1978, Nov.). *The informal support system of the "familyless" elderly: Who takes over?* Paper presented at the annual meeting of the Gerontological Society, Dallas, TX.

15. Brotman, H. (1982). *Every ninth American.* Special report prepared for the U.S. Special Committee on Aging. Washington, DC.

16. Shanas, E. (1979). Social myth as hypothesis: The case of the family relations of old people. *Gerontologist, 19:*3–9; and Shanas, E. (1979). The family as a social support system in old age. *Gerontologist, 19:*169–174.

17. Brody, Johnsen, Fulcomer et al., Women's changing roles and help for elderly parents; Brody and Schoonover, Patterns of parent-care when adult daughters work and when they do not; and Marks, M. (1987). The family dimension in long term care: An assessment of stress and intervention. *PRIDE Inst J, 6*(2): in press.

18. Cantor, M. (1984, Jan. 24). The family: A basic source of long-term care for the elderly. In P. H. Feinstein, M. Gornick, and J. N. Greenberg (Eds.), Long-term care financing and delivery systems: Exploring some alternatives [Conference Proceedings]. Washington, DC: Health Care Financing Administration, U.S. Dept. of Health and Human Services, p. 110.

19. Menken, J. (1985). Age and fertility: How late can you wait? *Demography, 22:*469–483;

20. Cantor, The family, p. 108.

21. Sheehan, N. W. (1986). Informal support among the elderly in public senior housing. *Gerontologist, 26*(2):171–175; and Ingersoll, B., and Antonucci, R. (1983, Aug.). Support networks among the middle aged and elderly: Asset or liability? Paper presented at the American Psychological Association meeting, Anaheim, CA.

22. Antonucci, R. (1984). Personal characteristics, social support and social behavior. In R. Binstock and E. Shanas (Eds.), *The handbook of aging and social sciences,* pp. 94–128. 2nd ed. New York: Van Nostrand Reinhold.

23. Young, C. L., Goughler, D. H., and Larson, P. J. (1986). Organizational volunteers for the rural frail elderly: outreach, case finding, and service delivery. *Gerontologist, 26*(4):342–344.

24. Spiegel, A. D. (1983). *Home health care.* Owings Mills, MD: National Health Publishing; and Robinson, B. C. (1983, Nov.). Characteristics of the convalescing home bound elderly. Paper presented at the annual meeting of the Gerontological Society of America, San Francisco, CA.

25. Cantor, M., and Little, V. (1984). Social care and the aging. In Binstock and Shanas, *Handbook of aging and social science,* pp. 745–781.

26. Lombardi, T. (1980, June 2). *Long term home health care in New York State: The experience of the Lombardi Program to date* [report of the symposium]. New York: St. Vincent's Hospital and Medical Center; Lombardi, T. (1986, Sept.). *Nursing Home Without Walls. Long term care at home.* Albany, NY: NY State Senate Health Committee; and New York State Senate Health Committee. (1985, Sept. 1). *Nursing Home Without Walls: An Update* (Health Bulletin #75-E). Albany, NY: NY State Senate Health Committee.

27. Koff, T. (1982). *Long-term care: An approach to serving the frail elderly.* Boston: Little Brown.

28. Shanas, the family as a social support system.

29. Ibid.

30. Fine, D. (1986). The home as workplace: Prejudice and inequity in home health care. *Caring, 5:*(4)12–20. Quote from p. 13.

31. Poulshock and Deimling, families caring for elders in residence.

32. Frankfather, D. L., Smith, M. J., and Caro, F. G. (1981). *Family care of the elderly: Public initiatives and private obligations.* Lexington, MA: Lexington Books/D.C. Heath.

33. Choi, T., LaVohn, J., and Christensen, M. (1983). Health specific family coping index for non-institutional care. *Am J Pub Health, 73:*1275–1277.

34. Robinson, B. C. (1983). Validity of a caregivers strain index. *J Gerontology, 38:*344–348.

35. Senator Bill Bradley [D-NJ]. Respite Care Training. 99th Congress, S.2586.

36. Eustis, N. N., Greenberg, J. N., and Patten, S. K. (1984). *Long-term care for older persons: A policy perspective.* Monterey, CA: Brooks/Cole.

37. Bregman, A. (1980). Living with progressive childhood illness: Parental management of neuromuscular disease. *Social Work in Health Care, 5:*387–408.

38. Koff, *Long-term care.*

39. Eustis, Greenberg, and Patten, *Long-term care for older persons;* Callahan, J. J., and Wallack, S. S. (1981). *Reforming the long-term care system.* Lexington, MA: Lexington Books/D.C. Health; and Meltzer, J., Farrow, F., and Richman H. (1981). *Policy options in long-term care.* Chicago: Univ. of Chicago Press.

40. Wetle, T., and Evans, L. (1984). Serving the family of the elder veteran. In T. Wetle and J. Rowe (Eds.), *Older veterans: Linking VA and community resources,* pp. 231–259. Cambridge, MA: Harvard Univ. Press.

41. Maryland Office on Aging. (1977). *Caring for elderly relatives.* Baltimore MD: Maryland Office on Aging.

42. Whitfield, S. (1981). *Report to the General Assembly on the family support demonstration project.* Baltimore: Maryland Office on Aging.

43. Wetle and Evans, Serving the family of the elder veteran.

44. Ibid.

45. Frankfather, Smith, and Caro, *Family care of the elderly.*

46. Barnes, R. F., Raskind, M. A., Scott, M., et al. (1981). Problems of families caring for Alzheimer's patients: Use of a support group. *J Am Geriatric Soc, 29:*80–85.

47. Spiegel, *Home health care;* and Hartford, M. E., and Parsons R. (1982). Groups with relatives of dependent adults. *Gerontologist, 22:*394–398.

48. Lonergan, E. C. (1982). *Group intervention.* New York: Jason Aronson.

49. Hartford and Parsons, Groups with relatives of dependent adults.

50. Department of Community Medicine. (1987). *Long term home health care at St. Vincent's Hospital: 14-year report.* New York: St. Vincent's Hospital; and Quirke, E., and Stahl, I. (1978). The social worker. In P. W. Brickner, *Home health care for the aged.* New York: Appleton-Century-Crofts.

51. Brickner, Home health care for the aged, pp. 120–123.

52. Ibid.

53. Cantor, The family.

54. Quam, J. K. (1983). Older women and informal supports: Impact on prevention. In J. Simson, L. B. Wilson, J. Hermalin, and R. Hess (Eds.), *Aging and prevention,* pp. 119–133. New York: Haworth Press. Quote from p. 128.

55. Blau, Z. (1983). *Old age in a changing society.* New York: Franklin Watts.

56. Hess, B. B. (1979). Sex roles, friendship and the life course. *Research on Aging, 1:*494–515.

57. Sheehan, Informal support among the elderly.

58. Cantor, The family.

59. Brody, S. J., Poulshock, W., and Maschiocchi, C. (1978). The family caring unit: A major consideration in the long-term support system. *Gerontologist, 18:*556–561.

60. Brody, E. (1966, Nov.). *Aging family.* Paper presented at the 19th annual meeting of the Gerontological Society, New York.

61. Zimmer, A. H., and Sainer, J. S. (1978, Nov.). *Strengthening the family as an informal support for their aged: Implications for social policy and planning.* Paper presented at the 31st annual scientific meeting of the Gerontological Society, Dallas, TX.

62. Frankfather, Smith, and Caro, *Family care of the elderly,* p. 72.

63. Glasse, Family caregiving and the elderly.

64. The 1983 Gallup Survey on Volunteering, Voluntary Action Leadership, winter 1984.

65. Crooks, J. B. (1981, summer). The role of women in volunteerism. *Voluntary Action Leadership,* pp. 22–28.

66. Cantor, The family; and Davis and Rawland, *Medicare policy.*

67. Spiegel, *Home health care.*

68. Netting, F. F., and Hinds, H. (1984). Volunteer advocates in long term care: Local implementation of a federal mandate. *Gerontologist, 24:*3–15.

69. Brickner, *Home health care for the aged.* Personal communication: Robin McCarty, CSW, Project Director, Village Visiting Neighbors, 371 Avenue of the Americas, New York, NY, 10014; July 1986.

70. History of Volunteer Chore Ministry. (1986). *Coordinators' Handbook.* Seattle, WA: Volunteer Chore Ministry; Caldwell, M. J. (1986, July 17). *Report to board of directors on volunteer chore ministry.* Seattle, WA: Catholic Community Services; and Chaffee, M. L. (1987). Volunteer chore ministry. *PRIDE Inst J, 6*(2): in press.

71. Cohen, A., Bertram, D. A., and Solomon, L. (1982). *A study of the feasibility of using senior volunteers in long term care.* Baltimore, MD: The Center for Hospital Finance and Management, The Johns Hopkins Medical Institutions.

72. Hillman, D. J. (1986). *Senior Volunteers: Project HELP* [Robert Wood Johnson Grant No. 08542] *Final Report.* New York: PRIDE Institute, St. Vincent's Hospital and Medical Center.

73. Cantor, The family.

74. Ibid., p. 111.

CHAPTER 9

1. U.S. Congress. Senate Subcommittee on Health, Committee on Finance. (1983, Nov. 3, 14). *Report of hearings on long-term care.* Washington, DC.

2. Report. Kansas Department of Social and Rehabilitation Services. Administrative Services. Information Services Section. Home and Community Board Services. Topeka, Kansas. September, 1986.

3. Carton, B. (1984, Sept. 9). Day care for elderly is an affordable alternative. *Washington Post.*

4. Weissert, W. G. (1979). Rationales for public health insurance coverage of geriatric day care: Issues, options, and impacts. *Journal of Health Politics, Policy and Law, 3:*555.

5. O'Brien, C. L. (1982). *Adult day care—a practical guide.* Monterey, CA: Wadsworth Health Sciences Division, p. 3.

6. U.S. Department of Health and Human Services, Health Care Financing Administration. (1981, Jan.). *Long term care: background and future directions.* Washington, DC: U.S. Dept. of Health and Human Services.

7. O'Brien, *Adult day care,* p. vi.

8. Weissert, Rationales for public health insurance coverage of geriatric day care.

9. Cohen, D., and Eisdorfer, C. (1986). *The loss of self: A family resource for the care of Alzheimer's disease and related disorders.* New York: W. W. Norton.

10. Mace, N. (1984). Report of a survey of day care centers. *PRIDE Institute J, 3*(3):38–43.

11. Carton, Day care for elderly; Mace, Report of a survey of day care centers; and U.S. House of Representatives, Subcommittee on Health and Long-Term Care, Select Committee on Aging. (1980, Apr. 23). *Adult day care programs.* Washington, DC: U.S. House of Representatives.

12. Abel, N. E. (1976). Daytime care lets elderly people stay home at night. *Modern Healthcare, 6:*23.

13. O'Brien, *Adult day care.*

14. Ibid.; and Greenblatt, M., and Chien, C. P. (1983). Depression in the elderly: Use of external support systems. In L. D. Breslau and M. R. Haug (Eds.), *Depression and aging: Causes, care and consequences,* pp. 193–207. New York: Springer.

15. Goupille, V. T. British geriatric day hospitals: Implications for America. In O'Brien, *Adult day care,* pp. 181–194. Quote from p. 181.

16. Greenblatt and Chien, Depression in the elderly.

17. O'Brien, *Adult day care;* and Weissert, W. G., Wan, T. T., and Livieratos, B. B. (1980, Feb.). *Effects and costs of day care and homemaker services for the chronically ill: A random experiment.* Washington, DC: Department of Health, Education and Welfare, National Center for Health Services Research.

18. Ibid.; U.S. Senate, Special Committee on Aging. (1977, Sept. 21). *Health care for older Americans: The alternatives issue, Part 5.* Washington, DC: U.S. Senate; and Weissert, W. G. (1978). Costs of adult day care: A comparison to nursing homes. *Inquiry, 15:*10.

19. O'Brien, *Adult day care;* U.S. House of Representatives, *Adult day care programs;* Weissert, Wan, and Livieratos, *Effects and costs of day care and homemaker services;* and Weissert, Costs of adult day care.

20. O'Brien, *Adult day care;* and U.S. House of Representatives, *Adult day care programs.*

21. O'Brien, *Adult day care.*

22. Weissert, Costs of adult day care.

23. O'Brien, *Adult day care.*

24. Ibid.; and U.S. House of Representatives, *Adult day care programs.*

25. O'Brien, *Adult day care.*

26. Sands, D. (1984). The Harbor Area adult day care center: A model program. *PRIDE Institute J, 3*(4):44–50.

27. Housing Authority of the Birmingham District (1986, Oct.). *Day Care for Adults.* Birmingham, AL.

28. O'Brien, *Adult day care.*

29. Ibid.

30. Ibid.; U.S. Dept. of Health and Human Services, *Long term care;* and U.S. House of Representatives, *Adult day care programs.*

31. O'Brien, *Adult day care.*

32. Gurewitsch, E. (1982, July–Aug.). Geriatric day care: The options reconsidered. *Aging,* pp. 21–26.

33. Weissert, Rationales for public health insurance coverage of geriatric day care.

34. Weissert, Wan, and Livieratos, *Effects and costs of day care and homemaker services.*

35. U.S. House of Representatives, *Adult day care programs.*

36. Gurewitsch, Geriatric day care.

37. U.S. House of Representatives, *Adult day care programs.*

38. Briefings. (Fall 1986). Center for Health Services and Policy Research, Northwestern University, Evanston, IL.

39. Ibid.

40. McCoin, J. M. (1983). *Adult foster homes.* New York: Human Sciences Press.

41. Steinhauser, M. B. (1978, Nov.). *Family home care program: A study of geriatric foster care services as an alternative housing environment in Illinois.* Springfield, IL: Sangamon State University.

42. Ibid.

43. Ibid.

44. U.S. Dept. of Health and Human Services, *Long term care.*

45. Greenblatt and Chien, Depression in the elderly.

46. Sherman, S. R., and Newman, E. S. (1979, July). Role of the caseworker in adult foster care. *Social Work,* pp. 324–328.

47. McCoin, *Adult foster homes.*

48. Roecker, M. A., and Dillon, P. W. (1971, Dec.). *Foster family homes for adults.* Olympia, WA: State of Washington Social and Health Services Department.

49. Volland, P. J. (1983). *Final report. The Johns Hopkins Hospital Community Care Program.* The Robert Wood Johnson Foundation. November 1, 1978–December 31, 1982. Baltimore, MD: Johns Hopkins Hospital; and Gottdenker, A. J. (1983, June). *A review of the methodology of the cost analysis performed by the community care program project.* Report issued by Laventhol & Horwath, CPAs, New York.

50. Volland, *Final report.*

51. Ibid., p. 44.

52. State of North Dakota Legislative Assembly, House Bill Number 1314, signed by the Governor March 7, 1983.

53. North Dakota Department of Human Services. Data obtained June 1, 1984.

54. State of North Dakota, House Bill no. 1314.

55. Steinhauser, *Family home care program.*

56. Ibid.

57. Newman, E. S., and Sherman, S. R. (1979–80). Foster-family care for the elderly: Surrogate family or mini-institution? *International Journal of Aging and Human Development, 10:*165.

58. Ibid.

59. Roecker and Dillon, *Foster family homes for adults.*

60. McCoin, *Adult foster homes.*

61. Sherman and Newman, Role of the caseworker in adult foster care.

62. McNulty, E. G., and Holderby, R. A. (1983). *Hospice—a caring challenge.* Springfield, IL: Charles C Thomas, p. vii.

63. Ibid.

64. Munley, A. (1983). *The hospice alternative.* New York: Basic Books, p. xi.

65. Ibid.; McNulty and Holderby, *Hospice;* and Saunders, C. (1981, June). The hospice: Its meaning to patients and their physicians. *Hospital Practice,* pp. 93–108.

66. Munley, *The hospice alternative.*

67. Ibid.

68. McNulty and Holderby, *Hospice.*

69. Reiss, K. (1982, Mar. 22). *Hospice care: A federal role?* Washington, DC: Congressional Research Service; and Enck, R. E. (1987). The role of physicians in hospice care. *J. for Physicians in Home Care, 1*(1):52–53.

70. New York State Senate, Committee on Aging. (1982, Sept.). *Hospice: Its concept and legislative development.* Albany, NY: NY State Senate.

71. Gibson, D. E. (1984). Hospice: Morality and economics. *Gerontologist, 24:*4.

72. Data obtained from the National Hospice Organization, 1985.

73. Saunders, The hospice; and Gibson, Hospice.

74. McNulty and Holderby, *Hospice.*

75. NY State Senate, *Hospice.*

76. Reiss, *Hospice care;* and Gibson, Hospice.

77. Greer, D. S., Mor, V., Birnbaum, H., et al. (1983, Nov.). *National Hospice Study Preliminary Final Report Extended Executive Summary.* McLean, VA: National Hospice Organization; and Kane,

R., Bernstein, L., Wales, J., et al. (1984). A randomized controlled trial of hospice care. *Lancet,* pp. 890–894.

78. Kane, Bernstein, Wales et al., A randomized controlled trial of hospice care.

79. Gwyther, L. (1986). What is respite care? *PRIDE Inst J, 5*(3):4–6. Quote from p. 4.

80. Ibid.; and Marks, R. (1987). The family dimension in long term care: An assessment of stress and intervention. *PRIDE Inst. J, 6*(2): in press.

81. O'Brien, *Adult day care;* New York State Senate, Committee on Aging and Select Committee on Interstate Cooperation. (1981, July). *Perspectives on respite care for the elderly.* Albany, NY: NY State Senate; and Perdue, J. (1984). Respite care for the frailer disabled elderly. *PRIDE Inst J, 3*(4):31–37.

82. NY State Senate, *Perspectives on respite care for the elderly;* and Foundation for Long Term Care. (1982, Feb.). *Respite care for the frail elderly, final report.*

83. Wilson, D., and Ellis, V. (1984, Apr.–June). Respite care. *Long Term Care Currents, 7:*7.

84. Crozier, M. C. (1982, Sept.–Oct.). Respite care keeps elders at home longer. *Perspectives on Aging,* pp. 11–13.

85. Foundation for Long Term Care, *Respite care for the frail elderly.*

86. Ibid.

87. Tysboula, S. (1984). Housing options for the elderly in France: Creative responses in the face of economic and demographic changes. *PRIDE Inst J, 3*(3):25–30.

88. NY State Senate, *Perspectives on respite care for the elderly.*

89. Hasselkus, B. R., and Brown, M. (1983). Respite care for community elderly. *American Journal of Occupational Therapy, 37:*83.

90. Crozier, Respite care keeps elders at home longer.

91. Wilson and Ellis, Respite care.

92. Ibid.

93. Dunn, L. (1986). Senior respite care program. *PRIDE Inst J, 5*(3):7–12.

94. Foundation for Long Term Care, *Respite care for the frail elderly.*

95. NY State Senate, *Perspectives on respite care for the elderly.*

96. Foundation for Long Term Care, *Respite care for the frail elderly.*

97. Wilson and Ellis, Respite care.

98. Rossman, I. (1977, March). Options for Care of the Aged Sick. *Hospital Practice,* pp. 107–116.

99. New hospital units found to help elderly at home. (1984, Dec. 27). *Boston Globe,* p. 10.

100. Folsom, J. C. (1980, July 16). Rehabilitation Psychiatry Offers Long-Range Payoffs. *Hospitals,* pp. 59–61.

101. Gwyther, What is respite care?; Dunn, Senior respite care program; French, C. J. (1986). The development of special services for victims and families burdened by Alzheimer's disease. *PRIDE Inst J, 5*(3):19–27; and Sanborn, B. (1986). San Diego's Alzheimer's Family Center. *PRIDE Inst J, 5*(3):13–18.

102. Arling, G., and McAuley, W. J. (1983). The feasibility of public payments for family caregiving. *Gerontologist, 23:*300.

CHAPTER 10

1. Smith, B. K. (1977). *The pursuit of dignity.* Boston: Beacon Press.

2. Ibid.

3. Hubbard, L. (1984). *Housing options for older Americans.* Washington, DC: American Association of Retired Persons [AARP].

4. Report on the New York State Institute on State Housing Policy for the Elderly. Convened by the State Office for the Aging, Division of Housing and Community Renewal and Department of State, October 18–20, 1978.

5. Callahan, J., Jr. (1982). Selected issues in home health care. New York, United Hospital Fund Conference, April 6, 1982.

6. Lane, L. (1983). Understanding long term care policy and the consequences for reimbursement. In *New Dollars for Long Term Care: Proceedings from the PRIDE Institute Conference, December 1982. PRIDE Inst J, 2*(2):7–16. Quote from p. 7.

7. Chellis, R. D., Seagle, J. F., Jr., and Seagle, B. M. (1982). *Congregate housing for older people: A solution for the 1980's.* Lexington, MA: Lexington Books.

8. New York State Senate Committee on Aging. (1982, Nov.) *Shared housing for the elderly.* Albany: NY State Senate; and Woodard, A. (1982). Housing the elderly. *Society, 19:*52.

9. American Public Health Association, Subcommittee on Standards for Housing the Aged and Infirm. (1953). *Housing an aging population.* Lancaster, PA: Lancaster Press.

10. Data provided by the U.S. Census Bureau based on the 1980 Census Report.

11. Chellis, Seagle, and Seagle, *Congregate housing for older people;* and Lawton, H. P., and Hoover, S. L. (1981). *Community housing choices for older Americans.* New York: Springer (1981).

12. Weiner, J. M. (1986). Financing and organizational options for long-term care reform: Background and issues. *Bull NY Academy of Medicine, 62:*75–86. Quote from p. 77.

13. Ramian, K.M.S. (1982). The needs for housing of the elderly. *Danish Med Bull, 29:*119.

14. Montgomery, J. E., Stubbs, A. C., and Daly, S. S. (1980). The housing environment of the rural elderly. *Gerontologist, 20:*444.

15. Ibid.; New York State Office for the Aging. (N.D.). *Building crime prevention into community development.* Albany, NY: NY State Office for the Aging; and Nofz, M. P. (1986). Social services for older rural Americans: Some policy concerns. *J Natl Assn of Social Workers, 31:*85–91.

16. Mayer, N. S., and Lee, O. (1981). Federal home repair programs and elderly homeowners' needs. *Gerontologist, 21:*312.

17. Callahan, Selected issues in home health care.

18. Woodard, Housing the elderly.

19. Sumichrast, M., Shafer, R. G., and Sumichrast, M. (1984). *Planning your retirement housing.* Washington, DC: AARP.

20. Parson, H. M. (1981). Residential design for the aging. *Human Factors, 23:*39.

21. Lawton, M. P. (1981). An ecological view of living arrangements. *Gerontologist, 21:*59.

22. Byerts, T. O., and Heller, T. (1985, Apr. 15). *Longitudinal research on congregate public housing.* Chicago, IL: Art and Urban Planning, College of Architecture, Univ. of Illinois.

23. Chellis, Seagle, and Seagle, *Congregate housing for older people.*

24. Lawton, An ecological view of living arrangements.

25. Byerts and Heller, *Longitudinal research on congregate public housing;* Csank, J. Z., and Zweig, J. P. (1980). Relative mortality of chronically ill geriatric patients with organic brain syndrome, before and after relocation. *J Am Geriat Soc, 28:*76; and Henig, J. R. (1981). Gentrification and displacement of the elderly: An empirical analysis. *Gerontologist, 21:*67.

26. Tissue, T., and McCoy, J. L. (1981). Income and living arrangements among poor aged singles. *Soc Sec Bull, 44:*3.

27. Brown, R., and Lieff, J. D. (1982). A program for treating isolated elderly patients living in a housing project. *Hosp & Comm Psych, 33:*147.

28. Lawton, An ecological view of living arrangements.

29. Ibid.

30. Tissue and McCoy, Income and living arrangements among poor aged singles.

31. Ibid.

32. Somers, A. R. (1985, July-Aug.). Two decades later: A strange silence. *Health Progress,* p. 19.

33. New York State Office for the Aging, *Building crime prevention into community development.*

34. Chapman, N. J., and Lieff, J. D. (1982). A program for treating isolated elderly patients living in a housing project. *Hosp & Comm Psych, 33:*147.

35. Ibid.

36. Sumichrast, M., Shafer, R. G., and Sumichrast, M. (1984). *Planning Your Retirement Housing.* Washington, DC: AARP, p. 3.

37. Ramian, The needs for housing of the elderly.

38. Sumichrast, Shafer, and Sumichrast, *Planning your retirement housing.*

39. Tissue and McCoy, Income and living arrangements among poor aged singles; Collins, G. (1984, Jan. 5). Care for far-off elderly: Sources of help. *New York Times;* and Livingston, M. (Ed.). (1979, January). *Forum III: Housing for the retired. A report of the Federal National Mortgage Association Conference.* Washington, DC: Federal National Mortgage Assn.

40. Parson, Residential design for the aging.

41. Lawton, M. P. (1980). *Social and medical services in housing for the aged.* Rockville, MD: National Institute of Health.

42. Chellis, Seagle, and Seagle, *Congregate housing for older people;* Woodard, Housing the elderly; and Sumichrast, Shafer, and Sumichrast, *Planning your retirement housing.*

43. Livingston, *Forum III.*

44. Sumichrast, Shafer, and Sumichrast, *Planning your retirement housing.*

45. Nasar, J. L., and Farokhpay, M. (1985). Assessment of activity priorities and design preferences of elderly residents in public housing: A case study. *Gerontologist, 15:*251–257.

46. Mor, V., Sherwood, S., and Gutkin, C. (1986). A national study of residential care for the aged. *Gerontologist, 26:*405–417.

47. Chellis, Seagle, and Seagle, *Congregate housing for older people;* and Ruchlin, H. S., and Morris, J. N. (1987). The Congregate Housing services program. *Gerontologist, 27:*87–91.

48. Summary Reports of the Committee Chairmen. (1981, Dec.). 1981 White House Conference on Aging, Washington, DC.

49. Chellis, Seagle, and Seagle, *Congregate housing for older people.*

50. American Public Health Association, *Housing an aging population.*

51. Subcommittee on Housing, Committee on Banking and Currency, U.S. Senate. (1956, Jan. 4). *Housing for the aged.* Washington, DC: Committee on Banking and Currency.

52. American Public Health Association, *Housing an aging population;* and Subcommittee on Housing, *Housing for the aged.*

53. American Public Health Association, *Housing an aging population.*

54. Ibid.

55. Ibid.

56. Ibid.

57. Subcommittee on Housing, *Housing for the aged.*

58. Butler, R. N. (1975). *Why survive? Being old in America.* New York: Harper & Row.

59. Chellis, Seagle, and Seagle, *Congregate housing for older people.*

60. Bennett, N. E. (1982, July 1). Responsibility for long-term care rests with private sector. *Hospitals.*

61. Vladeck, F. (1986, Aug.). *Housing for the elderly.* Document prepared for the Department of Community Medicine, St. Vincent's Hospital, New York. Typescript.

62. Milgram, G. (1983, Dec. 6). *Housing assistance to low- and moderate-income households.* Washington, DC: Congressional Research Service.

63. Sumichrast, Shafer, and Sumichrast, *Where will you live tomorrow?*

64. Lawton and Hoover, *Community housing choices for older Americans.*

65. Montgomery, Stubbs, and Daly, The housing environment of the rural elderly; Nofz, Social services for older rural Americans; and Struyk, R. J. (1980). Housing adjustments of relocating elderly households. *Gerontologist, 20:*45.

66. Mayer and Lee, Federal home repair programs and elderly homeowners' needs.

67. Letter to Senate Special Committee on Aging, April 1983.

68. Spar, K. (1981, July 21). *Federal weatherization programs.* Washington, DC: Congressional Research Service.

69. *The Congressional Record.* (1984, Jan. 30). Washington, DC: Government Printing Office, p. 5472.

70. Data provided by the U.S. Census Bureau.

71. Hinrichsen, G. (1985). The impact of age-concentrated, publicly-assisted housing on older people's social and emotional well-being. *J Gerontology, 40:*758–760.

72. Vanhorenbeck, S. (1982, June 21). *Housing programs affecting the elderly: A history and alternatives for the future.* Washington, D.C: Congressional Research Service.

73. Section 202, Federal Housing Act of 1959.

74. U.S. Dept. of Housing and Urban Development. (1979, Jan.). *Housing for the elderly and handicapped: The experience of the Section 202 program from 1959 to 1977.* Washington, DC: HUD.

75. U.S. Dept. of Housing and Urban Development. (1982). *The costs of HUD multifamily programs.* Washington, DC: U.S. Government Printing Office, 1982.

76. Turner, M. A. (1985). Buildup housing for the low income elderly: Cost containment in the Section 202 Program. *Gerontologist, 25:*271–277.

77. U.S. Dept. of Housing and Urban Development, Notice H81-65, Nov. 12, 1981.

78. Perspective on Aging. National Council on the Aging. March-April 1986.

79. Section 8, Federal Housing Act of 1974.

80. DePalma, A. (1983, Sept. 4). Housing that cares about the elderly. *New York Times.*

81. Vladeck, *Housing for the elderly.*

82. Brickner, P. W. (1978). *Home health care for the aged.* New York: Appleton-Century-Crofts, p. 181.

83. Scholen, K. (1986). *The role of home equity in financing long term care: A preliminary exploration.* Madison, WI: National Center for Home Equity Conversion, and Waltham MA: The Health Policy Center of Brandeis University; Jacobs, B. (1986). The national potential of home equity conversion. *Gerontologist, 26:*496–504; and Kenny, K., and Belling, B. (1987). Home equity conversion: A counseling model. *Gerontologist, 27:*9–12.

84. Scholen, K. (1985, Sept.). *Homemade pension plans: Converting home equity into retirement income.* Madison, WI: National Center for Home Equity Conversion.

85. Sumichrast, Shafer, and Sumichrast, *Planning your retirement housing;* and Butler, *Why survive?*

86. Musson, N. (1982). *The national directory of retirement residences: Best places to live when you retire.* New York: Frederick Fell; and Dobkin, L. (1983). *Shared housing for older people: A planning manual for match-up programs.* Philadelphia, PA: National Shared Housing Resource Center.

87. Dobkin, *Shared housing for older people.*

88. Ibid.

89. Vladeck, *Housing for the elderly.*

90. Chellis, Seagle, and Seagle, *Congregate housing for older people;* and Malozemoff, I. K., Anderson, J. G., and Rosenbaum, L. V. (1978). *Housing for the elderly: An evaluation of the effectiveness of congregate residences.* Boulder, CO: Westview Press.

91. Chellis, Seagle, and Seagle, *Congregate housing for older people;* Lawton, M. P., Moss, M., and Grimes, M. (1985). The changing service needs of older tenants in planning housing. *Gerontologist, 25:*257–264; and Topics in corporate planning. *Hospitals,* (1980, Mar. 1), pp. 68–72.

92. Lawton and Hoover, *Community housing choices for older Americans.*

93. Ehrlich, P., Ehrlich, I., and Woehlke, P. (1982). Congregate housing for the elderly: Thirteen years later. *Gerontologist, 22:*399–403.

94. Malozemoff, Anderson, and Rosenbaum, *Housing for the elderly;* and Topics in corporate planning.

95. Regnier, V., and Gelwicks, L. E. (1981). Preferred supportive services for middle to higher income retirement housing. *Gerontologist, 21:*54.

96. U.S. Senate Special Committee on Aging. (1983, May 25). *Life care communities: Promises and problems.* Washington, DC: U.S. Government Printing Office.

97. Nofz, Social services for older rural Americans.

98. Turner, Buildup housing for the low income elderly.

99. Chellis, Seagle, and Seagle, *Congregate housing for older people;* Malozemoff, Anderson, and Rosenbaum, *Housing for the elderly;* and Regnier and Gelwicks, Preferred supportive services for middle to higher income retirement housing.

100. Chellis, Seagle, and Seagle, *Congregate housing for older people;* Lawton, *Social and medical services in housing for the aged;* and Malozemoff, Anderson, and Rosenbaum, *Housing for the elderly.*

101. Chellis, Seagle, and Seagle, *Congregate housing for older people;* and Malozemoff, Anderson, and Rosenbaum, *Housing for the elderly.*

102. Ehrlich, Ehrlich, and Woehlke, Congregate housing for the elderly.

103. Chellis, Seagle, and Seagle, *Congregate housing for older people;* Freister, K., and Mose, J. R. (1981). On the evaluation of health factors in high-rise buildings. *Zbl Bakt Hyg, I Abt Orig, B172:*332; and U.S. Senate Special Committee on Aging. (1984, March). *Developments in aging.* Washington, DC: U.S. Government Printing Office.

104. Vladeck, *Housing for the elderly.*

105. Data obtained from the New York State Department of Social Services, January 1984.

106. Rankin, N. (1985). Enriched housing: A program of home and care. *PRIDE Inst J, 4:*34–40.

107. DePalma, Housing that cares about the elderly.

108. Musson, *The national directory of retirement residences.*

109. Adelmann, N. E. (1981). *Directory of life care communities.* New York: H. W. Wilson Co.

110. Zibart, E. (1983, July 24). Development built around health services survives stormy start. *Washington Post.*

111. *Lifecare Industry, 1984.* Bulletin issued by Laventhol and Horwarth, Certified Public Accountants. Philadelphia, PA, 1984.

112. Hunt, M. E., Feldt, A. G., Marans, R. W., et al. (1984). *Retirement communities: An American original.* New York: Haworth Press.

113. Butler, *Why survive?*

114. Adelmann, *Directory of life care communities.*

115. Ibid.

116. Rudnitsky, H., and Konrad, W. (1983, Aug. 29). Trouble in the Elysian field. *Forbes,* pp. 58–59; and Thorpe, N. (1983, Sept. 2). Communities for retirees on rise again. *Wall Street Journal,* p. 1.

117. American Public Health Association, *Housing an aging population;* and Sumichrast, Shafer, and Sumichrast, *Planning your retirement housing.*

118. Rose, A. M. (1983, May). Continuing care retirement centers: An expansion opportunity. *Am Health Care Assoc J,* pp. 36–39.

119. Chapman and Lieff, A program for treating isolated elderly patients.

120. Branch, L. G. (1987). Continuing care retirement communities: Self-insuring for long-term care. *Gerontologist, 27:*4–8; and Streimer, R. A. (1986). Innovative financing and delivery options for long term care. In T. Fox (Ed.), *Long Term Care and the Law,* pp. 37–48. Owings Mills, MD: National Health Publishing.

121. Kane, J. E. (1986). Growth must meet diversified demand. *Provider, 12:*8–11.

122. Sumichrast, Shafer, and Sumichrast, *Planning your retirement housing;* Hartzler, J. E. (1981, winter). Life care: A new component in the health care delivery system. *Health Care Rev;* Rudnitsky and Konrad, Trouble in the Elysian field; and U.S. Senate Special Committee on Aging, *Life care communities.*

123. Adelmann, *Directory of life care communities.*

124. Winkle Voss, H. E., and Powell, A. V. (1984). *Continuing care retirement communities: An empirical, financial and legal analysis.* Homewood, IL: Irwin.

125. U.S. Senate Special Committee on Aging, *Life care communities;* Adelmann, *Directory of life care communities;* and Rudnitsky and Konrad, Trouble in the Elysian field.

126. Thorpe, Communities for retirees on rise again.

127. Weiner, Financing and organizational options for long-term care reform; and Kane, Growth must meet diversified demand.

128. Lanahan, M. B. (1983). Life care retirement centers: A concept in development. *PRIDE Inst J, 2*(2):41.

129. Foderaro, L. W. (1986, Oct. 19). Should Penn South co-ops go private? *New York Times.*

130. A college provides housing for elderly. (1983, May 5). *New York Times,* May 5, 1983.

131. Christensen, B. G. (1982, July 1). "Hospital apartments" afford security to area's elderly. *Hospitals,* pp. 74–76.

132. Woodard, Housing the elderly.

133. King, W. (1983, Dec. 12). Desegregation stirs dismay in two Texas housing projects. *New York Times.*

134. Churchill, W., cited in Woodard, Housing the elderly.

135. Sumichrast, Shafer, and Sumichrast, *Planning your retirement housing.*

CHAPTER 11

1. Committee on Nursing Home Regulations, Institute of Medicine. (1986). *Improving the quality of care in nursing homes.* Washington, DC: National Academy Press.

2. Health Care Financing Administration [HCFA]. (1983, June 13, and 1985, Oct. 31). Medicare and Medicaid programs long-term care survey. *Federal Register, 51:*21550–21558, and *Federal Register, 50:*45584; and Balcerzak, S. J. (1985, Winter). UPDATE: The new long-term care survey process. *J Long-Term Care Administration,* pp. 106–108.

3. HCF Administration. (1979, Jan.). *Title XIX, Grants to states for medical assistance programs.* Washington, DC: Medicaid Bureau, Department of Health, Education and Welfare, pp. 534, 535.

4. Division of Long Term Care, Health Resources Administration, Department of Health and Human Services.

5. Nightingale, F. (1970). *Florence Nightingale at Harley Street; Her reports to the governors of her nursing home 1854–4.* London: Dent.

6. Haber, C. (1983). *Beyond sixty-five.* New York: Cambridge University Press, p. 83.

7. Vladeck, B. C. (1980). *Unloving care.* New York: Basic Books.

8. Baltay, M. (1983, Sept. 21). *Nursing home legislation: Issues and policies* (Report no. 83-181 EPW) Washington, DC: Congressional Research Service, Library of Congress.

9. Haber, *Beyond sixty-five.*

10. Health Section, Education and Public Welfare Division. (1983, Apr. 1). *Nursing homes: An overview of the federal role including summary of major legislative proposals in the 97th Congress.* Washington, DC: Congressional Research Service, Library of Congress.

11. Vladeck, *Unloving care.*

12. Office of the Actuary, HCFA. (1985, Dec.). Data from the Medicaid Statistics Branch, *Health Care Financing Review, 1985 Supplement.* Baltimore, MD: HCFA.

13. Medicaid and nursing home care: Cost increases and the need for services are creating problems for the states and the elderly (GAO 1 PE-84-1 Report). Washington, DC: October 21, 1983, pp. 16–17; Branch, L., and Jette, A. M. (1982). A prospective study of long term care institutionalization among the aged. *Public Health, 72:*1373–1379; McCoy, J. L., and Edwards, B. E. (1981). Contextual sociodemographic antecedents of institutionalization among aged welfare recipients. *Medical Care, 19:*907–911; and Pepper, N. H. (1982). *Fundamentals of care of aging, disabled and handicapped in the nursing home.* Springfield, IL: Charles C Thomas.

14. Brody, J. A., and Foley, D. J. (1985). Epidemiologic considerations. In E. Schneider, C. J. Wendland; A. W. Zimmer, et al. (Eds.), *The teaching nursing home*, pp. 9–25. New York: Raven Press.

15. Long Term Care Case Mix Reimbursement Program. (1985, April). *PRI reference manual: RUG II Training Project.* Albany, NY: New York State Department of Health; Axelrod, D. (1986, Jan. 14). Letter regarding PRI. Albany, NY: New York State Department of Health; and *RUGS—Problems and recommendations.* (1987). Nursing Home Community Coalition of New York State.

16. Brody and Foley, Epidemiologic considerations.

17. Weissert, W., and Scanlon, W. (1982, Nov.). *Determinants of institutionalization of the aged.* Washington, DC: Urban Institute.

18. Branch and Jette, A prospective study of long term care institutionalization among the aged.

19. Vincent, L., Wiley, J. A., and Carrington, R. A. (1979). The risk of institutionalization before death. *Gerontologist, 19:*361–367.

20. Keeler, E. B., Kane, R. L., and Solomon, D. H. (1981). Short and long term residents in nursing homes. *Medical Care, 19:*363–369;

21. Medicaid and nursing home care.

22. Liu, K., and Manton, K. G. (1984). The characteristics and utilization pattern of an existing cohort of nursing home patients. *Gerontologist, 24:*70–76; and Adelman, R. D., Marron, K., Libow, L. S., et al. (1987). A community-oriented geriatric rehabilitation unit in a nursing home. *Gerontologist, 27:*143–146.

23. Kasl, S. V. (1972). Physical and mental health effects of involuntary relocation and institutionalization on the elderly: A review. *Am J Public Health, 63:*377–384; Borup, J. H. (1981). Relocation process: Stress attitudes informational network and problems encountered. *Gerontologist, 21:*501–511; and Borup, J. H. (1982). The effects of varying degrees of interinstitutional environmental change on long term care patients. *Gerontologist, 22:*409–147.

24. Lieberman, M. A., and Tobin, S. S. (1983). *The experience of old age.* New York: Basic Books; and Hunt, M. E., and Roll, M. K. (1987). Simulation in familiarizing older people with an unknown building. *Gerontologist, 27:*169–175.

25. Blackmun, J. (1980). Concurring opinion on O'Bannon vs. Town Court. United States Supreme Court Ruling delivered June 23, 1980. *United States Law Week, 48:*4846–4850.

26. Lieberman and Tobin, *The experience of old age.*

27. Schultz, R., and Brenner, G. (1977). Relocation of the aged: A review and theoretical analysis. *Journal of Gerontology, 32:*323–333; Allison-Cooke, S. (1982). Deinstitutionalizing nursing home patients: Potential versus impediments. *Gerontologist, 22:*404–408; Barney, J. L. (1973). *Patients in Michigan nursing homes.* Ann Arbor, MI: Michigan and Wayne State University, Institute of Gerontology; and Kahn, K. A., Hines, W., Woodson, A. S., et al. (1977). A multi-disciplinary approach to assessing the quality of care in long term care facilities. *Gerontologist, 17:*61–65.

28. Kahn, Hines, Woodson et al., A multi-disciplinary approach to assessing the quality of care in long term care facilities.

29. Allison-Cooke, Deinstitutionalizing nursing home patients.

30. Hodgson, J. H., and Quinn, J. (1980). The impact of the Triage health care delivery system upon client morale, independent living and cost of care. *Gerontologist, 20:*364–371.

31. Falek, J. I. (1986). Ensuring delivery of care as chosen. *Provider, 12:*8–11.

32. Waxman, H. M., Carner, E. A., and Berkenstock, G. (1984). Job turnover and job satisfaction among nursing home aides. *Gerontologist, 24:*503–109.

33. Unpublished data based on "cleaned" 1984 Medicare/Medicaid data. Washington, DC: HCFA, 1985.

34. Committee on Nursing Home Regulations, *Improving the quality of care in nursing homes.*

35. Bureau of Labor Statistics. (1985). *Employment projections for 1995.* Washington, DC: HCFA.

36. Vladeck, *Unloving care.*

37. Chee, P., and Kane, R. (1983). Cultural factors affecting nursing home care for minorities: a study of Black American and Japanese-American groups. *J Amer Geriatrics Soc, 31:*109–112.

38. U.S. Department of Health and Human Services. (1980, Dec.). *How to select a nursing home.* Washington, DC: HCFA.

39. Waxman, H. M., Klein, M., Kennedy, R., et al. (1985). Insitutional drug abuse: The overprescribing of psychoactive medications in nursing homes. In E. Gottheil, K. A. Druley T. E. Skoloda, and H. M. Waxman (Eds.), *The combined problems of alcoholism, drug addiction and aging,* p. 179. Springfield, IL: Charles C Thomas.

40. Ibid., p. 189.

41. Nightingale, *Florence Nightingale at Harley Street;* Weber, G. H. (1981). *Assisting the elderly in long term care. A book of readings.* Springfield, IL: Charles C Thomas, pp. 73–93; and Winslow, G. R. (1984). From loyalty to advocacy. A new metaphor for nursing. *Hastings Report, 14*(3):32–40.

42. Harmer, B., and Henderson, V. (1955). *Textbook of the principles and practice of nursing,* 5th ed. New York: Macmillan, p. 14.

43. Greenlaw, J. (1986). Nursing: Matching solution with need. *Provider, 12:*11–14.

44. Feldman, A. (1982, Oct.). Transfer: Nursing home to hospital. *Geriatric Nursing,* pp. 307–310; and Chenitz, W. C. (1983, Mar./Apr.). Entry into a nursing home as status passage: A theory to guide nursing practice. *Geriatric Nursing, 4*(2): 92–97.

45. Mechanic, D., and Aiken, L. H. (1982). A cooperative agenda for medicine and nursing. *NEJM, 307:*747–750.

46. Vladeck, *Unloving care,* pp. 19–20.

47. Dawes, P. L. (1981). The nurse's aide and the team approach in the nursing home. *J Geriatric Psychiatry, 14*(2):265–276.

48. Brickner, P. W. (1971). *Care of the nursing home patient.* New York: Macmillan.

49. Weber, *Assisting the elderly in long term care.*

50. Barney, L. (1983, Jan./Feb.). A new perspective on nurse's aides training. *Geriatric Nursing,* pp. 44–48.

51. Public Health Law 2803, Chapter V Medical Facilities 1031-78, part 731, section 731.1, Medical Services 5713H.

52. Code of Federal Regulations No. 42, Public Health, part 400 to end, October 1978.

53. Birkitt, P. D. (1980). The medical director in the nursing home. *Aged Care and Services Review, 2*(3):13–23.

54. Public Health Law 2803.

55. Schwartz, T. B. (1982). For fun and profit: How to install a first-rate doctor in a third-rate nursing home. *NEJM, 306:*743–744.

56. Butler, R. N. (1981). The teaching nursing home. *JAMA, 245:*1435–1437.

57. Libow, L. S., and Waife, M. M. (1985, Oct.). Geriatric medicine: A mechanism for quality care. *Business and Health,* pp. 38–40; and Riesenberg, D. (1987). The teaching nursing home: a golden annex to the ivory tower. *JAMA, 257:*3119–3120.

58. Ahronheim, J. C. (1983). Pitfalls of the teaching nursing home: A case for balanced geriatric education. *NEJM, 308:*334–336; and Schneider, E. L. (1983). Teaching nursing homes. *NEJM, 308:*336–337.

59. Rumsey, H. (1982). Gerontological nursing: A pleasant surprise. *Imprint, 29*(5):34–35.

60. Mezey, M. D., and McGivern, D. O. (1986). *Nursing, nurse practitioners: The evaluation of primary care.* Boston: Little, Brown.

61. Schneider, E., Wendland, C. J., Zimmer, A. W., List, N., and Ory, M. (Eds.). (1985). *The teaching nursing home.* New York: Raven Press.

62. Cohen, E. S. (1986). Sound ethics must balance programs. *Provider, 12:*4–7.

63. Hoffman, P. P., Marron, K. R., Fillet, H., et al. (1983). Obtaining informed consent in the teaching nursing home. *J Amer Geriatric Soc, 31:*565–596.

64. Dubler, N. N. (1986). Honoring preference for the right to die. *Provider, 12:*30–23.

65. Ratza, R. M. (1984). Informed consent in clinical geriatrics. *J Amer Geriatrics Soc, 32:*175–176.

66. Curran, W. J. (1983). Medical standards and medical ethics in utilization review for nursing homes. *NEJM, 308:*435–436.

67. Besdine, R. W. (1983). Decisions to withhold treatment from nursing home residents. *J Amer Geriatrics Soc, 31:*602–606; Annas, G. J. (1983). Nonfeeding: Lawful killing in California, homicide in New Jersey. *Hastings Center Report, 13:*19–20; Cassel, C. K., and Harrison, R. L. (1986). Views on use of life support methods. *Provider, 12:*24–28; Shannon, M., Spicuzza, T., and Rango, N. (1986). Issues in caring the elders with dementia. *Provider, 12:*30–34; and Wanzer, S. H., Adelstein, S. J., Cranford, R. E., et al. (1984). The physician's responsibility toward hopelessly ill patients. *NEJM, 310:*955–959.

68. Bayer, R., Callahan, D., Fletcher, J., et al. (1983). The care of the terminally ill: Morality and economics. *NEJM, 309:*1490–1494; Uhlmann, R.F., Clark, H., Pearlman, R.A., et al. (1987). Medical management decisions in nursing home patients. *Ann Intern Med, 106:*879–885.

69. Steinberg, A., Fitten, L., and Kachuck, B. A. (1986). Patient participation in treatment decision-making in the nursing home: The issue of competence. *Gerontologist, 26:*362–366; and Meier, D. E., and Cassel, C. K. (1986). Nursing home placement and the demented patient. *Ann Intern Med, 104:*98–105.

70. Spelder, L. A., and Strickland, A. L. (1983). *The last dance: Encountering death and dying.* Palo Alto, CA: Mayfield; Fisher, R. H., Nadon, G. W., Shedletsky, R., et al. (1983). Management of the dying elderly patient. *J Amer Geriatrics Soc, 31:*563–564; Hilfiker, D. (1983). Allowing the debilitated to die: Facing our ethical choices. *NEJM, 308:*716–719; Portnow, J., and Miller, G. (1983). Allowing the debilitated to die [Letter to the editor]. *NEJM, 309:*862–63; Saunders, C., and Baines, M. (1983). *Living with dying: The management of terminal diseases.* New York: Oxford University Press; and Wilkes, E. (Ed.). (1982). *The dying patient: The medical management of incurable and terminal illness.* Ridgewood, NJ: George A. Bogden.

71. Patient's right to starve upheld. (1984, Feb. 5). *New York Times;* Gov. Lamm asserts elderly, if very ill, have a "duty to die." (1984, March 29). *New York Times;* and U.S. program offers dying as alternative to hospital care. (1983, Nov. 6). *New York Times.*

72. Fisher, Nadon, Shedletsky, et al., Management of the dying elderly patient, p. 563.

73. Doherty, K., Stein, S., and Linn, M. (1982). *Gerontology and Geriatrics Education, 2:*191–197.

74. Department of Community Medicine. (1987). *Chelsea-Village Program, 14-Year Report.* New York: St. Vincent's Hospital.

75. Hilfiker, Allowing the debilitated to die, p. 718.

76. Gatza, G. A. (1986, Sept.). Living wills. *New York Medicine;* Living Will Declaration. New York: Society for the Right to Die; and Newsletter (1987, summer). New York: Society for the Right to Die.

CHAPTER 12

1. U.S. Dept of Commerce, Bureau of the Census. (1984, May). Decennial censuses of the population 1900–1980 and projections of the population of the United States by age, sex, and race: 1983 to 2080 [Advance Report]. *Current Population Reports,* ser. P-25, no. 952; and Rosenwaike, I., and Logue B. (1985). *The extreme aged in America.* Westport, CT: Greenwood Press.

2. O'Shaughnessy, C., Price, R., and Griffith, J. (1985, Oct. 17). *Financing and delivery of long-term care services for the elderly* (Doc. 85-1033 EPW). Washington, DC: Congressional Research Service, Library of Congress, p. 6.

3. National Center for Health Statistics, Dept. of Health and Human Services, (1983, Sept.). *Changing mortality patterns. Health services utilization and health care expenditures: United States 1978–2003* (Analytical and Epidemiological Studies Series 3, no. 23, Pub. no. [PHS] 83-1407). Washington, DC: Dept. of Health and Human Services.

4. Doty, P., Liu, K., and Weiner, J. (1985). An overview of long-term care. *Health Care Financing Review, 6:*70.

5. Health Care Financing Administration, Dept. of Health and Human Services (1981, Jan.). *Long term care: background and future directions.* (HCFA Pub. no. 81-20047). Washington, DC: U.S. Dept. of Health and Human Services; and Marks, R. (1987). The family dimension in long term care. *PRIDE Inst J, 6*(1): in press.

6. Soldo, B. J., and Manton, K. G. (1985). Health status and service needs of the oldest old: Current patterns and future trends. *Millbank Memorial Fund Q/Health and Society, 63:*210.

7. Kotranski, L., and Halbert, J. (1986, May). *Philadelphia's elderly: Their health and social status, utilization and access to services.* Philadelphia, PA: Philadelphia Health Management Corp.

8. Rowe, J. (1985). Health care of the elderly. *NEJM, 312:*827–835.

9. Kanin, G. (1966). *Remembering Mr. Maugham.* New York: Atheneum. p. 16.

10. U.S. Bureau of the Census. (1985). *Current Population Reports.* ser. P-60, no. 149. *Money income and poverty status of families and persons in the United States: 1984* [Advance data from the March 1985 Current Populations Survey]. Washington, DC: U.S. Govt. Printing Office; and Estes, C. L., and Lee, P. R. (1986). Health problems and policy issues of old age. In L. H. Aiken and D. Mechanic (Eds.), *Applications of social science to clinical medicine and health policy,* pp. 335–355. New Brunswick, NJ: Rutgers Univ. Press.

11. O'Shaughnessy, Price, and Griffith, *Financing and delivery of long-term care services for the elderly,* pp. 7–8.

12. Rosenwaike and Logue, *The extreme aged in America;* and Davis, K., and Butler, R.N. (1987). *Old, Alone and Poor.* Report of the Commonwealth Fund Commission on Elderly People Living Alone in New York.

13. (1985). Summary of the 1985 Federal and State Legislative Policy. Washington, DC: American Association of Retired Persons; and Korcok, M. (1985). Medical schools face challenge of preparing physicians to care for fast-growing elderly population. Medical news. *JAMA, 253:*1225–1231.

14. Barry, P. B., and Ham, R. J. (1985). Geriatric education: What the medical schools are doing now. *J Am Geriatrics Soc, 33:*133–135; and Tideiksaar, R., Libow, L. S., and Chalmers, M. (1985). House calls to older patients: The medical student experience. *PRIDE Inst J, 4*(3): 3–8.

15. *Gerontological Nurse Practitioner Educational Directory.* (1985). Boise, ID: Mountain State Health Corp.

16. Rogers, T., Metzger, L., and Bauman, L. (1984). Geriatric nurse practitioners: How are they doing? *Geriatric Nursing, 5:*51; and Capezuti, E. (1985). Geriatric nurse practitioners: Their education, experience, and future in home care. *PRIDE Inst J, 4*(3):9–14.

17. Scanlan, B. (1985). *Primary care tracks in long term home health care at Saint Vincent's Hospital. Chelsea-Village Program 13-year report.* New York: Dept. of Community Medicine, St. Vincent's Hospital.

18. *Chelsea-Village Program 14-year report.* (1987). New York: Dept. of Community Medicine, St. Vincent's Hospital.

19. Arenth, L. M., and Mamon, J. A. (1985). Determining patient needs after discharge. *Nursing Management, 16:*20–24.

20. Dronska, H. (1983). Focus: The role of case management in long term home health care. *PRIDE Inst J, 2*(4):19–20.

21. Thurow, L. C. (1985). Medicine versus economics. *NEJM, 313:*611–614. Quote from p. 612.

22. Addis, S. S. (1985). Setting goals and priorities. *Am J Public Health, 75:*1276–1280.

23. Ibid.

24. Kübler-Ross, E. (1969). *On death and dying.* New York: Macmillan.

25. Quirke, E., and Stahl, I. (1978). The social worker. In P. W. Brickner, *Long term home health care for the aged.* New York: Appleton-Century-Crofts, p. 69.

26. *Home Health Line, 11:*273–284, 1986; Blumenthal, D., Schlesinger, M., Drumheller, P. B., et al. (1986). The future of Medicare. *NEJM, 314:*722–728; and Iglehart, J.K. (1987). Second thoughts about HMOs for Medicare patients. *NEJM, 316:*1487–1492.

27. Hospital Research and Educational Trust. (1986). *Emerging trends in aging and long-term care services.* Chicago, IL: American Hospital Assn.

28. Wolf, R. (1983). Medicare policy and regulatory control. *PRIDE Inst J, 2:*3–6.

29. Dept. of Health and Human Services report to the President. (1986, Nov. 19). *Catastrophic illness expenses.* Washington, DC; Senator Edward Kennedy (D-MA). (1987, Jan. 6). Health insurance coverage against catastrophic illness. S. 210; and Pear, R. A. Medicare shield for costly illness is voted by house. *The New York Times,* July 23, 1987.

30. Feder, J. (1987). Background on financial perspectives. Medicare's skilled nursing benefit. In B. C. Vladeck and G. J. Alfano (Eds.), *Medicare and extended care,* pp. 131–136. Owings Mills, MD: National Health Publ.

31. The other catastrophic cost (Editorial). *New York Times,* March 4, 1987; and Rovner, J. (1986, May 31). Long-term care: The true 'catastrophe'? *Congressional Quarterly Weekly Report,* pp. 1227–1231.

32. Sundwall, D. (1986). Federal legislation and initiatives in long term care. *PRIDE Inst J, 5:*7–13; and Fuchs, V. R. (1987). The counter revolution in health care financing. *NEJM, 316:*1154–1156.

33. Collier, E. (1986) Shaping a national policy for long term care. *PRIDE Inst J, 5:*5–6.

34. Ibid., p. 6.

35. Ibid., pp. 5–6.

36. Whitcomb, M. E. (1986). Health care for the poor—a public policy imperative. *NEJM, 315:*1220–1222; and Nutter, D. O. (1987). Medical indigency and the public health care crisis. *NEJM, 316:*1156–1158.

37. Sundwall, Federal legislation and initiatives in long term care.

38. Vladeck, B. (1983). Two steps forward, one back: The changing agenda of long term care reform. *PRIDE Inst J, 2*(3):3–10.

39. Sen. Lloyd Bentsen, The Home and Family Services Health Care Act of 1975. S. 2591; Rep. Claude Pepper, H. R. 12676; Rep. Dan Rostenkowski, Committee on Ways and Means Proposal of April 6, 1976; and Rep. Edward I. Koch, The National Home Health Care Act of 1975. H. R. 9829.

40. Docksai, R. F. (1984). Federally-funded demonstration projects: Following the path of S.234. *PRIDE Inst J, 3*(3):3–7.

41. *Home Health Line, 4* (1981) 15–16.

42. Letter, Senator Orrin Hatch to Mayor Edward I. Koch, April 22, 1982.

43. Sen. Orrin Hatch. (1981, Jan. 22). Community Home Health Services Act of 1981. 97th Cong., 1st sess. S.234, pp. 5–6.

44. Letter, Hatch to Koch.

45. *Home Health Line* (1981).

46. *Home Health Line, 3* (1980): 158–159

47. Grazier, K. L. (1985). The impact of reimbursement policy on home health care. *PRIDE Inst J, 5*(1):12–16. Quote from p. 13.

48. Van Gelder, S., and Bernstein, J. (1986). Home health care in the era of hospital prospective payment. *PRIDE Inst J, 5*(1):3–11; and U.S. Government Accounting Office. (1985, Feb. 21). Information requirements for evaluating the impacts of Medicare prospective payment on post-hospital long-term care services: preliminary report (PEMD-85-8). Washington, DC: GAO.

49. Bishop, C. E., and Stassen, M. (1986). Prospective reimbursement for home health care: context for an evolving policy. *PRIDE Inst J, 5*(1):17–26.

50. National Center for Health Statistics, *Changing mortality patterns;* and Spitler, B.J.C. (1981). Policies affecting older Americans. In R. H. Davis (Ed.), *Aging: Prospects and issues,* pp. 260–273. Davis, CA: Univ. of California Press.

51. O'Shaugnessy, Price, and Griffith, *Financing and delivery of long-term care services for the elderly,* p. ix.

52. Somers, A. (1982). Long-term care for the elderly and disabled. A new health priority. *NEJM, 307:*221–226.

53. Spitler, Policies affecting older Americans, p. 260.

54. Thurow, L. C. (1985). Medicine versus economics. *NEJM, 313:*611–614. Quote from p. 611.

55. Ruchlin, H. S., Morris, J. N., and Eggert, G. M. (1982). Management and financing of long-term care services. A new approach to a chronic problem. *NEJM, 306:*101–106. Quote from p. 102.

56. Willging, P. R., and Neuschler, E. (1982, July 1). Long-term care. Debate continues on future of federal financing of long-term care. *Hospitals,* pp. 61–66.

57. Thurow, Medicine versus economics, p. 612.

58. Doyle, A.C. (1907). Through the magic door. Tauchnitz Edition, p. 241.

Name Index

Aalberts, N., 340*n*2
Abel, N.E., 347*n*12
Abrahams, R., 312*n*49
Abramowitz, L., 329*n*176
Abrass, I.B., 320*n*29
Adami, H., 321*n*45
Adams, R.D., 327*n*140
Addams, Jane, 212
Addis, S.S., 358*nn*22, 23
Adelman, R.D., 355*n*22
Adelmann, N.E.,
    353*nn*109, 114, 115, 123;
    354*n*125
Adelstein, S.J., 357*n*67
Agre, J.C., 319*n*12
Ahronheim, J.C., 356*n*58
Aiken, L.H., 312*n*42;
    317*n*64; 356*n*45; 358*n*10
Albano, W.A., 112*n*;
    328*n*158
Albert, M.L., 326*n*120;
    327*n*124
Alfano, G.J., 313*n*57,
    315*n*13; 316*n*54;
    336*n*14; 337*n*23; 359*n*30
Alfrey, A.C., 326*n*101
Alibrandi, L.A., 334*n*135
Alksne, H., 331*nn*39, 52
Allison-Cooke, S., 314*n*69;
    355*nn*27, 29

Aloia, J.F., 320*n*33
Alzheimer, Alois, 85;
    322*n*14
Amaducci, L., 112*n*;
    326*n*108; 328*n*165
Anderson, G.F., 315*n*33
Anderson, J.G., 352*nn*90,
    94; 353*nn*99, 100, 101
Anderson, W.F., 321*n*3
Annas, G.J., 321*n*52;
    357*n*67
Ansak, M.L., 340*nn*54, 56
Antonucci, R., 344*nn*21,
    22
Antuono, P., 112*n*;
    326*n*108; 328*n*165
Aoki, F.Y., 332*n*88
Applebaum, R.A., 337*n*21;
    339*n*40
Applegate, W.B., 320*n*36
Arbogast, R.J., 49*n*
Arenth, L.M., 358*n*19
Arling, Greg, 241; 349*n*102
Armbrecht, H.J., 333*n*93
Aron, J.M., 112*n*
Aronson, M.K., 329*n*176
Artmann, H., 333*n*103
Asher, D.M., 325*n*78
Axelrod, D., 315*n*23;
    355*n*15

Babor, T.F., 335*n*143
Bach-Peterson, J., 336*n*7
Bahmanyar, S., 324*n*54
Bahr, Howard M., 124;
    331*n*48
Bailey, M.P., 331*nn*39, 52
Baines, M., 357*n*70
Baker, H., 321*n*46
Bal, D.G., 324*n*62
Balcerzak, S.J., 354*n*2
Ball, M.J., 324*n*54
Baltay, M., 354*n*8
Balter, M.B., 332*n*88
Bang, A., 314*n*68; 317*n*56;
    320*n*24; 343*n*73
Baranovsky, A., 321*n*45
Barberis, M., 310*n*1
Barboriak, J.J., 334*n*113
Barhydt, N.R., 339*n*39
Barnes, R.F., 329*n*174;
    345*n*46
Barnett, R.N., 320*n*32
Barney, J.L., 355*n*27
Barney, L., 356*n*50
Barry, P.B., 358*n*14
Barter, C.E., 319*n*16
Baum, A., 320*n*40
Bauman, L., 358*n*16
Baxter, R.J., 337*n*21;
    339*n*40

Bayer, R., 357n68
Bays, K.D., 312n42
Beck, J.C., 322n8; 323n48;
   326nn103, 113
Becker, H., 333n103
Becker, P.M., 318n1
Beckett, Katie, 196
Beckman, B., 319n23
Begg, T.B., 320n37
Beirne, K., 317n69
Belling, B., 313n53;
   352n83
Bennett, N.E., 351n60
Benson, D.F., 83–84; 112n;
   322n8; 323n47; 328n159
Bentsen, Sen. Lloyd,
   359n39
Bergmann, K., 321n3
Berkenstock, G., 355n32
Berman, D.E., 312n49;
   338n28
Bernstein, J., 316nn33, 48;
   339n42; 359n48
Bernstein, L., 349nn77, 78
Bertram, D.A., 346n71
Besdine, R.W., 316n53;
   318n3; 319n17; 357n67
Bick, K.L., 322nn3, 22
Binstock, R.H., 310n5;
   344n22
Birkitt, P.D., 356n53
Birnbaum, H., 338nn26,
   32; 339nn35, 37; 348n77
Bishop, C.E., 316nn37, 38,
   39–40; 359n49
Bissell, C., 332n85
Black, J., 191n; 192n
Blackmun, J., 355n25
Blake, Eubie, *xvi*
Blank, A., 336n6; 342n52
Blass, J.P., 112n; 328n165
Blau, Z., 345n55
Blazer, Dan G., 128;
   331nn61, 63
Blendon, R.J., 315n17;
   316n39
Blessed, G., 325n81
Block, L.H., 328n160
Blose, Irvin L., 119;
   329n2; 330nn12, 17, 33;
   332n70
Bluestone, E.M., 13;
   338n33

Blume, S.B., 334nn133, 135
Blumenthal, D., 358n26
Blusewicz, M.J., 333n101
Bockman, J.M., 325n72
Boller, F., 327nn122, 125,
   128
Bonanno, J.B., 319n24;
   343n72
Bondareff, W., 324n56
Bonstelle, S., 320nn40, 41
Borup, J.H., 314n69;
   335n4; 355n23
Bosman, H.B., 333n90;
   334n114
Botwinick, J., 333n97
Bourestom, N., 314n69;
   335n4
Bourn, P.G., 335n135
Bowen, D.M., 324n59;
   325nn81, 82
Bowen, F.P., 327n124
Bowen, Otis R., 300
Bradley, Sen. Bill, 205,
   305
Branch, L.G., 311n20;
   353n120; 354n13;
   355n18
Branson, M.H., 311n20
Braun, N., 337n16
Breckenridge, M.B.,
   322n23; 323n26
Bregman, A., 205; 345n37
Breitner, J.C.S., 325nn85,
   93
Brenner, G., 335n4;
   355n27
Breslau, L.D., 347n14
Brewer, V., 320n33
Brewster, Mary, 13
Brickfield, C.F., 311n16;
   318n87
Brickner, P.W., 311nn17,
   23; 319nn8, 14;
   327n139; 331n41;
   335nn1, 5; 336nn7, 10;
   340nn67, 69, 72;
   342n41; 343nn5, 6;
   345nn50, 51, 52;
   346n69; 352n82;
   356n48; 358n25
Brickner, R.M., 333n104
Bristow, L.R., 314n6;
   315n28

Brodows, B.S., 336n12;
   338n26
Brody, Elaine M., 203;
   211; 335n6; 336n7;
   343n7; 344nn9, 11, 17;
   346n60
Brody, H., 324n53
Brody, J.A., 311n18;
   355nn14, 16
Brody, J.E., 319n19
Brody, S.J., 310n2;
   312n34; 314n3; 346n59
Brotman, H., 344n15
Browdie, R., 342n42;
   343n1
Brown, B.B., 330n21
Brown, M., 349n89
Brown, P., 324nn65, 66,
   70
Brown, R., 324n65;
   325n76; 350n27
Brown, R.S., 339n40
Brown, T.E., 336n12;
   338n26
Brun, A., 323nn44, 46
Brunner, D., 314n11
Buchtel, H.A., 333n101
Budnick, L.D., 318n82
Buhler-Wilkerson, K.,
   311n32
Burack-Weiss, A., 336n7
Burger, M.C., 333n97
Burgio, K.L., 320n30
Burwell, B., 315n21
Butler, Robert N., 118;
   280; 315n26; 330n10;
   351n58; 353n113;
   356n56; 358n12
Butters, N., 333nn97, 102
Byerts, T.O., 350nn22, 25

Cahalan, D., 125n;
   331nn43, 56
Cala, L.A., 333nn101, 103,
   106
Caldwell, M.J., 346n70
Callahan, D., 357n68
Callahan, J.J., Jr., 312n49;
   337n21; 338n28;
   339n40; 350nn5, 17
Calne, D.B., 327n121

Camargo, C., 332*nn*75, 77
Campanini, T., 333*n*101
Campbell, A.H., 319*n*16
Campbell, A.J., 322*nn*17, 23; 323*n*25
Campion, E.W., 314*n*68; 317*n*56; 319*n*23; 320*n*24; 343*n*73
Cantor, Marjorie, 200, 202, 203, 210, 219; 335*n*6; 343*n*1; 344*nn*14, 18, 20, 25; 345*nn*53, 58; 346*nn*66, 73, 74
Caper, P., 313*n*54
Capezuti, E., 358*n*16
Capitman, J.A., 337*n*21; 339*nn*40, 42
Carey, Gov. Hugh, 156
Carner, E.A., 355*n*32
Caro, Frances G., 211; 335*n*6; 342*nn*52, 53, 55, 56, 57, 58; 345*nn*32, 45; 346*n*62
Carrington, R.A., 355*n*19
Carruth, B., 331*n*38
Carton, B., 346*n*3; 347*n*11
Caserta, M.S., 328*n*171
Cassel, C.K., 321*nn*43, 51; 357*nn*67, 69
Catalano, D.J., 336*n*6
Cato, 4
Cerf, J.J., 339*n*40
Chaffee, M.L., 314*n*70; 346*n*70
Chalmers, M., 358*n*14
Chapman, N.J., 350*n*34; 353*n*119
Charatan, F.B., 328*n*149
Chase, G.A., 325*n*85
Chatters, L.M., 336*n*7
Chee, P., 356*n*37
Chellis, R.D., 350*nn*7, 11, 23; 351*nn*42, 47, 49, 59; 352*nn*90, 91; 353*nn*99, 100, 101, 103
Chenitz, W.C., 356*n*44
Cherkasky, Martin, 13; 312*nn*34, 35, 36, 37; 338*n*33; 341*n*5
Chien, C.P., 347*nn*14, 16; 348*n*45
Choi, T., 345*n*33
Chow, W.S., 310*n*5

Christensen, B.G., 345*n*33; 354*n*131
Chumlea, W.C., 319*n*9
Churchill, W., 354*n*134
Cicero, 4
Ciompi, L., 334*nn*126, 127; 335*n*136
Cisin, H., 125*n*; 331*nn*43, 56
Claasen, R., 323*n*30
Clark, A.N.G., 341*n*17
Clark, E.O., 336*n*7
Clark, L.L., 312*n*33
Clark, R.F., 339*n*40
Clark, W.F., 342*n*42; 343*n*1
Coan, R.E., 337*n*23
Cohen, A., 346*n*71
Cohen, C., 312*n*34
Cohen, Donna, 98; 325*n*96; 326*n*98; 328*n*171; 346*n*9
Cohen, E.L., 325*n*81
Cohen, E.S., 321*n*51; 356*n*62
Cohen, G.D., 84; 322*n*13
Cohen, H.J., 318*n*1
Cohen, J., 342*n*49
Cohen, Wilbur J., 35–36; 315*nn*27, 29
Cohn, D., 329*n*187
Cohn, S.H., 320*n*33
Coke, Lord, 242
Coker-Vann, M., 324*nn*65, 70
Collier, Earl, 301; 359*nn*33, 34, 35
Collier, Merrick W., 229*n*
Collins, T., 320*n*36
Conney, T.G., 330*n*26
Coolidge, C.P., 320*n*26
Coppel, D., 328*n*171
Corrigan, E.M., 331*n*37
Corsellin, J.A.N., 326*n*109
Courtice, K., 329*n*174
Courville, C.B., 333*n*107
Coven, Carol R., 189–90; 329*n*180; 342*nn*44, 45, 47
Cox, M., 329*n*6
Coyle, J.T., 325*n*82
Cranford, R.E., 357*n*67
Crapper, D.R., 326*n*100

Creasey, H., 323*n*42
Cress, E.M., 319*n*12
Crooks, J.B., 346*n*65
Cross, P.S., 322*n*17
Crossley, H.M., 125*n*; 331*nn*43, 56
Crozier, M.C., 349*nn*84, 90
Crystal, S., 341*n*6
Csank, J.Z., 323*n*27; 350*n*25
Cummings, J., 112*n*; 323*n*47; 328*n*159
Curran, W.J., 357*n*66
Cutler, R.N., 325*n*95

Dahl, David S., 107; 328*nn*154, 155
Daly, S.S., 350*nn*14, 15; 351*n*65
Damasio, A.R., 112*n*; 324*nn*57, 58; 328*n*164
Damon, L.E., 335*n*4
Davies, Peter, 96; 325*nn*82, 83, 84, 86; 356*n*47
Davis, F.A., 328*n*148
Davis, J.S., 332*n*73
Davis, Karen, 28*n*; 53–54; 199; 310*n*4; 315*nn*25, 26; 316*nn*43, 55; 317*n*64; 318*nn*94, 95; 322*nn*17, 18, 19; 342*n*49; 343*nn*69, 74, 3; 344*n*10; 358*n*12
Davis, R.H., 359*n*50
Davison, A.N., 112*n*; 324*n*59; 326*n*108; 328*n*165
Deimling, G.T., 336*n*7; 344*n*7; 345*n*31
DeLong, M.R., 325*n*82
Demeter, S., 112*n*; 328*n*164
DePalma, A., 352*n*80; 353*n*107
Diamond, J., 329*n*176
Diamond, L.M., 312*n*49; 338*n*28
DiCicco-Bloom, Barbara, 189–90; 329*n*180;

DiCicco-Bloom (*Continued*)
334*n*121; 342*nn*44, 45,
47, 48
Dickens, Charles, 149;
335*n*2
Dickson, R., 327*n*138
DiClemente, Carlo C.,
140; 334*n*120
Dillon, P.W., 348*nn*48, 59
Dix, Dorothea, 212
Dobkin, L., 352*nn*86, 87, 88
Dobrof, Rose, 329*n*177;
336*n*6
Dobson, A., 315*n*31;
337*n*22
Docksai, R.F., 359*n*40
Doherty, K., 357*n*73
Domanowski, Gerard F.,
12; 311*n*29; 340*n*2;
341*nn*4, 5
Dono, J.E., 339*n*40
Donovan, D.M., 335*n*140
Dornbrand, L., 321*n*51
Doty, P., 357*n*4
Doyle, Sir Arthur Conan,
309; 360*n*58
Drinan, Cong. Robert F.,
224
Dronska, Harriet, 23–24;
314*n*71; 358*n*20
Droszcz, C.P., 112*n*;
328*n*158
Druley, K.A., 321*n*48;
329*n*181; 356*nn*39, 40
Drumheiler, P.B., 358*n*26
Dubler, N.N., 321*n*51;
328*n*167; 357*n*64
Dunn, D.D., 322*nn*17, 18,
19
Dunn, L., 329*n*186; 349*n*93
Duque, Sister Teresita,
323*n*24; 340*n*67
Durenberger, Sen. Dave,
318*n*93
Dustman, R.E., 333*n*101
Duthie, E.H., Jr., 332*n*81;
334*n*113

Eaton, S.B., 319*n*7; 321*n*46
Eckardt, M.J., 327*nn*135,
136, 137

Edwards, B.E., 354*n*13
Eggers, P.W., 28*n*; 313*n*56;
315*n*22; 343*n*61
Eggert, G.M., 336*n*12;
338*n*26; 360*n*55
Ehrlich, I., 352*n*93;
353*n*102
Ehrlich, P., 352*n*93;
353*n*102
Eidus, R., 336*n*6
Eisdorfer, Carl, 98;
312*n*34; 321*n*3; 325*n*96;
326*n*98; 328*n*171; 346*n*9
Eisert, M., 334*nn*126, 127;
335*n*136
Elizan, T.S., 327*nn*123,
125
Ellis, V., 349*nn*83, 91, 92,
97
Elston, R.C., 322*n*20
Enck, R.E., 348*n*69
Engel, B.T., 320*n*30
Engle, G.L., 318*n*1
English, J.T., 313*n*54
Epstein, A.M., 316*n*33
Esiri, M.M., 323*n*45
Esquirol, J.E.D., 84;
322*n*12
Estes, C.L., 315*n*24;
317*n*64; 358*n*10
Eustis, N.N., 345*nn*36, 39
Evan, L., 345*nn*40, 43, 44
Evashwick, C., 337*n*16

Fabian, D.R., 322*nn*7, 23;
335*n*3; 336*n*6; 343*n*7
Fahn, S., 327*n*130
Falek, J.I., 321*n*51; 355*n*31
Farley, Hugh T., 239
Farokhpay, Mitra, 248;
351*n*45
Farrow, F., 313*n*52;
318*n*99; 345*n*39
Featherstone, H.J., 112*n*;
327*n*125
Feder, J., 313*n*60; 336*n*14;
337*nn*20, 23; 359*n*30
Feifel, H., 311*n*22; 336*n*9
Feigenbaum, L.Z., 112*n*
Feinstein, P.H., 314*n*70;
317*n*71; 344*n*18

Feldman, A., 356*n*44
Feldman, R.G., 112*n*
Feldt, A.G., 353*n*112
Feller, B.A., 338*n*25
Ferris, S.H., 333*nn*93, 108
Fillenbaum, G.G., 319*n*23;
320*n*41
Fillet, H., 356*n*63
Fine, Doris R., 203–4;
341*n*19; 342*n*43; 345*n*30
Finkle, B.S., 334*n*116
Firman, J., 317*n*73
Fischer, C.M., 327*n*140
Fischer, W., 334*n*124
Fisher, R.H., 284;
357*nn*70, 72
Fisman, M., 324*n*54
Fitten, L., 321*n*43; 357*n*69
Fletcher, J., 357*n*68
Flinn, G.A., 333*nn*93, 108
Foderaro, L.W., 354*n*129
Foley, D.J., 355*nn*14, 16
Foley, W., 316*n*35
Folsom, J.C., 116;
329*nn*183, 185; 349*n*100
Folstein, Marshall F., 97;
325*nn*85, 93
Forbes, G.B., 332*n*79
Fordham, C., 311*n*25
Foster, S., 320*n*39
Fox, J.H., 323*n*30
Fox, Peter D., 14; 312*n*40
Fox, T., 318*n*97; 353*n*120
Francis, P.T., 324*nn*60, 63
Frank, O., 321*n*46
Frankfather, Dwight L.,
211; 345*nn*32, 45; 346*n*62
Freister, K., 353*n*103
French, C.J., 329*n*186;
349*n*101
Frengley, J.D., 320*nn*40,
41
Freudenheim, M., 318*n*81
Freund, Gerhard, 135;
333*n*94
Friedel, R.O., 321–22*n*3
Friesen, A.D.J., 328*n*157
Fuchs, V.R., 359*n*32
Fulcomer, M.C., 335*n*6;
343*n*7; 344*n*17
Fuld, P.A., 326*n*119
Fullerton, W., 313*n*52;
318*n*99

Gaitz, C.M., 322*n*20
Gajdusek, D.C., 323*n*49; 324*nn*61, 66, 69
Galanter, M., 333*n*96; 334*n*115; 335*nn*140, 143
Galen, 131
Gallego, D.T., 314*n*69; 335*n*4
Gambert, S.R., 319*n*23; 332*n*81; 334*n*113
Garraway, M., 327*n*138
Garry, P.J., 319*n*8
Garver, D.L., 329*n*4; 332*n*82; 334*nn*109, 110
Garvey, M., 337*n*16
Gatza, G.A., 321*n*50; 357*n*76
Gauner, G., 338*nn*26, 32; 339*nn*35, 37
Gaus, C.R., 316*n*39
Gelwicks, L.E., 352*n*95; 353*n*99
Gentry, D., 320*n*39
George, L.K., 319*n*23; 320*n*41
Georgeson, G., 316*n*54
Gershon, S., 112*n*; 328*n*159
Gibson, D.E., 348*nn*71, 73, 76
Gibson, P.H., 324*n*53
Gibson, R.E., 324*n*60
Gibson, R.M., 318*n*90
Gill, J.S., 333*n*91
Gilmore, A.J.J., 321*n*3
Girard, D.E., 330*n*26
Glasse, L., 344*n*13; 346*n*63
Glatt, M.M., 139; 330*nn*7, 25; 334*n*112
Glenn, N.D., 330*n*14
Go, R.C.P., 322*n*20
Goldfield, N., 312*n*49; 337*n*16; 338*n*28
Goldgaber, D., 324*n*54
Goldman, C.M., 314*n*3; 316*n*47
Goldman, P., 337*n*16
Goldsmith, M.F., 325*n*91
Goldsmith, S.B., 312*n*49; 337*n*16; 338*n*28
Goldstein, D.B., 329*n*1; 330*nn*19, 23; 331*n*51; 334*n*130

Goldstein, S., 318*n*2
Gomberg, Edith, 126, 127, 140, 141; 331*nn*35, 36, 40, 50, 59, 64; 332*nn*74, 83, 87; 334*nn*117, 122, 124
Goodspeed, N.B.H., 337*n*16
Goodwin, J.S., 319*n*8
Goodwin, M., 342*n*30
Gordon, Jack (J.R.), 140; 334*n*120
Gorelick, D.A., 333*n*96; 334*n*115
Gornick, J.N., 314*n*70
Gornick, M., 28*n*; 313*n*56; 315*n*22; 317*n*71; 343*n*61; 344*n*18
Gottesman, L.E., 313*n*63
Gottheil, E., 321*n*48; 329*n*181; 356*n*39
Goudsmit, J., 325*n*78
Goughler, D.H., 344*n*23
Gould, D.A., 315*n*13
Goupille, V.T., 347*n*15
Gowan, A.E., 310*n*4
Grahams, R., 338*n*28
Graves, S., 320*n*36
Grazier, Kyle L., 306; 316*n*34; 359*n*47
Green, B.R., 311*n*22; 336*n*9
Greenberg, George, 28*n*; 32*n*; 33*n*; 50*n*; 191*n*; 193*n*; 194*n*
Greenberg, J.N., 28*n*; 312*n*49; 313*n*56; 315*n*22; 317*n*71; 338*n*28; 343*n*61; 344*n*18; 345*nn*36, 39
Greenblatt, M., 347*nn*14, 16; 348*n*45
Greene, J.G., 329*n*184
Greenlaw, J., 321*n*51; 329*n*177; 356*n*43
Greer, D.S., 348*n*77
Grey, I., 341*n*17
Griffin, M.R., 319*n*11
Griffith, J., 314*nn*2, 8; 315*n*30; 316*nn*40, 42, 45, 49, 50; 317*nn*57, 67, 75; 342*nn*51, 59; 343*nn*63, 65, 66, 67, 68,

2; 357*n*2; 358*n*11; 359*n*51
Grimes, M., 352*n*91
Gross, H.W., 335*n*139
Groth-Junker, A., 336*n*12
Growdon, J.H., 325*n*81
Gruenberg, E.M., 321*n*3; 322*n*22
Grumme, T., 333*n*104
Gumb, Jackson, 223
Gupta, K.L., 319*n*23
Gurewitch, E., 347*nn*32, 36
Gurioli, C., 331*n*55
Gurland, B.J., 322*n*17
Gusella, J.F., 327*n*130
Guterman, S., 315*n*31; 337*n*22
Gutkin, C., 351*n*46
Gwyther, L., 349*nn*79, 81, 101

Haber, Carole, 268; 311*n*28; 354*nn*6, 9
Haberman, M.P., 331*nn*39, 52
Hachinski, Vladimir C., 100; 324*n*54; 326*nn*109, 112, 116, 117
Haddad, A.M., 321*n*51
Haddow, C.M., 53; 318*n*92
Hadley, E.C., 319*n*6
Haggerty, E.C., 340*n*66
Hakim, S., 327*n*140
Halamandaris, V.J., 175*n*
Halbert, J., 358*n*7
Hall, H.D., 177, 178, 179; 341*nn*14, 15, 16, 18
Hall, P., 331*n*42
Haltia, M., 323*n*30
Ham, R.J., 332*n*80; 335*n*4; 358*n*14
Hammerschmidt, J.P., 322*n*16
Hammond, J., 337*n*23
Haney, T., 320*n*39
Hansen, J.C., 340*nn*55, 57, 60, 61, 62, 63
Harford, T.C., 327*nn*135, 136, 137

Harmer, B., 356*n*42
Harrill, I., 321*n*46
Harrington, C., 312*n*49;
315*n*24; 338*n*28
Harrison, M.J.G.,
328*nn*148, 152
Harrison, R.L., 321*n*51;
357*n*67
Hartford, J.T., 327*n*134;
329*n*4; 330*n*27; 331*n*61;
332*nn*81, 85; 333*nn*90,
92, 93, 94, 95;
334*nn*120, 132, 134
Hartford, M.E., 336*n*7;
345*nn*47, 49
Hartzler, J.E., 353*n*122
Haskell, William L., 131;
332*nn*75, 77
Haskins, B., 339*n*42
Haslanger, K., 342*n*54
Hasselkus, B.R., 349*n*89
Hatch, Sen. Orrin G.,
303–5; 359*nn*42, 43, 44
Haug, M.R., 347*n*14
Havia, T., 321*n*44
Hay, A.W.M., 319*n*10
Haycox, J.A., 329*n*174
Heffernan, P.G., 314*n*69;
335*n*4
Heinrich, J., 311*n*32
Heinz, Sen. John, 38;
315*n*32; 316*n*48
Heller, T., 350*nn*22, 25
Hemsi, Loic, 113;
328*nn*168, 169, 170;
329*nn*175, 178, 182
Henderson, G., 324*n*53
Henderson, V., 356*n*42
Henig, J.R., 350*n*25
Hennekens, C.H.,
332*nn*75, 76
Hermalin, J., 345*n*54
Herman, S.P., 112*n*;
328*n*159
Heros, R.C., 326*n*111
Hess, B.B., 345*n*56
Hess, R., 345*n*54
Hesselbrock, M.N.,
335*n*140
Heston, Leonard L.,
97–98; 325*n*90; 326*n*97
Higgins, A., 324*n*54
Hildahl, V.K., 332*n*88

Hilfiker, David, 285;
357*nn*70, 75
Hill, T.C., 324*n*60
Hillman, Deborah, 216;
346*n*72
Hinchman, A., 329*n*179
Hinds, H., 346*n*68
Hines, W., 355*nn*27, 28
Hinrichsen, G., 352*n*71
Hodgson, J.H., 339*nn*45,
49; 355*n*30
Hoffman, P.P., 356*n*63
Hoffman, S., 319*n*11
Hoffmann, J.C., 312*n*44
Holderby, Robert A., 237;
348*nn*62, 63, 65, 68, 74
Holman, B.L., 324*n*60
Holmberg, L., 321*n*45
Holtzman, J.M., 335*n*4
Hoover, S.L., 350*n*11;
351*n*64; 352*n*92
Horn, J.L., 335*n*140
Horowitz, A., 336*n*6;
339*n*40
Horr, N.K., 328*n*166
Howard, J.T., 324*n*62
Hubbard, L., 349*n*3
Hughes, S., 336*n*12;
338*n*26
Hunt, M.E., 353*n*112;
355*n*24
Hunt, W.C., 319*n*8
Hyman, Bradley T., 91;
324*nn*57, 58
Hyman, M.M., 331*n*38

Igbal, K., 324*n*51
Iglehart, J.K., 313*n*54;
358*n*26
Ihara, Y., 323*n*47
Inberg, M.V., 321*n*44
Ingersoll, B., 344*n*21
Irish, D.P., 311*n*22; 336*n*9
Isenberg, Y., 331*n*41
Isreal, Y., 334*n*111

Jackson, J.S., 336*n*7
Jacobs, B., 317*n*71; 352*n*83
Jacobson, G., 325*n*87

Jahnigen, D.W., 329*n*177
Jansen, C., 321*n*46
Jarvik, Lissy F., 97; 112*n*;
322*n*20; 325*n*89;
328*nn*147, 149
Jaslow, S.P., 321*n*46
Javanovic, L., 337*n*16
Jellinek, E.M., 145;
335*n*142
Jellinger, K., 327*n*142
Jenkins, W.J., 332*nn*75, 78
Jennings, M.C., 316*n*48;
341*n*13
Jensen, F., 339*n*33
Jeremy, J., 332*nn*75, 78
Jette, A:M., 319*n*23;
354*n*13; 355*n*18
Johnsen, P.T., 335*n*6;
343*n*7; 344*nn*11, 17
Johnson, C.L., 336*n*6
Johnson, Jeffrey, 200;
344*n*14
Johnson, K.G., 314*n*70
Johnson, Pres. Lyndon, 35
Johnson-Pawlson, J.,
342*n*30
Jones, B., 333*n*98; 333*n*101
Josephson, K.R., 319*n*23;
320*nn*27, 41, 42
Judd, B.W., 326*nn*110,
115; 327*n*131
Judge, T.G., 321*n*3

Kachuck, N., 321*n*43;
357*n*69
Kaebler, C.T., 327*nn*135,
136, 137
Kaehny, W.D., 326*n*101
Kafetz, K., 329*n*6
Kahn, K.A., 355*nn*27, 28
Kalant, H., 334*n*111
Kallmann, F.J., 97; 325*n*88
Kane, E., 313*nn*57, 59
Kane, J.E., 353*n*121
Kane, R.L., and Kane,
R.A., 153; 310*n*9;
319*n*23; 320*n*29;
337*nn*19, 20; 338*n*29;
348–49*nn*77, 78; 355*n*20;
356*n*37
Kanin, Garson, 288; 358*n*9

Kanoti, George, 184; 342n36
Kasl, S.V., 355n23
Kastenbaum, R., 330nn8, 9, 20; 331n49; 334nn119, 127
Katz, S., 311n20
Katzman, Robert, 88; 112n; 322nn3, 4, 22; 323n37; 323n45; 324n61; 325nn80, 94; 326n102; 327nn121, 122, 145; 328n146
Kaufman, A., 340n67
Kay, D.W.K., 321n3; 322n20
Keele, M.S., 320n33
Keeler, E.B., 355n20
Keller, M., 331n55
Kelly, J.T., 315n31
Kelsey, J.L., 319n11
Kennedy, Pres. John F., 225
Kennedy, Sen. Edward, 359n29
Kennedy, R., 321n48; 329n181; 356nn39, 40
Kenny, K., 313n53; 352n83
Kessler, D., 312n34
Khadraturan, Z.S., 324n52
Khanna, J.M., 334n111
Kilmartin, T., 330n15
Kiloh, L.G., 327n133
King, L., 312n34
King, M.B., 327n134; 333n92
King, W., 354n133
Kingsbury, D.T., 325n72
Kistler, J.P., 326n111
Kitagawa, Y., 327n143
Kivlahan, D.R., 335n140
Klatzo, I., 326n99
Kleban, M.H., 344n7
Klein, M., 321n48; 329n181; 356nn39, 40
Kling, A., 322n7
Kluge, W., 333n104
Koch, Edward I., 303; 359nn39, 42, 44
Kodner, D.L., 310n10; 312n49; 318n89; 338n28; 339n51

Koff, 345n38
Kondo, J., 323n47
Konner, M., 319n7; 321n46
Konrad, W., 353nn116, 122; 354n125
Korcok, M., 358n13
Koren, M.J., 340n68
Kosterlitz, J., 317n62
Kotranski, L., 358n7
Kral, V.A., 87; 323n34
Kramer, M., 313n61
Krentz, S.E., 316n48; 341n13
Krishman, S.S., 326n100
Kro, Marlowe, 234n
Kübler-Ross, E., 358n24

Lambert, A., 332n72
Lanahan, M.B., 128
Lander, R., 321n1; 323n35
Lane, Laurence F., 49, 50; 317nn80, 81; 318nn84, 85, 86; 350n6
Langendorf, R., 312n34; 338n26
Large, G.W., 332n88
Largen, J.W., 327nn134, 136; 333n92
Larson, E.B., 112n; 327n125
Larson, P.J., 344n23
Larsson, T., 325n87
Lassen, N.A., 326nn109, 112
Lauerman, R.J., 335n143
LaVohn, J., 345n33
Lawton, M. Powell, 246; 350nn21, 24, 28, 29; 351nn41, 64; 352nn91, 92
Laxton, C., 337n17
Layzer, Emily, 183; 337n15; 341nn8, 9; 342nn31, 32
Lazenby, H., 317n65
Leach, B., 334n135
Leader, S., 316n36; 337n22
Leal-Sotello, M., 313n54
Learner, R.M., 336n12; 338n26

Lechich, A., 103n; 319n8; 337n18
Ledingham, J.G.G., 319n20
Lee, O., 350n16; 351n66
Lee, P.R., 315n24; 317n64; 358n10
Lefkowitz, Pearl, 122–23; 331n41
Lefton, E., 320nn40, 41
LeGendre, F.R., 326n101
LeGrain, P.M., 335n141
Leitschuh, T.H., 334n113
Lenke, B., 313n54
Lentz, W.N., 312n49; 338n28
Lerea, L. Eliezer, 186; 342nn38, 39
Levenson, D., 312n34
Leverenz, J., 325n96; 326n98
Levit, K.R., 318n90
Levkoff, S.E., 316n53
Lewis, M.A., 313n54
Libow, L.S., 321nn43, 53; 328n149; 355n22; 356n57; 358n14
Lichtig, L.K., 313n54
Lieberman, A.N., 326n118; 327nn126, 127, 129, 141
Lieberman, M.A., 319n13; 355nn24, 26
Lieff, J.D., 350nn27, 34; 353n119
Lifson, Art, 52; 318n91
LiMauro, Barbara F., 186; 342nn38, 39
Lind, S.E., 313n55
Linn, B.S., 335n4
Linn, M., 357n73
Linn, N.W., 335n4
Lipkowitz, R., 329n176
Lipman, A., 344n12
Lipsman, R., 312n50
List, N., 356n61
Little, V., 344n25
Liu, B., 341n21; 343n2
Liu, Korbin, 273; 341n21; 343n2; 355n22; 357n4
Livieratos, B.B., 337n23; 347nn17, 18, 19, 34
Livingston, M., 351nn39, 43
Lo, B., 321n51

Loeb, C., 326*nn*108, 110
Lofthouse, R., 324*n*65;
    325*n*76
Logue, B., 310*n*4; 311*n*18;
    357*n*1; 358*n*12
Lokich, J.J., 337*n*16
Lombardi, Tarky, Jr., 20,
    155–58, 158*n*; 338*n*30;
    344*n*26
Lonergan, E.C., 342*n*46;
    345*n*48
Long, C., 332*n*80
Lossinsky, 324*n*71
Love, A.H.G., 321*n*46
LoVerne, S., 112*n*;
    328*n*159
Luchi, R.J., 320*nn*40, 41
Lund, D.A., 328*n*171
Lundin, D.V., 332*n*86
Luxenberg, J., 112*n*
Lynch, H.T., 112*n*; 328*n*158

MacAdam, M.A., 316*n*54;
    320*n*24; 343*n*73
Mace, N.L., 328*n*166;
    346*n*10; 347*n*11
Maddox, George, 4;
    310*n*5; 330*n*13
Madigan, D., 315*n*21
Magno, Josefina B., 235,
    237
Majovski, L.V., 324*n*64
Malken, B., 321*n*45
Maloney, T.W., 315*n*17;
    316*n*39
Malozemoff, I.K.,
    352*nn*90, 94; 353*nn*99,
    100, 101
Mamon, J.A., 358*n*19
Mangiaracina, A.J.,
    312*n*44
Manheimer, D.I., 332*n*88
Mankikar, G.D., 341*n*17
Mann, D.M.A., 326*nn*103,
    105
Mann, T., 331*n*62
Manton, Kenneth G., 273;
    318*n*5; 341*n*21; 343*n*2;
    355*n*22; 358*n*6
Manuelidis, L., 324*n*65;
    325*n*76

Marans, R.W., 353*n*112
Marcy, M.L., 335*n*4
Marks, M., 344*n*17
Marks, R., 336*n*6; 349*n*80;
    358*n*5
Markson, E.W., 313*nn*57,
    59
Marron, K.R., 355*n*22;
    356*n*63
Marsden, C.E., 328*nn*148,
    152
Marsh, G.M., 324*n*64
Marshall, E., 336*n*6
Marshall, J., 326*nn*109,
    112
Martin, D.C., 319*n*23
Martin, J.B., 327*n*130
Maschiocchi, C., 346*n*59
Mastaglia, F.L., 333*nn*101,
    103, 106
Mather, J.H., 316*n*51
Mathis, Evelyn, 272*n*
Matsuyama, S.S., 322*n*20;
    325*n*89
Matsuzawa, Taiju, 89;
    323*n*43
Matusz, W., 318*n*88
Maugham, W. Somerset,
    288
May, M.I., 314*n*68
Mayer, J., 331*nn*44, 45, 60
Mayer, N.S., 350*n*16;
    351*n*66
Mayfield, D., 331*n*42
Mazziotta, J.C., 327*n*130
McAuley, Willing J., 241;
    349*n*102
McCaffrey, K., 312*n*49
McCarty, Robin, 213*n*;
    346*n*69
McCoin, J.M., 347*n*40;
    348*nn*47, 60
McCormack, J.J., 313*n*57
McCosh, L.M., 322*nn*17,
    23; 323*n*25
McCoy, J.L., 30, 31;
    350*nn*26; 351*n*39;
    354*n*13
McCusker, J., 336*n*12
McDowell, J.B., 319*n*23
McGivern, D.O., 356*n*60
McGuire, E.A., 332*n*82
McKinley, M.P., 325*n*72

McLeod, G., 331*n*42
McMahon, M., 260*n*
McNerney, W.J., 317*n*61;
    318*n*96
McNulty, Elizabeth G.,
    237; 348*nn*62, 63, 65,
    68, 74
McPherson, K., 313*n*54
McTernan, M.T., 314*n*3;
    316*n*47
Mechanic, D., 317*n*64;
    356*n*45; 358*n*10
Meese, W., 333*n*104
Meier, D.E., 321*n*43;
    357*n*69
Meiners, M., 318*n*82
Mellinger, G.E., 332*n*88
Melnic, V.L., 328*n*167
Meltzer, J., 313*n*52;
    318*n*99; 345*n*39
Menken, J., 201; 344*n*19
Mesulam, M., 326*n*114;
    327*n*131
Metzger, L., 358*n*16
Meyer, B.M., 320*n*33
Meyer, J.S., 326*nn*110,
    115; 327*nn*131, 134, 136,
    143; 333*n*92
Mezey, M.D., 356*n*60
Michal, M.H., 318*n*97
Migiolo, M., 333*n*101
Mikhailidis, D.P.,
    332*nn*75, 78
Milgram, G., 351*n*62
Miller, G., 357*n*70
Miller, M., 330*n*30
Mills, Wilbur, 35
Mishara, Brian L., 118;
    330*nn*8, 9, 20; 331*n*49;
    334*nn*119, 127
Mitteness, L.S., 320*n*29
Mobley, G.M., 337*n*23
Moerman, E.J., 318*n*2
Mohs, R.C., 322*nn*17, 18,
    19
Mold, J.W., 320*nn*34, 35
Montgomery, J.E.,
    350*nn*14, 15; 351*n*65
Moore, Florence, 183;
    337*n*15; 341*nn*8, 9;
    342*nn*31, 32
Mootz, Ann, 181; 341*n*27
Mor, V., 348*n*77; 351*n*46

Moretz, R.C., 324*n*71
Mori, H., 323*n*47
Morlock, M., 341*n*24
Morris, J.N., 337*n*16;
  360*n*55
Morrow, C.H., 325*n*78
Morscheck, P., 323*n*28
Morse, J.H., 317*n*56;
  320*n*24; 343*n*73
Mortimer, J.A., 322*nn*19, 20
Morycz, R.K., 319*n*23
Mose, J.R., 353*n*103
Moser, K., 337*n*16
Moss, M., 352*n*91
Mossel, P.A., 339*n*40
Moynihan, D.P., 311*n*30
Mozar, H.N., 324*n*62
Mukherjee, D., 319*n*9
Muller, E.M., 338*n*29
Munley, A., 348*nn*64, 65,
  66, 67
Musson, N., 352*n*86;
  353*n*108
Myers, M.H., 321*n*45

Nadon, G.W., 357*nn*70, 72
Naranjo, C.A., 334*n*129
Nasar, Jack (J.L.), 248;
  351*n*45
Nerviano, V.J., 335*n*139
Netting, F.F., 346*n*68
Neuschler, E., 360*n*56
Newacheck, P., 312*n*49;
  338*n*28
Newald, J., 316*n*35
Newcomer, R., 312*n*49;
  338*n*28
Newman, E.S., 348*nn*57,
  58, 61
Newton, M., 332*n*81;
  334*n*113
Nightingale, Florence, 268;
  354*n*5; 356*n*41
Nofz, M.P., 350*n*15;
  353*n*97
Nutter, D.O., 359*n*36

O'Brien, Carol Lium, 224;
  346*nn*5, 7; 347*nn*13, 14,

17, 18, 19, 20, 21, 23,
  24, 25, 28, 29, 30, 31;
  349*n*81
Oldstone, M.B.A.,
  324*nn*65, 70
Ollstein, R., 340*n*66
O'Rourke, B., 338*n*26
Ory, M., 356*n*61
O'Shaughnessy, Carol, 26,
  44, 193, 289, 307;
  314*nn*2, 8; 315*n*30;
  316*nn*40, 42, 45, 49, 50;
  317*nn*57, 67, 75;
  342*nn*51, 59; 343*nn*63,
  65, 66, 67, 68, 2; 357*n*2;
  358*n*11; 359*n*51
Ostuni, J.A., 320*n*33
Ouslander, J.G., 320*n*29

Packwood, Sen. Bob, 305
Paetau, A., 323*n*30
Pagan-Bertucci, A., 314*n*4
Pagliaro, A.M., 328*nn*157,
  160, 161; 330*n*28; 332*n*86
Pagliaro, L.A., 328*nn*157,
  160, 161; 330*n*28;
  332*n*86
Pahl, J.J., 327*n*130
Pakkenberg, H., 326*n*109
Palmer, A.M., 324*nn*60, 63
Parkinson, J., 102;
  327*n*123
Parrish, J., 335*n*141
Parson, H.M., 350*n*20;
  351*n*40
Parsons, O.A., 333*n*98
Parsons, R., 336*n*7;
  345*nn*47, 49
Partanen, J.V., 323*n*42
Pascarelli, E.F., 334*n*124
Pastalan, L., 314*n*69;
  335*n*4
Pastor, Paul A., 127;
  331*nn*47, 57; 332*n*71
Patten, S.K., 345*nn*36, 39
Pawlson, L.G., 335*n*4
Peachey, J.E., 334*n*129
Pear, R.A., 359*n*29
Pelham, A.O., 342*n*42;
  343*n*1
Penn, R., 323*n*30

Pennybacker, Margaret R.,
  128; 331*nn*61, 63
Pepper, Rep. Claude,
  359*n*39
Pepper, N.H., 354*n*13
Perkel, R.L., 336*n*12;
  338*n*26
Perl, D.R., 326*n*100
Perry, E., 324*n*61; 325*n*81
Perry, R.H., 324*n*61;
  325*n*81
Perry, S., 337*n*16
Persily, N.A., 310*n*2;
  312*n*34; 314*n*3
Persson, K., 332*n*85
Peto, J.J., 328*n*161
Pettengill, J., 313*n*54
Phelps, M.E., 327*n*130
Phillip, P.A., 319*n*20
Phillips, B.R., 339*n*40
Pickett, N.A., Jr., 318*n*82
Piktialis, D.S., 316*n*54;
  320*n*24; 343*n*73
Pitt, William, 242
Plato, 131
Plumb, J.D., 336*n*12;
  338*n*26
Plutarch, 127
Pollack, E.S., 313*n*61
Pomeroy, K., 324*nn*65, 70
Portnoi, V.A., 313*n*62
Portnow, J., 357*n*70
Poulshock, S.W., 336*n*7;
  344*n*7; 345*n*31; 346*n*59
Powell, A.V., 353*n*124
Powell, F., 319*n*23
Powell, L.S., 329*n*174
Pratter, F., 338*nn*26, 32;
  339*nn*35, 37
Preston, G.A.N., 322*n*3
Price, D.L., 325*n*82
Price, R., 314*nn*2, 8;
  315*n*30; 316*nn*40, 42, 45,
  49, 50; 317*nn*57, 67, 75;
  342*nn*51, 59; 343*nn*63,
  65, 66, 67, 68, 2; 357*n*2;
  358*n*11; 359*n*51
Prioleau, M., 337*n*16
Proust, M., 330*n*15
Prusiner, Stanley B.,
  94–95; 325*nn*72, 73, 74,
  75, 77, 79, 81
Puranen, M., 323*n*42

Quam, J.K., 345*n*54
Quinn, J., 159–62;
  339*nn*44, 45, 47, 48, 49,
  50; 340*n*53; 355*n*30
Quirke, E., 336*n*7; 337*n*15;
  345*n*50; 358*n*25
Quittkat, S., 326*n*100

Rabinowitz, E., 330*n*16
Raisz, H., 338*n*26
Ramian, K.M.S., 350*n*13;
  351*n*37
Rango, N., 323*n*29; 357*n*67
Rankin, N., 353*n*106
Rantakokko, V., 321*n*44
Rapoport, S.I., 323*n*42
Raskind, M.A., 329*n*174;
  345*n*46
Rathbone-McCuan, Eloise,
  126, 126*n*; 331*n*54;
  334*n*131
Ratza, R.M., 357*n*65
Ravenna, P., 312*n*34;
  338*n*26
Ray, W.A., 319*n*11
Reagan, Ronald, 300–301
Redick, R.W., 313*n*61
Reever, K.E., 336*n*7
Regnier, V., 352*n*95;
  353*n*99
Reifler, B.V., 112*n*;
  327*n*125
Reina, J.C., 332*n*79
Reinken, J., 322*nn*17, 23;
  323*n*25
Reisberg, Barry, 86, 87–88;
  322*nn*6, 7, 9, 10, 13, 15,
  19, 21, 22, 23; 323*nn*32,
  33, 36, 39, 44; 324*nn*51,
  61, 66, 67, 68; 325*n*81;
  326*nn*100, 103, 116, 117,
  118, 119; 327*n*122;
  328*n*171; 329*n*174;
  333*nn*93, 108
Reiss, K., 348*nn*69, 76
Resnick, N.M., 320*n*29
Reuler, J., 330*n*26
Richman, H., 313*n*52;
  318*n*99; 345*n*39
Richmond, Julius B., 133;
  332*n*89

Rifkind, B., 320*n*38
Riley, M.W., 320*n*31;
  330*n*13
Robbins, F.D., 313*n*57
Roberds, L.A., 126*n*;
  331*n*54
Roberts, D.E., 311*n*32
Roberts, G.W., 324*n*65;
  325*n*76
Robins, L.N., 330*n*13;
  332*n*67
Robinson, B.C., 344*n*24;
  345*n*34
Robinson, N., 341*nn*11,
  29; 342*n*35
Roche, A.F., 319*n*9
Roecker, M.A., 348*nn*48,
  59
Rogers, R.L., 326*n*110;
  333*n*92
Rogers, T., 358*n*16
Roland, L.P., 327*n*130
Roll, M.K., 355*n*24
Rolls, B.J., 319*n*20
Rooney, C.B., 334*n*113
Ropper, A.H., 326*n*111
Ropschlau, W.H.E.,
  334*n*111
Rosato, F.E., 337*n*16
Rose, A.M., 353*n*118
Rosenbaum, L.V.,
  352*nn*90, 94; 353*nn*99,
  100, 101
Rosenberg, N., 330*n*13
Rosenthal, P., 340*n*66
Rosenwaike, I., 310*n*4;
  311*n*18; 357*n*1; 358*n*12
Rosin, A.J., 329*n*176;
  330*n*25
Rosner, B., 332*nn*75, 76
Ross, J.H., 315*n*31
Rossman, I., 349*n*98
Rostenkowski, Rep. Dan,
  359*n*39
Roth, M., 322*n*3; 323*n*35
Rovner, J., 340*n*68;
  359*n*31
Rowe, J., 316*nn*51, 53, 54;
  317*n*56; 318*n*3; 319*n*17;
  319–20*n*24; 343*nn*72, 73;
  345*n*40; 358*n*8
Rowland, Diane, 28*n*;
  53–54; 199; 310*n*4;

315*nn*25, 26; 316*nn*39,
  43, 55; 317*n*64;
  318*nn*94, 95; 342*n*49;
  343*nn*69, 74, 3; 344*n*10
Rubenstein, Laurence Z.,
  103; 319*n*23; 320*nn*27,
  41, 42; 326*n*113;
  327*nn*131, 132; 328*n*156
Ruchlin, Hirsch S., 308;
  337*n*16; 360*n*55
Rudder, C., 319*n*22
Rudnitsky, H., 353*nn*116,
  122; 354*n*125
Rumsey, H., 356*n*59
Ruth, V., 322*n*20; 325*n*89
Ruther, M., 314*n*4
Rutstein, D.D., 330*n*18
Ryan, C., 333*nn*97, 102
Rymer, M., 315*n*21

Sainer, J.S., 346*n*61
St. George, J., 342*n*48
Salazar, Andres M., 93;
  324*n*66
Salzman, H., 312*n*34;
  338*n*26
Samorajski, T., 327*n*134;
  329*n*4; 330*n*27; 331*n*61;
  332*nn*81, 85; 333*nn*90,
  92, 93, 94, 95, 99, 100;
  334*n*120
Sanborn, B., 329*n*186;
  349*n*101
Sands, Daniel, 228*n*;
  347*n*26
Saunders, C., 348*nn*65, 73;
  357*n*70
Sawyer, D., 314*n*4
Scanlan, B., 358*n*17
Scanlon, W.J., 313*n*60;
  337*nn*20, 23; 355*n*17
Schaffner, W., 319*n*11
Scharer, L.K., 314*n*70
Scharf, Joan, 228*n*
Scheibel, A.B., 323*n*48;
  324*n*61
Schenkenberg, T.,
  333*n*101
Scherl, D.J., 313*n*54
Schimel, David, 31;
  315*n*15

Schlesinger, M., 358n26
Schneider, D., 312n49;
　338n28
Schneider, E., 311n18;
　319n6; 355n14; 356n61
Schoenberg, B.S., 321n3
Scholen, K., 255n; 313n53;
　317nn68, 70, 74, 77, 78;
　352nn83, 84
Schoonover, C.B., 343n7;
　344n17
Schorah, C.J., 319n10
Schore, J., 339n40
Schreiber, M.S., 336n12;
　338n26
Schuckit, Marc A., 127;
　329n3; 330nn18, 31, 32,
　34; 331nn47, 57, 58;
　332n71; 334n125
Schultz, E., 319n12
Schultz, R., 355n27
Schulz, J.H., 310n5
Schulz, R., 335n4
Schwartz, T.B., 321n49;
　356n55
Schweiker, R.S., 313n54
Scialli, A.R., 320n34
Scott, M., 329n174; 345n46
Seagle, B.M., 350nn7, 11,
　23; 351nn42, 47, 49, 59;
　352nn90, 91; 353nn99,
　100, 101, 103
Seagle, J.F., Jr., 350nn7,
　11, 23; 351nn42, 47, 49,
　59; 352nn90, 91;
　353nn99, 100, 101, 103
Seeman, P., 334n111
Segal, J., 338n26
Segal, P., 320n38
Segerberg, O., 319n15
Seixas, F.A., 329n5;
　334n116
Sellers, E.M., 334nn111,
　129
Semple, T., 320n37
Serfass, R.C., 319n12
Seshagiri, V., 338n29
Shafer, R.G., 350n19;
　351nn36, 38, 44, 63;
　352n85; 353nn117, 122;
　354n135
Shanas, Ethel, 203; 336n7;
　344nn16, 22; 345nn28, 29

Shannon, M., 357n67
Sharfstein, S.S., 313n54
Shaw, T., 327nn134, 136;
　333n92
Shea, M.A., 315n31
Shealy, M.J., 339n46
Shedletsky, R., 357nn70,
　72
Sheehan, N.W., 344n21;
　345n57
Sheldon, F., 328n172
Shen, J., 338n26; 340nn55,
　57, 58, 59, 60, 61, 62, 63
Sherman, F.T., 328n149
Sherman, M.N., 319n8
Sherman, S.R., 348nn57,
　58, 61
Sherwood, S., 351n46
Shipley, J.M., 333n91
Shuman, L., 320nn40, 41
Shuttleworth, E.C., 88;
　323nn40, 41
Silverstone, B., 336n7
Sims, N.R., 324nn60, 63;
　325nn81, 82
Simson, J., 345n54
Singer, J.E., 320n40
Sjogren, T., 325n87
Skellie, F.A., 336nn12, 13;
　337n23
Skelton, D., 328n161;
　330n28
Sklar, B.W., 336nn12, 26
Skoloda, T.E., 321n48;
　329n181; 356nn39, 40
Small, G.N., 112n
Small, G.W., 328nn147,
　149
Smith, B.K., 349nn1, 2
Smith, E., 319n12
Smith, J.P., 337n16
Smith, J.S., 327n133
Smith, Michael J., 211;
　345nn32, 45; 346n62
Smith, M.R., 332n80;
　335n4
Smith, R., 329n184
Snope, F.C., 335n3; 336n7;
　343n7; 344n8
Soeldner, J.S., 318n2
Soininen, H., 323n42
Soldo, B.J., 310nn2, 3;
　336n7; 358n6

Solomon, D.H., 355n20
Solomon, L., 346n71
Solon, 84
Somers, Anne (A.R.), 246,
　307; 318n82; 322nn7,
　23; 335n3; 336nn6, 7;
　343n7; 350n32; 360n52
Southern, P., 324nn65, 70
Space, S., 334n121
Spar, J.E., 326nn103, 104,
　107; 328n148
Spar, K., 352n68
Spelder, L.A., 357n70
Spicuzza, T., 357n67
Spiegel, Allen D., 12,
　212–13; 311n29; 335n4;
　336nn13, 14; 339nn47,
　49; 340n2; 341nn4, 5;
　343nn62, 64, 70;
　344n24; 345n47; 346n67
Spillane, J.A., 325n81
Spitler, B.J. Curry, 307;
　359n50; 360n53
Sroka, H., 327nn123, 125
Stahl, I., 336n7; 337n15;
　345n50; 358n25
Starr, Janet, 181, 182;
　341nn26, 28
Stassen, Margaret, 39–40;
　316nn37, 38; 359n49
Stead, W.W., 321n47
Steel, K., 112n; 313nn57,
　59
Steele, R., 311n26
Stein, H.F., 320nn34, 35
Stein, S., 357n73
Steinberg, A., 321n43;
　357n69
Steinberg, E.P., 315n33
Steinberg, G., 329n174
Steinhauser, M.B., 347n41;
　348nn42, 43, 55, 56
Stephens, S.A., 339n40
Stern, R.S., 316n33
Steuer, J.L., 336n7
Stevens, R., 312n41;
　315n13
Steward, J.E., 311n32;
　312n33
Stiedmann, M., 321n46
Stone, J., 322nn4, 19;
　323n31
Storandt, M., 333n97

Streicher, E., 326n99
Streimer, R.A., 353n120
Strickland, A.L., 357n70
Strong, J., 322n5
Stuart, M.R., 335n3;
   336n7; 343n7; 344n8
Stubbs, A.C., 350nn14, 15;
   351n65
Sulkava, R., 323n30
Sumichrast, M., 350n19;
   351nn36, 38, 44, 63;
   352n85; 353nn117, 122;
   354n135
Summers, William K., 93;
   324n64
Sun, A.Y., 333nn99, 100
Sundwall, D., 359nn32, 37
Swick, T., 321n57

Takeda, Shumpei, 89;
   323n43
Tanahashi, N., 327n143
Tateishi, J., 324n65
Tawaklna, T., 326nn110,
   115; 327n131
Taylor, R.J., 336n7
Taylor, S.E., 320n40
Teasdale, T.A., 320nn40,
   41
Tedesco, J., 316n48;
   317n61
Teravainen, H., 327n121
Terry, Robert, 88; 322nn3,
   22; 323n38; 327nn121,
   122, 145
Thienhaus, O., 330n27;
   334nn132, 134
Thomas, Charles C.,
   356n41
Thomas, J., 332n84
Thomas, L., 322n16
Thomas, M.A., 339n33
Thompson, R.H., 338n29
Thorpe, N., 353n116;
   354n126
Thurow, Lester, 293;
   358n21; 360nn54, 57
Tideiksaar, R., 358n14
Tietz, M.W., 320n32
Tilly, J., 314n11
Timbury, J.C., 329n184

Timms, D., 337n16
Tissue, T., 350nn26, 30,
   31; 351n39
Tobin, J.D., 332n82
Tobin, S.S., 319n13;
   355nn24, 26
Todorov, A.B., 322n20
Tomlinson, B.E., 324n53
Torack, Richard M., 84;
   322nn9, 14
Trager, B., 341n23;
   337n23
Triegaardt, J., 334n131
Turner, M.A., 352n76;
   353n98
Turner, N., 337n16
Turner, P.A., 337n15
Turwoski, A., 342n42;
   343n1
Tysboula, S., 349n87

Uhlenberg, P., 310n6

Vaillant, G., 334n118
Van Gelder, S., 316nn33,
   48; 359n48
Van Hoesen, G.W.,
   324nn57, 58
Vanhorenbeck, S., 352n72
Vaupel, J.W., 310n4
Veech, R.L., 330n18
Vertrees, J., 313n54
Vestal, R.E., 332n82
Vincent, L., 355n19
Vining, E.M., 319n6
Vir, S.C., 321n46
Vladeck, Bruce, 16, 278,
   56, 312nn41, 43, 47;
   313nn54, 57; 315n13;
   316n54; 318n101;
   336nn8, 14; 337n23;
   339n34; 354nn7, 11;
   356nn36, 46; 359n30, 38
Vladeck, F., 351n61;
   352nn81, 89; 353n104
Volland, P.J., 233n;
   348nn49, 50, 51
Von Gall, M., 333n103

Waife, M.M., 321nn43,
   53; 356n57
Wald, Lillian, 13, 174, 212
Waldman, J., 340n54
Waldo, D., 317n65;
   318n90
Wales, J., 349nn77, 78
Walker, R.D., 335n140
Wallace, J., 334nn133, 135
Wallack, Stanley, 45, 56;
   312nn49, 51; 317nn58,
   68; 318nn98, 100; 338n28
Walsh, M.L.W., Sr.,
   340n66
Wan, T.T.H., 337n23;
   347nn17, 18, 19, 34
Wanberg, K.W., 335n140
Wanzer, S.H., 357n67
Wasow, M., 328n173
Waxman, Howard M.,
   276; 321n48; 329n181;
   355n32; 356nn39, 40
Webb, M., 261n
Weber, G.H., 356nn41, 49
Wehr, E., 312n45
Weiner, Joshua, 243–44;
   350n12; 354n127; 357n4
Weisbard, A., 328n167
Weiskottch, H.G., 339n33
Weiss, Kenneth, 124;
   331n46
Weiss, L.J., 336n12;
   338n26
Weiss, S.M., 337n16
Weissert, William G., 226,
   229–30; 310n7; 311n14;
   317n71; 337n23;
   346nn4, 8; 347nn17, 18,
   19, 22, 33, 34; 355n17
Wells, Charles E., 107;
   112n; 322n6; 327nn133,
   144; 328nn148, 150, 151,
   153
Welte, T., 316nn51, 53,
   54; 317n56; 319n24;
   321n53; 343nn72, 73;
   345nn40, 43, 44
Wendland, C.J., 355n14;
   356n61
Wennberg, J.E., 313n54
Werner, A.A., 340n2
Wessel, Peter, 48–49;
   317nn76, 79

West, Rebecca, 12
Whisnant, J., 327n138
Whitcomb, M.E., 359n36
White, J., 325n90; 326n97
White, J.S., 322n11
White, P., 325n81
Whitehead, W.E., 320n30
Whitfield, S., 345n42
Wieland, G.D., 319n23;
  320nn27, 41, 42
Wilcock, G.K., 323n45
Wiley, J.A., 355n19
Wilkes, E., 357n70
Wilkins, J.N., 333n96;
  334n115
Wilks, S., 85
Willett, W., 332nn75, 76
Willging, Paul, 23;
  314n67; 360n56
Williams, B.O., 320n37
Williams, E.P., 330n24;
  331n38
Williams, M.E., 319n23;
  320n41
Williams, P.T., 332nn75, 77
Williams, T.T., 319n23;
  320n41
Wilson, D., 349nn83, 91,
  92, 97

Wilson, L.B., 345n54
Winkle Voss, H.E.,
  353n124
Winn, S., 312n49
Winslow, G.R., 356n41
Winston, E., 340n1
Wise, R.W., 333n93
Wisniewski, H.M.,
  324nn51, 71; 326n99
Woehlke, P., 352n93;
  353n102
Wolf, P.A., 333n91
Wolf, R., 359n28
Wolfson, L.I., 327n145
Wood, W.G., 333n93
Woodard, A., 350nn8, 18;
  354nn132, 134
Woodson, A.S., 355nn27,
  28
Worm-Peterson, J.,
  326n109
Worthington, P.H., 337n16
Wright, S.D., 328n171
Wurtman, Richard J., 91,
  97; 323n50; 324n55;
  325nn73, 81, 92;
  326n106
Wyden, Cong. Ron,
  318n93

Yahr, M.D., 327nn123,
  124, 125
Yalla, S.V., 320n29
Yordi, C., 338n26;
  340nn54, 55, 57, 60, 61,
  62, 63
Young, C.L., 344n23

Zahourek, R.P., 334n121
Zarit, J.M., 328n166
Zarit, S.H., 328n166;
  336n7
Zawadski, R.T., 336n12;
  338n26; 339n43;
  340nn54, 55, 56, 57, 58,
  59, 60, 61, 62, 63
Zezulka, A.V., 333n91
Zibart, E., 353n110
Zimberg, Sheldon, 129,
  130n; 331n61; 332nn68,
  69; 334nn133, 135
Zimmer, A.H., 346n61
Zimmer, A.W., 355n14;
  356n61
Zimmer, J.G., 336n12
Zweig, J.P., 323n27;
  350n25

Subject Index

AARP/Prudential, 52
abuse, potential for, 186–88
ACTION, 212, 215
Activities of daily living (ADL), 7
acute auditory hallucinosis, 104
Adams House, 225
Administration on Aging, 162, 163, 251, 258
adult day care, 296; *see also* day care
Adult Day Care—A Practical Guide (O'Brien), 224
adult foster homes, 230–34
Aetna insurance, 52
age, concept of benefits on basis of, 35
aged people, varying concepts of, 12
Agencies on Aging, 42–43
aging, as process, 71–80
Aid to Families with Dependent Children, 29
Alabama, day care centers in, 228
Alaska: Medicaid costs in, 29; SSI payment in, 41
alcohol abuse, 130
alcohol intake, 125
Alcoholics Anonymous (AA): older people in, 120; use of group therapy, 144
alcoholism: approaches to treatment of, 140–44; consequences of in older people, 131–39; and definition of terms, 129–30; diagnosis of, 120–22; effects of on other organs, 137–38; among elderly, 75, 117–45; and health-related problems, 132–33; tar-

get organs for, 133–37; therapeutic nihilism in treatment of, 140; as treatable dementia, 104–5
almshouses, 12, 249, 268
aluminum toxicity, and AD, 98–99
Alzheimer's disease (AD), 83, 85–99; adult day care and, 224, 228; brain alterations in, 89–93; cause of, 93–99; defining, 87–89; genetic origin of, 96–98; prevalence of, 86–87; respite care and, 239
American Association of Homes for the Aging, 261
American Association of Professional Standards Review Organizations, 22
American Association of Retired Persons (AARP), 51
American Hospital Association, 51
American Medical Association, 35
American Public Health Association, 243
American Red Cross, 216
amyloid: and AD, 90–91; and prions, 94–95
anhedonia, 107
anthropomorphic indices, 61
AOA, *see* Administration on Aging
Arizona: and beds for elderly, 16; as only non-Medicaid state, 22
As You Like It (Shakespeare), 85
assessment, need for comprehensive, 67–68, 73, 76

Association for the Improvement of the Poor, Family Services Bureau of, 174
ataxia, 94, 112

Balanced Budget and Deficit Control Act of 1985 (Gramm-Rudman-Hollings Act), 11
Baucas Amendment of 1980 (PL 96-265), 49
benign senescent forgetfulness, 87
Beverly Foundation, 281
block grants, 20, 43–44
Blue Cross of North America, 52
body, as health factor, 60, 71, 74, 78
body mass, changes in and aging, 131–32
Boston, adult day care centers in, 225
Boston Dispensary, 12
brain: effects of alcoholism on, 134; models for, 135–37
brain tumors, as treatable, 105

California: adult day health care centers in, 162, 227–28; Medicaid in, 29, 32; and Title XX, 194
cannibalism, ritual, 94
capitation plans, 20
cardiovascular system, and alcoholism, 138
caregivers: impact of health care on, 204–6; importance of needs of, 238, 239; responsibilities of, 282
Caregivers Strain Index, 204
cascade effect, 320nn34, 35
case management, and discharge planning, 23–24, 292–93
Catastrophic Health Insurance, legislation, 300
catecholamine functions, brain's, 135
"categorically needy," 29
Catholic Community Services of Seattle, 215
cerebral hemorrhage, 99, 106
cerebrovascular accidents (CVAs), 99–100
Certificates of Need, 31
certification, virtues of, 13–14
Certified Home Care Agencies, and HMOs, 297–98
certified home care programs, 151–52
checklist, nursing home, 275–76
Chelsea-Village program, 165–71; on alcoholism, 119, 142–43; characteristics of cli-

ents of, 168, 169, 170, 171; financing of, 165; fourteen-year report of, 14; physician involvement in, 166–69; results, 169
choline acetyltransferase (CAT): and AD, 92, 95–96; and HD, 103
Church Council of Greater Seattle, 215
cirrhosis, definition of, 137
City of Chicago Housing Authority, 249
class distinction, and alcohol intake, 126
climate, as health factor, 65–66, 72
cognitive restructuring, 63
community, characteristics of and housing, 246–47
community psychiatry movement, 22
Community Care for Elderly program, 228–29
Community Care Organization for Dependent Adults (CCODA), 163–65
Community Home Health Services Act of 1980 (S.3211), 303, 305
Community Home Health Services Act of 1981 (S.234), 303–4, 305
Community Service Society of New York, 211
Comprehensive Employment and Training Act (CETA), 252
computed tomography (CT), 89, 136
confabulation, 105
congregate housing, 258–60
Congressional Research Service, Library of Congress, 26
Connecticut: Medicaid costs in, 29; respite care in, 239
Consolidated Omnibus Reconciliation Act of 1985 (COBRA), 11
"convoy of social support," 201
coping skills: as health factor, 72, 75, 78; importance of, 63–64
cortical dementias, 83
cost control, 19–21, 54
cost sharing, 164
Cowley Royal Hospital, 225
Creutzfeldt-Jakob disease (CJD), and AD, 93–95
CT, *see* computed tomography

daughters, as primary caregivers, 200–201
day care: adult, 223–30; as component in long term care, 116; and funding issues, 229–30; growth of (in U.S.), 225–26; history of, 225; model programs, 227–29; pro-

day care (*Continued*)
    gram components, 226–27; purpose, 224–25
Deficit Reduction Act of 1984, 11
dehydration, 319n20
Delaware, Medicaid costs in, 29
delerium tremens (DTs), 104–5
dementia, 81–116; adult day care centers and, 224; defining, 83–84; and environmental change, 109–10; epidemiology of, 81–83; historical background of, 84–85; medical diseases and, 110–12; multi-infarct, 99–101; reversible in elderly, 111–12; therapeutic approaches to, 112–16; treatable, 103–12
demographic imperative, 4
dendritic destruction, and AD, 90, 92, 96
denial, as main defense mechanism, 143–44
Denmark, elderly housing in, 244, 249
Department of Health, Education and Welfare, (PL 92-603, Sec. 222), and adult day care, 225–26
Department of Health and Human Services (HHS): channeling demonstration of, 161–62; and home improvement funding, 252; on long term care insurance policies, 50; on numbers of candidates for nursing homes, 154; and research on aging, 69
Department of Housing and Urban Development (HUD), 250; community development funding of, 251; and On Lok, 163; and Section 8, 163, 254–55; and Section 202, 253, 258
depression, as treatable, 107–8
Deregulation Task Force, 16
Diagnosis-Related Group (DRG), 21, 38; *see also* DRGs
Diagnostic and Statistical Manual of Mental Disorders (DSM-III), 81
dialysis dementia, 98
digitalis delirium, 108
discharge, barriers to, 274
discharge planning: and case management, 23–24, 292–93; and DRGs, 21
disease, 60–61; chronic, 61; definition of, 60; as health factor, 60–61, 71, 74, 78
disorders, psychiatric, as treatable dementias, 107–8
diuresis, and alcoholism, 138
domestic chores, 178–79
Domestic Volunteer Service Act, 212, 215
Down's syndrome, 97; and AD, 97–98
DRGs, 67, 301, 306

drug therapy, alcoholism and, 143
DTs, 139

East Tennessee Advocacy Assistance Program, 213
economics, and alcohol intake, 126
elderly: and burden of health care expenses, 46–47; as home owners, 243–44; increased income for, 20; special importance of home to, 242
elderly poor, double jeopardy of, 32
eligibility, 291–92
emergency response systems, 152
Employee Retirement Income Security Act of 1974 (ERISA), 46
England, elderly housing in, 249; *see also* Great Britain
Enriched Housing, 259–60
entitlement programs, 20
environment, and housing, 244–45
Eryximachus (Plato), 131
ethics, question of, 281–85

falls, studies on, 65
family: needs of in dementia situations, 114–15; reimbursement to, 206–7; social services for, 207–10
family abandonment, myth of, 201
Family Coping Index, 204
family status, housing and, 245–46
family support network, 203
Family Support Program, 211
family therapy, alcoholism and, 143
Farmers Home Administration (FmHA), 250, 251, 252; and Section 202 housing, 254, 258
Federal Council on Aging, 7
Federal Housing Administration, 250, 269
Federal National Mortgage Association, Forum III of, 248
fibroblasts, 60
finances, as health factor, 66–67, 72, 76
financing, innovative models of, 292
fitness: effects of on functioning ability, 62; as health factor, 72
5-fluorouracil, 108
Florida: adult day care funding in, 229; Community Care for Elderly, program of, 228–29; respite care in, 239

Fort Greene (houses), 249
foster care, 296
Foundation for Long Term Care, 240
foundations: and geriatric nursing, 281; and
   volunteer programs, 216
frail elderly: foster care for, 230–34; France,
   238–39; guide for home care of, 205–6;
   housing options for, 255–63; and informal
   supports, 198–219; needs of, 180; and
   placement in nursing home, 298; requirements of, 200; *see also* elderly; old-old
France, respite care in, 238–39
friends, as caregivers, 210–11
fringe benefits, employee, 20, 55
frontal - limbic - diencephalic disruption
   model, 136–37

Gamma-aminobutyric acid (GABA), 103
gastrointestinal tract, 138
gender, and alcohol intake, 125–26
General Accounting Office, 18, 30
genetic basis, and alcohol intake, 127
"Geriatric evaluation," VA, 241
Geriatric evaluation units (GEUs), 45, 67–68
geriatric research, education, and clinical
   centers (GRECS), 45
Gerontological Society, 247
gerontology, training in, 290–91
gout, and alcoholism, 138
government: and changes in financing, 54–
   55; an evolutionary role for, 10; and expenditures for care of elderly, 27–28; and
   other sources of funds, 40–45; responsibility of for long term care insurance, 53
Gramm-Rudman Hollings Act, 29, 34, 41
granny-bashing, 115
Group Home Project, 259
group therapy, alcoholism and, 144
Great Britain: hospices in, 236; National
   Health Service of, 225, 229
grief, study of, 186

Harbor Area Adult Day Care Center, 227–28
Hawaii: adult day care in, 234; Medicaid in,
   32
health: extrinsic factors affecting, 64–71; intrinsic factors affecting, 60–64; relation of
   to disease, 59–80; relation of to functional
   ability, 59–80

health care, and home health aides, 179–80
Health Care Financing Administration
   (HCFA): on nursing home regulations,
   265–66; and Nursing Home Without
   Walls, 156; and On Lok Senior Health Services, 163; and long term care insurance,
   53; and skilled nursing requirement, 36
Health maintenance organizations (HMOs),
   20
health workers, attitude of toward alcoholics, 120
health-related facilities (HRFs), 267
HELP, *see* Project HELP
hematoma, subdural, 105–6, 138–39
hepatic encephalopathy, 105
hepatitis, acute alcoholic, 137–38
high-technology services, 152–53
Hill-Burton Act, 14, 269
hip fracture, 319n11
home care: and HMOs, 297–98; under Medicare, 39–40; for poor, 12
Home and Community Based Services Act of
   1987, 304
Home and Community Based Services for
   the Elderly Act of 1985, 304
home dialysis, 337n16
home equity conversion, 47–49, 255; *see also*
   reverse mortgage
home health aide, 176
home health care: early programs of, 13; emphasis of, 150–51; home improvement,
   251–52; Medicare coverage of, 37; support
   groups for workers in, 189–90
home visits, Medicare expenditures on,
   39–40
homeboundedness, 170
homemaker, 175
homesharing, requirements of, 256–58
hospice care, 235–37; Medicare coverage of,
   37, 296–97
Hospice—A Caring Challenge (McNulty and
   Holderby), 237
Hospital Survey and Construction Act, 269
hospital-based home care (HBHC), 45,
   196–97
hospitals: as home health care sponsors, 298;
   overstay in, 21–22; as pesthouses, 12
hotels, for elderly, 256
housekeeper/chore service worker, 175
housekeeper aides, 174
housing, 242–64; history of for elderly, 249–
   50; and long term care, 292; rural policy on,
   251; significance of, 243–47; solutions for

housing (*Continued*)
  elderly, 247–48, 251–63; spectrum, 248;
  substandard, 244
Housing Act of 1970, 250
Housing Authority (Birmingham, Ala.), day
  care centers of, 228
Housing and Community Development Act
  of 1974, 250
Human Resources Administration (HRA)
  (NYC), home attendant program of,
  191–93
Huntington Valley, adult day care center,
  227–28
Huntington's disease (HD), 102–3
hydrocephalus, normal pressure, 106–7

Ida B. Culver (house), 249
Idaho, Medicaid in, 32
Illinois: study of geriatric foster care in, 231;
  licensing of adult care homes in, 234
income, major sources of, 46
indemnity payouts, 50
independence, importance of maintaining, 4
Individual Retirement Account (IRA), and
  long term care costs, 55
Individual retirement mortgage account
  (IRMA), 48–49
individual rights, validity of asserting, 10–11
infantilization, 149
infection, and AD, 93–95
informal supports, 180, 198–219; families
  and friends as, 203–4, 210–11; giving help
  to natural supporters, 206–10; impact of on
  caregivers, 204–6; overview of, 211–12;
  and volunteers, 212–19
in-home services, tax deductions for, 55
Institute of Medicine, 265
institutional programs, alcoholism and, 144
insulin therapy, 337*n*16
intermediate care facilities (ICFs), 267, 269
International Ladies Garment Workers
  Union, 263
Iowa: adult day care in, 234; elderly housing
  in, 251
isolation, as lifelong tendency, 201; problem
  of, 188–89

John Hancock Insurance Company, 13
Johns Hopkins Hospital Community Care
  Project, 232–33

Johns Hopkins University Department of
  Health Policy and Management, 53–54

Kansas, community-based services of, 223
Kellogg, W.K., Foundation, 281
Kerr-Mills amendments, 14–15, 269
King Lear (Shakespeare), 85
kinship network, thinning out of, 199
Korsakoff's psychosis, 105
Kuru, and AD, 93–95

lacunar state, 100–101
Laennec's cirrhosis, 105
legislation, and long term health care, 299–
  307
Levodopa, 102
life care, 260–63
Lifecare Industry, 261
iife care retirement centers, 51
Life Care Services, Inc., 262
life expectancy, increased, 5–8
life goals, and elderly people, 171–72
liver, and alcoholism, 137–38
living space, as health factor, 64–65, 72, 78
Living Will, 79
lobbying, value of, 18–19
long term care: alternative funding for,
  20–21; approaches to financing, 53–56;
  changes in meaning of, 301; definition of,
  10; ethical and moral considerations of,
  79–80; federal government's definition of,
  267; financing, 25–56; impact of DRGs
  on, 38–39; and Medicare changes, 36–37;
  planning for, 23; private financing of,
  45–53
long term care insurance, 49–53; and home
  equity conversion, 47
Long Term Care Insurance Promotion and
  Protection Act, 53
long term care spectrum, 8–10, 286–309; aberration in, 156; and access to services,
  291–93; and allocation of resources, 293–
  94; and attitudes on aging, 288–89; creation of, 3–4; and demographic imperative,
  287–88; financing of, 307–9; and legislation, 299–306; and program development,
  294–99; and training in gerontology, 290
Long Term Care Survey, 180
Long Term Home Care Demonstrations,
  158–62; Chelsea-Village Program, 165–71;

On Lok Senior Health Services, 162–65; Triage program, 159–62; types of, 159

long term home health care: definition of terms, 151–53; demonstrations of, 158–72; exemplary programs of, 154–55; Nursing Home Without Walls, 155–58; values and significance of, 153–54

Long Term Home Health Care Programs (LTHHCPs), 156

Louisiana, and nursing home residents, 32

Low-Income Home Energy Assistance Program, 252

lungs, effect of alcoholism on, 138

Luria-Nebraska, neuropsychological battery, 333n97

major activity, loss of ability in, 8

malnutrition, 139

Maryland: congregate housing in, 259; and RUGS, 33

Massachusetts: ADL study of, 7; adult day care services in, 230; study of on nursing home costs, 29

Meals-on-Wheels, 42

Medicaid (Title XIX), 11, 26–34; and adult day care, 225, 226, 229, 233, 234; and adult day health care centers, 162; and chronic care needs, 301; and cost sharing, 164; decrease in federal funding of, 34; distinctions in, 16; distribution of expenditures of, 32; as fifty different programs, 32; financial effect of, 66–67; and home health aides, 177, 183, 191–93; impact of on distribution of patients, 30–31; and NYC home attendant program, 191–93; and 1981 waivers, 193; and nursing home reimbursement, 269–70; pro-institutional bias of, 30, 55; and respite care, 240; summary, 33–34; and support of long term care, 156; waivers, 158, 162, 164–65

Medicaid-Medicare Anti-Fraud and Abuse Amendments (PL 95-142), 270

Medicaid patients, discrimination against, 30–31

medical care, 68–71; definition of, 68; as health factor, 68–71, 73, 76, 79

medical director, 279–80

medical indigency, 15

medical practice, ethical, 184

medical procedures, risk-benefit ratio of, 68–69, 73

medical reactions, 108–9

medically needy, 29

Medicare (Title XVIII), 11, 35–40, 64; and adult day care, 225; and conditions of participation, 123; and home health aides, 177, 191, 193–94; hospice benefit in, 235; and long term care, 36–37; and neglect of chronic needs, 298, 302; and nursing home reimbursement, 269; Parts A&B, 64–65; Part C, 305; revision of as key, 299; skilled nursing requirement of, 152; structure for reform of, 54–55; and Title XXI, 305; waivers, 158, 160, 163, 164–65

Medicare Supplemental Insurance, 49

Medi-gap policies, 49

memory, short term, 62–63

memory loss: and alcohol abuse, 121; and Alzheimer's disease, 87–88, 91

Menorah Park (Cleveland, OH), 228

mentally ill, fate of chronically, 22

Metropolitan Life Insurance Company, 13

Michael Reese Hospital, 13

Michigan, adult day care in, 234

MID (multi-infarct dementia), and AD, 99–100

Minnesota: and Medicaid regulations, 31; Medicaid reimbursement in, 33

Mississippi, Medicaid costs in, 29

Mitchell-Lama program, 253

mobile homes, 256

Model Project on Aging grant, 163

Mongolism, 97

Montefiore Hospital, 13, 156, 174, 241

Moosehaven, 249

Moreland Commission, 156

Mount Vernon House, 260

Munley, Sister Anne, 236

National Association of Home Builders, 247

National Citizens Coalition of Nursing Home Reform, 213

National Committee on Homemaker Service, 175

National Council on Aging, 226, 254

National Council on Alcoholism, 129

National Council for Homemaker Services, 181

National Foundation for Hospice and Home Care, 175

National Health Service (Great Britain), 225, 229

National Home Health Care Act of 1975, 303, 305

National HomeCaring Council, 175, 181, 183; accreditation program of, 184

National Hospice Organization, 235

National Institute on Adult Day Care, 226

National Long Term Channeling Demonstration, 161–62

National Nursing Home Survey (NNHS), 272–73

natural support system: groups for, 208–10; in urban area, 201

Nebraska, adult day care in, 234

neurofibrillary tangles (NFTs), and AD, 90–91, 99

neurotransmitters: abnormalities of, 95–96; metabolism of, 92–93

New Jersey, Medicaid in, 29, 31

New Jersey Housing Authority, and elderly housing, 249

New Jersey Society of Architects, 260

New Mexico, elderly housing in, 251

New York (City): adult day care funding in, 229; alcoholism studies in, 122; Department for the Aging, 216, 217; home attendant program, 191–93; Medicare expenditures in, 191

New York State: adult day care funding in, 234, 235; congregate housing in, 259–60; elderly housing in, 244, 250; and licensing, 181–82; Medicaid in, 33, 191; Nursing Home Without Walls, 18, 20, 155–58; Office on Aging, report of, 200, 212; and paraprofessional workers, 175; respite care in, 238, 240; and RUGS, 67

New York State Health Department, 165

New York Times, 32, 132

Nevada, Medicaid costs in, 29

1981 White House Conference on Aging, 69, 248

normal-pressure hydrocephalus (NPH), 106–7

North Dakota Foster Care, 233–34

Northwestern University Center for Health Services and Policy Research, 230

nurse practitioner, geriatric, 290–91

nurse's aides, 278–79

nursing, 277, 281

nursing care: chronic, 37; skilled, 36–37, 152

Nursing Home Without Walls, 18, 20, 155–58, 298; case management of, 157; eligibility for, 157; enrollment in, 157–58; history of, 155–56; services provided by, 157

nursing homes, 265–85; administration of, 276, 279; alcoholism in, 144; beds per 1,000, 17; expansion of, 153–54; future requirements for, 5; and Hill-Burton Act, 14; history of, 268–73; as "houses of death," 118–19; as last resort, 299; liberal entry standards of, 18–19; and medical director, 279–80; organization of, 276–79; quality of life in, 275–76; question of ethics in, 281–85; teaching, 280–81; and transfer trauma, 274

nutrition, and aging, 61–62, 71, 75, 78

Office of Human Development Services, 163

Ohio, SSI payment in, 41

Oklahoma, and Title XX, 194

Old Age XI (Cicero), 4

Older Americans Act (Title XX), 11, 42–43; and adult day care funding, 226, 229; and home health aides, 177, 183, 191, 194–95

older drinkers: age of onset, 123–25; characteristics of, 122–28; class distinction in, 126; economics of, 126; gender, 125–26; genetic basis of, 127; numbers of, 122–23; understanding the problem, 127–28

old-old, increase in numbers of, 287

ombudsman programs, 43

Omnibus Budget Reconciliation Act of 1981 (PL 97-35), 193; and Section 2176, 32–33; and SSBG, 43–44

Omnibus Reconciliation Act of 1980 (PL 96-499), 37, 270, 305–6

On Lok Senior Health Services, 162–65

open-ended funding, 18

Oriental people, and reaction to alcohol, 119–20

oxygen therapy, 337n16

palliation, 236

paraprofessional services, 152, 295

paraprofessional workers, 173–97; building morale of, 188–90; definition of terms, 176; ethical matters and, 184–88; historical background of, 174–76; importance of, 173; sources of funding for, 190–97; specific functions of, 178–81; standards for, 181–82; training of, 182–84

Parkinson, Dr. James, 102

Parkinson's disease (PD), 101–2, 239; *see also* PD
patient: and AD, 113–14; barriers between worker and, 185–86; Medicaid influence on distributions of, 30–31; as primary interest, 115
PD, and NPH, 106–7
pensions, and long term care costs, 46
Performing Arts for Crisis Training, Inc., 190
pernicious anemia, 110–12
personal care worker, 175, 179
Philadelphia Jewish Welfare Society, 174
physical dependence, and alcoholism, 139
physicians: in nursing homes, 278; role of in long term care, 68–69; and training in gerontology, 290; as volunteers in CVP, 166–69
Plains Indians, 119
Planning Your Retirement Housing (Sumichrast, Shafer, and Sumichrast), 247
polypharmacy, 120
poor laws, English, 249
population, nursing home, 270–73
poverty, and advanced age, 46, 289
premature aging model, 135–36
PRIDE Institute Journal of Long Term Home Health Care, 224
prions, and AD, 94–95
private payments, 190–91
professional narcissism, 10
Project HELP, 216–18
Prospective Payment System (PPS), 38, 306
Prudential Insurance Company of America, 51
pseudodementia, 107
psychological strength: as health factor, 72, 74, 78; importance of nurturing, 63
psychosocial therapy, alcoholism and, 143
public housing, 252–53

quality of life, in nursing home, 275–76
Queen Nursing Home, 144
Quinn, Joan, 159–62

Reagan administration, housing policy of, 250, 254–55
reality orientation, 115–16
reimbursement, geographic variability in, 16
research: basic agenda for, 69; international, 70

Resource utilization groups (RUGS), 31; *see also* RUGS
respite care, 237–41, 295; controversies about, 240–41; history of, 239–40; as long term care component, 116; program purposes of, 238–39; training for, 204–5
resuscitation, guidelines for, 282
Retired Senior Volunteer Program, 212, 215
reverse mortgage concept, 48; growth of, 20–21
Rhode Island: Medicaid in, 32; spend-down provisions in, 26
right-hemisphere dysfunction model, 136
Robert Wood Johnson Foundation, 281; and adult foster care program funding, 232–33; and Project HELP, 216–18
RUGS, 271; financial effect of, 67; impact of, 38–39; as reimbursement approach, 33
Rural Policy Development Act, 251

St. Vincent's Hospital and Medical Center of New York, 165–71, 213; Department of Community Medicine, 165
Scotland, elderly housing in, 249
scrapie, and AD, 94–95
Section 8 housing program, 254–55
Section 202 housing, 253–54
Section 2176 (PL 97-35), 215
Senate Finance Committee Subcommittee on Health, 223
Senate Special Committee on Aging, 38
senile dementia, 83; Swedish studies on, 96
senile dementia of the Alzheimer type (SDAT), 83; phases of, 88–89
senile plaques, 90; and AD, 90–91, 95
senile squalor syndrome, 329n6
senility, and dementia, 82–83
senior citizen's housing, 255–56
Senior Companion Program, 212, 215
Senior Respite Care Program (Portland, OR), 239
sexual bias, in paraprofessional field, 181
shared housing, 256–57
Sheltered Housing Program, 259
Sisters of Charity of St. Vincent de Paul, 165
skilled nursing facilities (SDFs), 267, 269
skilled nursing requirement, elimination of, 303
Social/Health Maintenance Organizations (SHMOs), 51; as capitation program, 20; federal support of, 155

Social Security Act of 1935, 14
Social Security Act of 1974, 43, 268–69
Social Security Administration: payment adjustment of, 56; study of on coping, 64
Social Security Amendments of 1972, 269
Social Security Amendments of 1983, 11, 38–39
Social Services Block Grant (SSBG) program, 43–44; and home health aides, 177, 191, 194
Somerville / Cambridge (Massachusetts) Elder Services, 239
South Carolina: adult day care in, 234; respite care in, 239
South Coast Institute for Applied Gerontology, 228
South Dakota: elderly housing in, 251; Medicaid in, 32
spend down, 26, 29, 298
Spiritus frumenti, 131
SSI, *see* Supplemental Security Income
states: and Agencies on Aging, 42–43; and long term care insurance, 53; and nursing home expenses, 154; and paraprofessional workers, 175; role of in Medicaid, 34; and SSBG funds, 43; and SSI, 41
subcortical dementias, 83, 101–3
suicide, and alcohol abuse, 121–22
superannuation, notion of dependent, 12
Supplemental Security Income (SSI), 40–41; and congregate housing funding, 259; and Medicaid, 29; and paraprofessional workers, 191, 195–96
support persons, as health factor, 66, 72, 76, 79
supportive services, and OAA, 42–43
Sweden, senile dementia studies in, 96

Tax Equity and Fiscal Responsibility Act of 1982 (TEFRA), 11, 37, 306
Tennessee, spend-down provisions in, 26
Texas: Medicaid in, 32; respite care in, 239
therapeutic nihilism, 140; *see also* Health workers, attitude of
therapies, and chronically disabled, 152
thyroid disease, 110
Title XVI of Social Security amendments of 1972; *see* Supplemental Security Income
Title XVIII, *see* Medicare
Title XIX, *see* Medicaid
Title XX (Older Americans Act), 11, 42–43

Title XX: Social Services Block Grant, and adult day care, 226, 229, 234
Title XXI, 305; *see also* Medicare
Tompkins Square House, 249
transfer trauma, 274
transportation: and long term care, 292; and medical care, 69
treatment: alcoholism and methods of, 142–44; principles guiding, 73, 141–42
Triage program, 159–62; financing of, 160; and government support, 161; results of, 161–62; and transportation, 160–61; and waivers, 160
trisomy 21, 97
"2176 waivers," 33
twins, senile dementia studies on, 97

ubiquitin, 323*n* 47
United States Bureau of the Census, on nursing home population, 23
United States Special Committee on Aging, 200
University of North Carolina Program on Aging, 226
Urban Institute, 272
urinary incontinence, 70–71, 320*nn* 29, 30

very old people, clinical disorders of, 4; *see also* frail elderly; old-old
Veterans Administration Home Care Services, 191, 196–97
Veterans Administration Nursing Home Care Unit, 239
Veterans Administration programs, 44–45; GEUs of, 67–68
Village Nursing Home, 280, 282
Village Visiting Neighbors (VVN), 213–15
Virginia, elderly housing in, 251
Virginia Commonwealth University Center on Aging at, 241
Visiting Nurse Service (NYC), 13, 14, 174, 192, 213
Voluntary Chore Ministry, 215–16
volunteers, 212–19; advantages of, 218–19; current status of programs, 215–18; definition of, 212–13; disadvantages of, 218–19; and friendly visitor programs, 213–15